D0075956

SYMPTOM RELIEF IN PALLIATIVE CARE

Second Edition

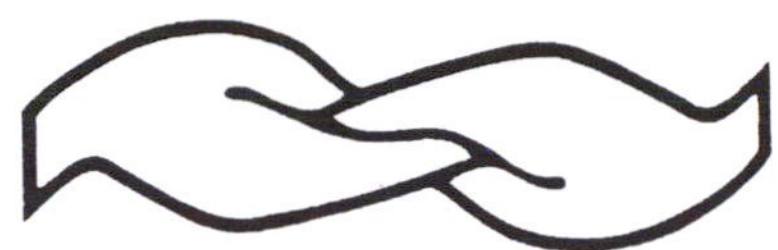

MERVYN DEAN
Palliative Care Physician
Western Memorial Regional Hospital
Corner Brook, NL, Canada

JUAN-DIEGO HARRIS
Director, Pain Medicine and Palliative Care
Claxton-Hepburn Medical Center
Richard E. Winter Cancer Treatment Center
Ogdensburg, NY, USA

and

CLAUD REGNARD
Consultant in Palliative Care Medicine
St Oswald's Hospice, Newcastle Hospitals NHS Trust
Visiting Professor of Research, Northumbria University
Newcastle upon Tyne, UK

Radcliffe Publishing
Oxford • New York

Radcliffe Publishing Ltd
18 Marcham Road
Abingdon
Oxon OX14 1AA
United Kingdom

www.radcliffepublishing.com
Electronic catalogue and worldwide online ordering facility.

UK editions:
First Edition 1983
Second Edition 1986
Third Edition 1992
Fourth Edition 1998
Fifth Edition 2004
Sixth Edition 2010

North American editions:
First Edition 2005
Second Edition 2011

British Library Cataloguing in Publication Data

A catalogue record for this book is available from the British Library.

ISBN-13: 978 184619 355 2

The paper used for the text pages of this book is FSC® certified. FSC (The Forest Stewardship Council®) is an international network to promote responsible management of the world's forests.

FSC
Mixed Sources
Product group from well-managed forests and other controlled sources
Cert no. SA-COC-001530
www.fsc.org
© 1996 Forest Stewardship Council

Typeset by Pindar New Zealand, Auckland, New Zealand
Printed and bound by Hobbs the Printers, Southampton, UK

FOREWORD TO SECOND EDITION

Palliative care continues to evolve as an academic discipline, with an increasing awareness of its significance in the comprehensive care of patients and their families and an expanding evidence base guiding practice. With continued development in treatment options for the management of pain and other symptoms, the clinician is challenged to keep current with new pharmaceutical agents and other therapeutic modalities, as well as to keep pace with the expansion of the practice of palliative care to address a growing spectrum of medical conditions and care settings.

The second edition of *Symptom Relief in Palliative Care* once again delivers in its commitment to serve as a clear, concise resource that can be quickly consulted to guide patient care. Its efficiency of use derives from the intuitive organization and layout of its information-dense content. The *Clinical Decision and Action Checklist* and *Key Points* leading each new clinical topic serve to focus the reader on the information that follows. The problem-oriented summary tables addressing clinical decisions and actions are driven by potential clinical scenarios, quickly guiding a pragmatic approach to a problem at hand.

The growing literature informing the practice of palliative care is reflected in the up-to-date references in this new edition. The number of references has doubled for the Pain chapter since the 2006 edition, and more than one-third of these are from 2007 and later. Where a solid evidence base is not yet available for a specific issue, this is acknowledged and a best-practice approach is presented, based on the extensive experience of the authors and the best information available.

The section addressing *Difficult Decisions* has been updated to reflect recent Joint Statements and publications regarding issues of making ethical choices, decision-making capacity, and cardiopulmonary resuscitation. These are some of the most challenging aspects of palliative and end-of-life care, encountered throughout daily patient care. Nonetheless, clear and practical guidance is difficult to glean from ethical and philosophical debates in the literature. The framework presented in *Symptom Relief in Palliative Care* is a valuable and welcome guide for such complex issues.

The second edition of *Symptom Relief in Palliative Care* continues to serve as a distinctly practical and problem-oriented resource for clinicians providing palliative and end-of-life care. The text has evolved to reflect continued developments in available treatments, changes in areas of policy and ethics, and the ever-broadening scope of the clinical practice of palliative care.

Mike Harlos MD, CCFP, FCFP
Professor, Faculty of Medicine
University of Manitoba
Medical Director
Palliative Care
Winnipeg Regional Health Authority
August 2010

PREFACE TO SECOND EDITION

Symptom Relief in Palliative Care describes the management of patients with advanced disease. Its foundation is a clinical decision approach based on what the patient has to tell us. It is our clear intention that the patient's information should guide the professional to appropriate management, rather than prescribe a specific approach. This provides a clearer framework and leaves the choice of route to the individual patient and professional. We are offering a map for guidance, not a route march! There is also no intention to provide a comprehensive palliative care text since there are many excellent examples available today. *Symptom Relief in Palliative Care* is not written to be read cover to cover, but is intended as a bedside aid, to be consulted when you feel you need additional help and advice. The information is divided into tables which are based on clinical algorithms and contain the management advice, and the text which provides additional information and advice.

This second edition is based on a UK text whose first edition was published just over 27 years ago in 1983. It has been written specifically for Canada and the United States. Mervyn Dean again brings his knowledge and enthusiasm as a palliative care physician, and Juan-Diego Harris shares his expertise in pain medicine and palliative care. Radcliffe Publishing are now well established with a range of palliative care books. As always, this edition has been rewritten and updated to take into account the advances in knowledge and care that have occurred since the last edition.

Symptom Relief in Palliative Care continues to apply to cancer and non-cancer patients with advanced disease. Throughout, the text continues to be relevant to children with life-threatening and life-limiting illness. Several sections have been modified to take into account people who have severe communication difficulties. The sections on symptoms other than pain and on emergencies are set out alphabetically. The *Emergencies* section is now easier to find at the end of the book. The *Drug information* section has been extensively updated.

With the publisher we further evolved the design to be easier to read with a second color for clarity and emphasis. Most of the tables containing management advice are now on right-hand pages. Over 1740 references have been categorized to make their evidence base clearer. The index has been revised to make it useful for a busy clinician.

We sincerely hope that *Symptom Relief in Palliative Care* will continue to support professionals in a wide cross-section of care teams palliating advanced disease.

Mervyn Dean
Juan-Diego Harris
Claud Regnard
August 2010

DEDICATION

This book is dedicated to the patients and families from whom we have learnt as much as, if not more than, from our mentors and colleagues.

ACKNOWLEDGMENTS

We are indebted to all our colleagues who kept us on the right track and so kindly gave us their time and advice. We are particularly grateful to these colleagues who advised, reviewed or helped to co-write specific sections:

Mary Beresford, Nurse Specialist Wound Care, Western Memorial Regional Hospital, Corner Brook, NL, Canada
Malignant ulcers and fistulae

Alison Gardner Biggs, Articled Student-at-law, 2008–2009 term, Canadian Medical Association
Advance care planning; capacity

Ellie Bond, Associate Specialist, Children's Unit, St. Oswald's Hospice, Newcastle-upon-Tyne, UK
Advice on pediatric palliative care throughout the book

Simon Chapman, Ethics Advisor, National Council for Palliative Care, London, UK.
Decisions around capacity

Kath Clark, Day Services Lead, St. Oswald's Hospice, Newcastle-upon-Tyne, UK
Edema and lymphedema

Ellen J. Darabaner, Circuit librarian Hunter-Rice Health Sciences Library, Watertown, New York, NY, USA
Library services

Mellar P. Davis, Professor of Medicine, Cleveland Clinic Lerner School of Medicine
Palliative Medicine and Supportive Oncology Services
Case Western Reserve University Cleveland, Ohio, USA
Review of some US non-pharmacological data

Maureen Field, Clinical Nurse Specialist in Palliative care and Liverpool Care Pathway Facilitator, Newcastle Hospitals NHS Trust, UK
Terminal phase

Lynn Gibson, Senior Physiotherapist, Northumberland, Tyne & Wear NHS Trust, UK
Identifying distress in the person with communication difficulties
Discussing preferred priorities of care
Nutrition and hydration problems
Issues around cardiopulmonary resuscitation

Judith Bedford Jones, Legal Counsel and Manager of Legal Services, Canadian Medical Association
Advance care planning; capacity

Andrew Hughes, Consultant in Palliative Medicine, St. Oswald's Hospice, Newcastle-upon-Tyne, UK
Edema and lymphedema

Fiona Thompson, Team Leader, Lymphedema Service, St. Oswald's Hospice, Newcastle-upon-Tyne, UK
Edema and lymphedema

Kathryn Mannix, Consultant in Palliative Medicine, Newcastle Hospitals NHS Trust, Newcastle-upon-Tyne, UK
Nausea and vomiting

Dorothy Matthews, Macmillan Nurse for People with Learning Disability, Northumberland, Tyne & Wear NHS Trust, UK
Identifying distress in the person with communication difficulties
Discussing preferred priorities of care
Nutrition and hydration problems
Issues around cardiopulmonary resuscitation

Robert Milch, Center of Hospice and Palliative Care, Buffalo, NY, USA
Delivery routes for medications in the US

Mary G. Mihalyo, Assistant Professor Pharmacy Practice, Duquesne University Mylan School of Pharmacy, Pittsburgh, PA, USA
Various US drug queries

Karen Power, Pharmacist, Western Memorial Regional Hospital, Corner Brook, NL, Canada
Various queries on drug availability throughout the book

Lyndia Quan, Registrar in Oncology and Palliative Care, Melbourne, Australia
Drug interactions

Fiona Randall, Consultant in Palliative Medicine, Royal Bournemouth and Christchurch NHS Trust, Dorset, UK
Discussing preferred priorities of care
Making ethical choices
Decisions around cardiopulmonary resuscitation

Nina Regnard, Clinical Nurse Specialist, Liverpool (Continence Advisor and Colorectal Screening Nurse Specialist)
Diarrhea
Urinary problems and sexual difficulties

Joanne Rodgerson, RCN, St. Oswald's Hospice, Newcastle-upon-Tyne, UK
Malignant ulcers and fistulae
Skin problems

Al Muto & staff, Pine Pharmacy, Williamsville, NY, USA
Medications from US compounding pharmacies

Bryan Vernon, Lecturer, Newcastle University, Newcastle-upon-Tyne, UK
Making ethical choices

Finally, we thank **Paul Stringer**, Graphic Designer, for the 'Hands' logo.

CONTENTS

Introduction

THE CONSEQUENCES OF ADVANCED DISEASE

In the past, palliative care centered around caring for patients at the end of life, most with cancer. However, as many life-threatening conditions are now treated more effectively, they have become more chronic with survival times of years or even decades. Although many such "life-limiting" conditions include non-cancer diseases, even cancer is becoming increasingly chronic with more effective treatment. The popular perception has been that different conditions have distinct disease trajectories. This is no longer true and many conditions overlap in prognosis and have a wide variety of disease trajectories.[1] For example, the average prognosis of Alzheimer's dementia (4.5 years) overlaps with many cancers.[2]

Whether the disease is life threatening or life limiting, it remains a creeping crisis that invades the lives of patients, families, partners and carers alike. From the time of diagnosis the patient, partner, and family face a series of multiple losses and adjustments just like a bereavement. Although some people will grow from the experience, it remains a distressing experience for all.

The distress of the patient

Patients already have to face the loss of their future life, and to this has to be added any loss of function as the illness progresses. Everyday activities can become a source of distress and irritation that may require so much effort that sleep, appetite, and concentration are affected, leaving the individual physically and emotionally drained. Activities which once gave life meaning and purpose are curtailed, reduced, or abandoned. A loss of control is an important cause of anxiety, depression and anger. These losses alter social interactions, reduce an individual's ability or desire to communicate with others, and cause that individual to become dissociated from life around them. Valued relationships suffer and may be lost. One woman explained:[3]

"I've come to hate the way I am towards my grandchildren. I love them to bits, I love to see them, but then I just couldn't be bothered with them. I'd get tired easily because of the pain and I didn't have the energy or patience left for them, and I'd be short. I'd never been like that. Their mother stopped bringing them to the house. Now when they visit they treat me like a stranger. It saddens me to think how they will remember me."

These multiple losses may make patients question their situation:

Why has this happened to me?
What is it all about?
What next?

How a person copes, and is helped to cope, with these big questions will have an impact on their distress, whatever its cause.

The distress of the partners and family

Siblings, parents, and partners also suffer losses. They try to be understanding, but often feel sidelined by all the care directed at the patient. Used to facing difficulties together, carers find it difficult to reach the patient, producing a feeling of powerlessness. A sense of injustice, anger, and guilt is particularly common in parents and siblings confronted with the reality of outliving a dying child or young adult.

Unprepared for their new role, carers learn by trial and error. Not surprisingly, they question their skills and may even question whether they were responsible for the patient's present suffering. They have little time for relaxation, reflection or for thinking about the future. Others may be drawing on their capacity to care, leaving little or no capacity to care for themselves. In long-term illnesses such as slowly progressive degenerative neurological disease and advancing dementia, carers have the additional burden of managing even the most basic daily needs over many months or years. A loss of privacy at home is common as families and partners adjust to the intrusive experience of new health professionals visiting and attending to the patient's intimate needs:

"I used to love the evenings together when the house would be locked up, and we would curl up to watch a movie. We can't really do that now, it's difficult to relax, it's always on our mind that they'll be coming to get him ready and put him to bed."[3]

The distress of the professional carers

The sense of isolation in patients and carers is reflected in professionals. They are faced with multiple physical, psychological, spiritual, and social issues and yet often have had little or no training in managing these problems. This sense of loss can cloud judgment so that sensible, caring professionals can make illogical and inappropriate decisions. The consequence is unrelieved distress. An example is an excessive concern about opioid adverse effects.[4] Unrelieved pain persists and surveys have shown that severe pain remains unrelieved in over half of cancer patients,[5,6] nearly one-third of renal failure patients,[7] and over 60% of AIDS patients.[8,9] Such distress seems insurmountable. But palliative care is now well established as an effective means of managing such distress.

PALLIATIVE CARE: A SAFE PLACE TO EXPRESS SUFFERING (A UNIQUE PARTNERSHIP)

The WHO states that palliative care:[10]

- Provides relief from pain and other distressing symptoms.
- Affirms life and regards dying as a normal process.
- Intends neither to hasten nor postpone death.
- Integrates the psychological and spiritual aspects of patient care.
- Offers a support system to help patients live as actively as possible until death.
- Offers a support system to help the family cope during the patient's illness and in their own bereavement.
- Uses a team approach to address the needs of patients and their families, including bereavement counseling, if indicated.
- Will enhance quality of life, and may also positively influence the course of illness.
- Is applicable early in the course of illness, in conjunction with other therapies that are intended to prolong life, such as chemotherapy or radiation therapy, and includes those investigations needed to better understand and manage distressing clinical complications.

Many specialties share these goals, but palliative care has several additional characteristics:

- It recognizes that it cannot remove all distress generated by loss, but that people can be helped to shift their focus of hope and cope with those losses.[11,12]
- It provides a path through the physical, psychological, spiritual, and social distress that helps the patient (adult or child), partner, family, and professional achieve a worthwhile quality of life.

- It provides a therapeutic environment in which the distress can be safely and effectively expressed.[13] With sufficient skills and experience this can be enabled anywhere.
- It does this in a therapeutic partnership with
  - the patient, partner and family
  - with professionals through direct help, support, advice, research, education, and policy or strategy development.

SHARING THE CONSEQUENCES OF ADVANCED DISEASE

Pain and other symptoms often cause psychological distress such as anxiety or a low mood, but these usually settle rapidly if the symptom is relieved. If, however, the symptom persists or there are fears and unresolved concerns about issues such as the disease, relationships, beliefs, money, or the home, the psychological distress will continue and is likely to delay attempts to manage the symptom. Indeed, it is unusual for a symptom to exist as the only cause of distress, and the phrase "total pain" was coined by Dame Cicely Saunders to stress the broad nature of such distress in advanced disease.[14]

Three essential human needs risk becoming blocked:[15,16]

- *choice* (to choose or be chosen)
- *understanding* (to understand or be understood)
- *love* (to love or be loved).

Symptoms such as pain can block choice by limiting actions and plans. Understanding can become blocked if information is not forthcoming or the nature and extent of the symptom is not believed. Love can become blocked by the effect of anger, irritability, or low mood on close relationships. The result of blocking choice is frustration, anger and bitterness; blocking understanding causes fear and anxiety; while blocking love causes isolation and loneliness. If any of the feelings persist, depression is often the result. Sometimes patients develop behaviors that further complicate treatment and recovery.

Issues around these needs must be addressed. For the majority of patients, this care will be provided by their usual carers. Such supportive care often uses the principles and practices of palliative care, but requires the professional carers to have an understanding of, and some training in, those principles and practices.

For some patients, however, the problems they face are severe or complex. For these patients, the specialist support of a palliative care team is necessary.[17] These teams can include nurses, doctors, social worker, physiotherapist, occupational therapist, pharmacist, and chaplain, all working interprofessionally.

Help starts with assessment and supportive communication. It is essential to reduce the distress of physical symptoms, but anxiety, anger, and depression also need to be identified and eased. The full range of additional treatments possible is wide and depends on the enthusiasm of the team, but includes touch,[18–20] hypnosis,[21] sensory stimulation, art therapy,[22,23] music therapy,[24,25] imagery,[26] and other complementary therapies.[27] When the psychological distress is severe, expert help will be required. The skills needed may be those of cognitive behavioral therapy, psychiatry, or family therapy, although the choice sometimes depends on availability of personnel rather than suitability of the approach.

PRINCIPLES OF SYMPTOM RELIEF IN PALLIATIVE CARE

- **Effective supportive care is the right of every patient, partner, and relative, and the duty of every health care professional.** Access to training, updating, and to specialist palliative care services should be widely available.
- **Ensure adequate team skills, knowledge, attitudes and communication.** Individuals and teams need basic skills in communication and diagnosis, together with the knowledge of symptoms in advanced disease, their effects and management.
- **Create a safe place to express suffering.** This is not a building, but the *relationship* between patient and carer (lay and professional), one that enables the patient and family to feel safe to express their distress.[13] Not all distress can be removed, but the expression and understanding of that distress are therapeutic.
- **Ensure the patient is at the center of treatment decisions.** This applies whether the patient has capacity for these decisions (in which case their opinion is paramount), or they do not have capacity (in which case decisions must be made in the patient's best interests).
- **Establish a relationship with the patient, the partner, and family.** The flow of information and treatment decisions should be controlled by the patient, not by the professional.
- **Do not wait for a patient to complain – ask and observe.** Patients with persistent distress do not always look distressed. They may be withdrawn, with poor sleep or mobility, and the effects of the pain may have spread to the partner or relative. Assessing the way the problem affects the patient gives a more patient-centered view of the problem than using severity scales or tools which are open to bias and often unhelpful in deciding treatment. The comments of the partner, parents or other relatives and carers are often helpful.
- **Accurately diagnose the cause of the problem.** A successful treatment is dependent on a clear diagnosis, together with the willingness to modify the choice depending on the response. This tailors the treatment to the individual person.
- **Patients often have multiple problems.** Problems are often multiple and mixed. In advanced cancer, for example, 85% of patients have more than one site of pain, and 40% have four or more pains.[28] Agreeing with the patient the order of priority of symptom relief builds trust through a working relationship.
- **Do not delay starting treatment.** Symptoms should be treated promptly since they become more difficult to treat the longer they are left. This is partly because their persistence makes it increasingly difficult for the patient to cope. Treatment must start as soon as the diagnosis is made.
- **Administer drugs regularly in doses titrated to each individual, that ensure the symptom does not return.** If a drug gives effective relief for 4 hours, then prescribe it 4 hourly, if it is effective for 12 hours, give it 12 hourly. "As required" or "PRN" administration on its own will not control continuous symptoms.
- **Set realistic goals.** Accept the patient's goals. If these seem overly optimistic, negotiate some additional *shorter*-term goals. If the patient's goals seem overly pessimistic then negotiate some additional *longer*-term goals. A clear plan of action based on negotiated goals helps the

patient, partner and family see a way out of their distress.

- **Reassess repeatedly and regularly.** Accurate titration of treatment demands reassessment.
- **Treat concurrent symptoms.** Patients with other symptoms such as nausea and breathlessness experience more pain than those without these symptoms.[29]
- **Empathy, understanding, diversion, and elevation of mood are essential adjuncts.** Drugs are only part of overall management. What matters most is the relationship between the patient, partner and family, and health professional.

REFERENCES: INTRODUCTION

B = book; C = comment; Ch = chapter; CS-n = case study-no. of cases; CT = controlled trial; E = editorial; GC = group consensus; I = interviews; LS = laboratory study; MC = multi-center; OS = open study; R = review; RCT = randomized controlled trial; RS = retrospective survey; SA = systematic or meta analysis.

1 Gott M, Barnes S, Payne S, Parker C, *et al.* (2007) Patient views of social service provision for older people with advanced heart failure. *Health and Social Care in the Community*. **15**(4): 333–42. (MC, OS-542)

2 Xie J, Brayne C, Matthews FE. (2008) Medical Research Council Cognitive Function and Ageing Study collaborators. Survival times in people with dementia: analysis from population based cohort study with 14-year follow up. *British Medical Journal*. **336**: 258–62. (MC, OS-438)

3 McKeever M, Regnard C. (1997) Qualitative interviews. In: *Palliative Crisis Response Service (PCRS) Needs Assessment. Final Report: February 1997.* Newcastle: St. Oswald's Hospice. (RT)

4 Jacobsen R, Sjogren P, Moldrup C, Christrup L. (2007) Physician-related barriers to cancer pain management with opioid analgesics: a systematic review. *Journal of Opioid Management*. **3**(4): 207–14. (SA-65)

5 Addington-Hall J, McCarthy M. (1995) Dying from cancer: results of a national population based investigation. *Palliative Medicine*. **9**: 295–305. (MC, OS, I)

6 van den Beuken-van Everdingen MH, de Rijke JM, Kessels AG, Schouten HC, van Kleef M, Patijn J. (2007) Prevalence of pain in patients with cancer: a systematic review of the past 40 years. *Annals of Oncology*. **18**(9): 1437–49. (SA-52)

7 Murtagh FE, Addington-Hall J, Higginson IJ. (2007) The prevalence of symptoms in end-stage renal disease: a systematic review. *Advances in Chronic Kidney Disease*. **14**(1): 82–99. (SA-59)

8 Breitbart W, Dibiase L. (2002) Current perspectives on pain in AIDS. *Oncology (Williston Park)*. **16**(7): 964–8 (R, 24 refs)

9 Breitbart W, Dibiase L. (2002) Current perspectives on pain in AIDS. *Oncology (Williston Park)*. **16**(6): 818–29, 834–5 (R, 95 refs)

10 *World Health Organization National Cancer Control Programmes: policies and managerial guidelines, 2nd ed.* (2002) Geneva: World Health Organization. pp. 1–4.

11 Kennedy V, Lloyd-Williams M. (2006) Maintaining hope: communication in palliative care. *Recent Results in Cancer Research*. **168**: 47–60.(R)

12 Duggleby WD, Degner L, Williams A, Wright K, Cooper D, Popkin D, Holtslander L. (2007) Living with hope: initial evaluation of a psychosocial hope intervention for older palliative home care patients. *Journal of Pain and Symptom Management*. **33**: 247–57. (RCT-60)

13 Stedeford A. (1987) Hospice: a safe place to suffer? *Palliative Medicine*. **1**: 73–4.

14 Saunders CM. (1967) In: *The Management of Terminal Illness*. London: Hospital Medicine Publications. (Ch)

15 Heron, J. (1996) *Co-operative Inquiry: research into the human condition*. London: Sage.

16 Liossi C, Mystakidou K. (1997) Heron's theory of human needs in palliative care. *European Journal of Palliative Care*. **4**: 32–5. (C)

17 Doyle D. (2003) Editorial. *Palliative Medicine*. **17**(1): 9–10. (E)

18 Sims S. (1988) The significance of touch in palliative care. *Palliative Medicine*. **2**: 58–61. (R)

19 Beider S, Mahrer NE, Gold JI. (2007) Pediatric massage therapy: an overview for clinicians. *Pediatric Clinics of North America*. **54**(6): 1025–41.

20 Lafferty WE, Downey L, McCarty RL, Standish LJ, Patrick DL. (2006) Evaluating CAM treatment at the end of life: a review of clinical trials for massage and meditation. *Complementary Therapies in Medicine*. **14**(2): 100–12. (SA-27)

21 James U. (2005) *Clinical Hypnosis Textbook: a guide for practical intervention*. Oxford: Radcliffe Publishing.

22 Connell C. (1992) Art therapy as part of a palliative care programme. *Palliative Medicine*. **6**: 18–25. (R)

23 Nainis N, Paice JA, Ratner J, Wirth JH, Lai J, Shott S. (2006) Relieving symptoms in cancer: innovative use of art therapy. *Journal of Pain and Symptom Management*. **31**(2): 162–9. (OS)

24 Mandel SE. (1992) Music therapy in the hospice: "Music alive". *Palliative Medicine*. **5**: 155–60. (R)

25 O'Kelly J, Koffman J. (2007) Multidisciplinary perspectives of music therapy in adult palliative care. *Palliative Medicine*. **21**: 235–41. (I, n=20)

26 Kearney M. (1996) In: *Mortally Wounded: stories of soul pain, death and healing*. Dublin: Mercier. (B)

27 Gatlin CG, Schulmeister L. (2007) When medication is not enough: nonpharmacologic management of pain. *Clinical Journal of Oncology Nursing*. **11**(5): 699–704. (R)

28 Twycross RG, Harcourt J, Bergl S. (1996) A survey of pain in patients with advanced cancer. *Journal of Pain and Symptom Management*. **12**: 273–82. (OS)

29 Desbiens NA, Mueller-Rizner N, Commors AF, Wenger NS. (1997) The relationship of nausea and dyspnoea to pain in seriously ill patients. *Pain*. **71**: 149–56. (MC, OS)

NOTES

Getting started

Setting the scene and starting the interview

CLINICAL DECISION AND ACTION CHECKLIST

1 Are you unfamiliar with the patient's details?
2 Is the location for the interview unsuitable?
3 Greet the person, introduce yourself.
4 Is the person accompanied?
5 Is only a short time available for the interview?
6 Does the person object to you being here?
7 Does the person object to the time available?
8 Does the person object to you taking notes?
9 Does the person object to you sharing information with the team?

KEY POINTS

- Spending time on "setting the scene" enables the person to share their concerns.
- This part of the interview is usually brief (a few minutes at most).
- Seeing the patient alone increases disclosure, but this does not have to be at the first meeting.
- Only a few major problems can be discussed in under 30 minutes.
- Taking notes shows the person you value their comments.
- Sharing information within the team is essential for effective care.
- In the case of children it is imperative to seek input from the parents and carers, as well as the child.

INTRODUCTION

In most situations, care starts with talking, and listening, to the patient, their partner or relative. Spending a little time in setting the scene for this discussion can make the experience more helpful for both the professional and the person in the discussion.

SETTING THE SCENE

Introducing yourself is surprisingly easy to forget, especially if you are on familiar territory, such as the hospital. It helps to explain your role and the reason for seeing them, and it is essential to have an understanding of the patient's details before starting an interview. It is distressing and irritating for a person to realize the professional does not know or understand the patient's illness and investigations.

Location: Ideally, find somewhere that is quiet and private enough to allow the person to feel safe enough to share their problems. If possible, switch off beepers and cell-phones, and disconnect telephones to minimize interruptions. When interviewing children and their families, choose a child-friendly environment and ensure that you have sufficient helpers and toys around to enable each person's needs to be disclosed, understood and addressed.

Seeing the person alone will result in more disclosure of the person's concerns.[1] This needs to be balanced against the important need to include partners and relatives in the care, if the patient wishes this. It is common practice in palliative care to see patients and partners together on the first meeting, and then to see individuals on their own at a later stage. Similarly, when looking after children and young people with life-limiting illness, it is usual to meet first with the family and child together, taking account of the child's age and competence. It is important to be vigilant for the undisclosed needs of the child and family members, and separate interviews can be planned with the child or young person alone, and with the parent(s) alone.

Time available for discussion: it is not possible to elicit the problems of a patient with advanced disease in less than 30 minutes. Less time than this only allows for a few major issues to be elicited. Nevertheless, it is important to make the time available, clear to the person. People disclose their problems more quickly knowing how much time is available. However, for an ill person, even 30 minutes may be exhausting and it is then important to prioritize on the issues that trouble the person most.

Setting roles and objectives: The person may have a very different objective to yours. For example, you may want to discuss their pain, but their most pressing concern is getting home. Insisting on discussing pain alone will frustrate the person and may even see them blocking your suggestions for pain relief. Planning with them the best way of managing their pain at home will be much more helpful.

Taking notes: it is essential to make notes of important cues and issues because it shows the person you are taking their problems seriously, it does not hinder disclosure, and gives you a record for the future. However, taking notes should not absorb you so much that there is prolonged loss of eye contact and empathy. It is also important to check if there are any details that the person does not wish to be recorded.

Sharing information: this is essential for effective team working and makes the best use of the team's pooled expertise. It also reduces the risk of over-dependency on the professional, or unrealistic expectations.[1] Holding "secrets" for

Clinical decision	If YES carry out the action below
1 Are you unfamiliar with the person's details?	• Read the chart before seeing the patient, partner or relative.
2 Is the location for the interview unsuitable?	• **If possible** — find somewhere that is quiet and private enough to allow the person to feel safe enough to share their problems. — switch off beepers and cell-phones, and disconnect telephones. • **When interviewing children and their families** choose a child-friendly environment and ensure that you have sufficient helpers and toys around to enable each person's needs to be disclosed, understood, and addressed.
3 Greet the person and introduce yourself by name – explain your role and objectives.	
4 Is the person accompanied?	• **Ask the patient if they want the other person or persons to come in with them.** *If person agrees:* ask who the other person is and see them both together. Arrange a time later to see the patient alone. *If person disagrees:* ask whether they would like to include the other person later in the interview or on another occasion. • With dying children and their families, consider who should most helpfully and appropriately be present at each stage of the interview.
5 Is only a short time available for discussion?	• **If less than 30 minutes are available or patient is too unwell for a full interview:** focus on recent changes or major problems only.
6 Does the person object to you being here?	• **Explore the reasons and renegotiate the objectives**, e.g. concentrate on main problem only. Ask if they would prefer you to return later or if they would like to see someone else.
7 Does person object to time available?	• **If time is too short:** explore the reasons and try to negotiate follow-up interviews. *If person objects to negotiation:* acknowledge this and end interview. *If person agrees to negotiation:* arrange longer interview for later. • **If time is too long:** explore reasons and negotiate more limited objectives, e.g. main problem only.
8 Does person object to you taking notes?	• **Explore the reasons:** *If person objects to negotiation:* agree not to take notes. *If person agrees to negotiation:* take notes of what has been agreed (person may ask for some information to be left unrecorded).
9 Does the person object to sharing information with team?	e.g. person insists that some or all information is kept secret • **Advise person that you cannot agree to secrecy** *If person objects:* offer to refer to a professionally supported counselor. *If person agrees:* go on to elicit the current problems.

Adapted from Maguire, Faulkner and Regnard[2]

patients is unhelpful for patients, divisive to teams and potentially harmful to professionals. The only exceptions are priests in a confessorial role or professionals who receive individualized professional support to fulfill their work, such as social workers or counselors.

A note about children: with ill children and their families there can be powerful dynamics of fear, guilt, protection, and counter-protection that can prevent good communication within the family. These can manifest verbally or non-verbally. They often cannot be dealt with immediately but need discussion with the care team. To protect their parents, dying children will often explore concerns and fears with outsiders such as siblings, other child patients or junior staff members. This is poignantly demonstrated by the way some children, on being told difficult news, apologize to their parents. It is important to anticipate, support, and manage such situations.

Helping the person to share their problems

CLINICAL DECISION AND ACTION CHECKLIST

1 Greet the person and introduce yourself by name and title.
2 Do you find it difficult to let the person do the talking?
3 Does the person have an obvious, overriding problem?
4 Is the person unable to prioritize?
5 Ask the person to list the most troublesome problems.
6 Clarify and specify each problem in turn.
7 Is the person obviously distressed?
8 Have the main problems been disclosed?
9 Is the agreed time for the interview almost at an end?

KEY POINTS

- Encouraging the person to tell their own story encourages them to share their problems and is itself therapeutic.[3]
- Avoid closed questions, focusing on physical problems or switching the subject.
- Withhold giving advice until the full story has unfolded.
- Avoid false reassurance.

INTRODUCTION

Advanced disease can create multiple problems for patients, partners and families[4–6] Despite this, nurses and doctors have difficulty enabling people to disclose their concerns.[5,7,8] Doctors and nurses commonly use behaviors that discourage a person from sharing their concerns, especially emotional issues.[7,9,10] Patients are *less* likely to disclose problems if the professional uses closed or leading questions, focuses on physical aspects, switches the subject to avoid a difficult question, or moves rapidly to give advice or reassurance.[9]

ELICITING THE PROBLEMS

Overriding problem: a patient may be in severe pain, or be vomiting or frightened. This needs to be addressed before any interview can continue.

Ask the person to list the problems: this is essential as professionals fail to pick up more than half of patients' concerns.[7]

Ask about feelings early in the interview: failing to ask about feelings early in an interview greatly reduces the likelihood that the patient will express those feelings.

Check each problem: use short and precise questions to detail the problems. Summarize your understanding with the person to make sure you have understood the issues correctly.

Distress: people who are obviously distressed would like this acknowledged, together with help to understand why they are feeling this way. Professionals often feel anxious when this distress is openly expressed, fearing that they have "upset" the person or caused psychological damage. In reality, it shows that the person feels safe enough to show distress.

People with severe communication difficulties pose a particular challenge in identifying the presence and cause of distress (*see* p. 31).

Summarize and explain: this is the time to discuss the plan for help and treatment, and to set realistic goals.

Concluding the interview: this is as important as starting the interview. If the professional does not finish within the agreed time the person may think they have unlimited time and demand more time, which prevents the professional spending time with other patients.

People are more likely to share their problems if:

- The professional is *actively listening* by:
  - enabling the person to tell the story their way with a minimum of interruptions.
  - asking open questions, e.g. "Can you tell me about any difficulties you're having?" rather than, "Is the pain better?"
  - using questions about emotions early in the interview, e.g. "How has this affected you emotionally?" This should be in the first 10 minutes of the interview.[9]
  - not avoiding a difficult question (*see Answering difficult questions*, p. 19).
- Reassurance is used wisely:
  - it must never be false reassurance
  - any information must be clear
  - the reassurance must not be used to avoid a difficult situation or question.
- You have received training: attending interactive workshops on communication improves communication skills,[11,12] especially if clinical supervision is available on returning to work.[13]

Children: young children may not understand the abstract concepts of death and dying, but this does not mean that they have no understanding of what they are facing. These understandings can be elicited, especially if the skills and tools of the whole team are used to enable the child to communicate through word, storytelling, art, or music. Children will test adults carefully before opening up. This may take the form of casual questions dropped into conversations in inappropriate places. The answers must be appropriate to the child (*see Answering difficult questions*, p. 19).

Spiritual issues: these are often overlooked when assessing patients and spiritual distress is present in many diseases and ages.[14–17] No spiritual tools or measures are suitable for palliative care,[18] and these issues must be elicited as part of an interview and care provided by the whole interdisciplinary team.[19,20] For some patients spirituality will be

Clinical decision	If YES carry out the action below
1 Greet person and introduce yourself by name and position.	
2 Do you find it difficult to let the person do the talking?	• **If you prevent the person saying things in their own way** at the beginning of the interview they are much less likely to tell you their problems. — ask the person to tell their story, e.g. "I've read your chart but I would like you to tell me what has happened since." — keep interruptions to a minimum — avoid early or false reassurance — ask about feelings early on in the interview (in the first 10 minutes) — check out spiritual issues (this may be about formal religious beliefs or enquiring if anything gives them a feeling of hope) — avoid explanations about disease process and treatment until the patient has presented all their current issues — be aware of your own embarrassment or awkwardness in some areas such as sexual issues. If this is difficult, arrange for training or for someone else to ask on your behalf. NB. Allowing the patient to talk in this way does not lengthen the interview.
3 Is there an obvious, overriding problem? e.g. severe pain	• **Agree this is a priority**, e.g. "It seems to me that your main problem is . . ." • **Check** if they want help with the problem now, e.g. "Do you want me to give you something now for the pain?" • **Manage the problem:** see the appropriate clinical decision table for guidance to management. • **Return later** to complete the interview.
4 Is the person unable to prioritize?	• **Focus on the most obvious problem** (e.g. pain) or the first problem chosen or mentioned.
5 Ask the person to list the most troublesome problems	
6 Check each problem using short and precise questions: — **clarify** its precise nature — **specify** when it started, its severity, duration, and pattern — **briefly summarize** your understanding of the problem.	
7 Is the person obviously distressed?	• **Acknowledge the distress**, e.g. "You seem anxious. Do you want to talk about it?" *If the person can bear to talk about it:* explore each emotion. *If the person cannot bear to talk about it:* agree that the person can discuss this later if they feel the need. • **If the person has a severe communication difficulty:** *see* p. 31.
8 Have the main problems been disclosed?	• **Explain** to the patient — what you think is the cause of each problem — what they can do to help themselves. • **Give an overview** of your short- and long-term plans. • **Provide a realistic goal** for treatment. • **Agree on future plans.**
9 Is the agreed time for the interview almost at an end?	• **Explain** that time is nearly up. • **Summarize** issues, e.g. "So the main problems are . . ." • **Check** if there is anything the person wants to add. • **Make concluding statement**, e.g. "I'd like to arrange the next appointment . . ." • **Arrange next interview.**

Adapted from Maguire, Faulkner, and Regnard[2]

formalized in religious practice and belief, but for others it will encompass a much wider belief in perceived support that goes beyond physical care. Whichever approach a person takes the key issue centers around fostering hope.[21,22]

Hope of realistically achieving something good in the future is at the heart of coping with advanced illness and enabling a good quality of life. Unlike denial or optimism, hope needs people to be realistic, since one can only successfully hope for something that is possible, not something that can never be achieved. It is about being open to possibilities.

Hope is a realistic desire for good in the face of uncertainty and it helps a person cope with tragedy and loss.

Hope shows itself in different ways at different stages of illness.

- Early in the disease there is hope of cure.
- As the illness progresses there is hope of control and hope for comfort.
- At the end of life the hope often changes to one for peace and a pain-free death.

Hope shows itself in different ways in different people. Some people are practical in their hope, e.g. hoping to avoid pain, tying up loose ends, or going home to die.

Others are more generalized in their hope, e.g. the hope to be at peace, to take "each day as it comes," hope that they are valued, and a hope of "letting go" at the end.

Fostering hope will need to be adapted to the individual:

Focus of hope: As an illness progresses the patient needs to be allowed to change the focus of his or her hope, e.g. from cure to comfort.

Action: Allowing the person to talk safely about their fears and hopes will help.

Abrupt change: Keep a lookout for patients whose pace of change has been abrupt, e.g. being told their illness cannot be cured or treated.

Action: Allow these people extra time to mull over this new information, with a trusting ear to listen.

Information overload: The person may make it clear they do not want more information at present, e.g. "I don't want to hear any more bad news." This shows they are in "reality overload" and cannot take any more information right now.

Action: Make sure the team knows of the person's wishes. Avoid misinterpreting this "reality overload" as a lack of knowledge – this can push professionals into loading even more information onto the person when they are already struggling with the knowledge they have!

Physical symptoms: Hope is soon damaged by persistent physical symptoms, e.g. pain, nausea, vomiting.

Action: Make sure the team knows about the problem and deals promptly with the symptom.

Psychological symptoms: Hope is very difficult to keep going in the presence of persistent psychological symptoms, e.g. anxiety, anger, or a clinical depression.

Action: Let the team know if the person seems anxious, angry, frightened, or withdrawn so these symptoms can be eased.

Difficult life: Hope is difficult to foster if a person's life has been one of neglect, rejection, or abuse.

Action: Allow the person time to talk over future possibilities. They may need specialist help.

Religious beliefs: these can be a source of comfort (e.g. believing in a peaceful afterlife), or distressing (e.g. fear of being judged unworthy, or a belief that the illness is a punishment).

Action: the involvement of a cleric from their religion can be helpful if that cleric has an open and adaptable understanding of helping people with advanced disease.

Answering difficult questions

CLINICAL DECISION AND ACTION CHECKLIST

1 Acknowledge the importance of the question
2 Is the setting inappropriate?
3 Position yourself correctly
4 Check why the question is being asked
5 Is the person reluctant to pursue the question?
6 Is a clear answer difficult?
7 Is a clear answer impossible?
8 Is the answer bad news?

KEY POINTS

- Difficult questions arise out of a person's uncertainty.
- Acknowledging the question is key.
- Answers may be unclear or impossible.
- Being honest about not knowing improves rather than hinders relationships.
- Some answers mean more bad news.

INTRODUCTION

People take time to adjust to the shock of advanced disease. During this time they will often seek clarification and information from health professionals, often asking different health care professionals the same questions. While some questions will be straightforward, other questions are more difficult to answer, e.g. "Why has this happened to me?"

WHY ARE QUESTIONS DIFFICULT?

Many factors can make some questions difficult.[23,24]

For the patient and partner there is a need for information to make rational choices, but this may conflict with the fears of advancing illness (treatment, symptoms, emotions, dying, relationships, and finances) and the need to maintain hope in the face of uncertainty[25] These factors inevitably generate difficult questions.

For the professional there are fears of being blamed, of eliciting an emotional reaction, of admitting ignorance, of expressing emotions, of medical hierarchy and of doing something for which they have received little or no training.[24] These factors make the questions from a patient or partner more difficult to answer.

CULTURAL ISSUES

Cultures have different views about what information should be exchanged, based on differing views of individualism.[26,27] This needs to be taken into account since open disclosure is a Western belief that is not shared universally.

THE FIRST STEPS

Acknowledge the importance of the question: acknowledging a person's concern is a recurring key action. It emphasizes that you have listened and are taking the issue seriously.

The setting: while a quiet, private setting seems ideal, difficult questions are often asked at the foot of the stairs or on busy wards. Remember that the person may be asking in that setting because they feel safe to do so. You can offer to go somewhere more private, but if they are comfortable where they are, accept the setting they have chosen.

Position yourself correctly: standing over a patient or positioning yourself with a desk in between you and the person will hinder communication and is disliked by people receiving difficult news.[28]

Check the question: it is important to ensure that you are both on the same wavelength. This is the opportunity to check through any problems with the person's understanding or any difficulties the professional is having with the question.

FINDING AN APPROPRIATE RESPONSE

Difficult answers: these are difficult because the answers are unclear, not known, or may make the person or professional distressed. If there is no clear answer, being honest about not knowing is respected and often increases rather than diminishes the relationship.

Impossible answers: professionals may find a question impossible to answer. If this is because of a lack of knowledge or experience, the person should be referred to someone who has the knowledge, or has the experience in answering such questions.

Children: a common error is to give an adult understanding to a child's question. For example, in answering a child's question, "Where will I go when I die?", an adult may launch into images of heaven, terrifying the child with images of a disconnected and faraway place full of walking dead people. In reality, motivated by his fear of closed spaces and the dark, the child may be asking if he will be buried like his grandmother. Therefore, checking why the child is asking that question is very important.

Clinical decision	If YES carry out the action below
1 Acknowledge the importance of the question, e.g. "That's an important question."	
2 Is the setting inappropriate?	Difficult questions are often asked in inappropriate places and dropped nonchalantly into conversations. Children are particularly likely to do this when checking out an adult before opening up, but adult patients can also do this. • **Offer to move somewhere quieter or more private.** • **If the person seems frightened or reluctant to go elsewhere:** accept the setting the person has chosen and continue with the conversation.
3 Position yourself correctly: position yourself at the same level as the person, ideally sitting without a desk between the two of you.	
4 Check why the question is being asked, e.g. "What makes you ask that?"	
5 Is the person reluctant to pursue the question?	• **Acknowledge the ambivalence** and check if they want to continue, e.g. "You seem uncertain whether you want to discuss this. Do you want to continue?" • **If they misunderstood:** — check for deafness, drowsiness or confusion — ask again in a different way. • **Were you unprepared for the question?** — apologize for the inattention — show that you are listening by acknowledging the importance of the question — check if they want to continue. • **Are you uncomfortable with the question?** Be prepared to describe your feelings, e.g. "I don't know what to say." • **If the person is clear about stopping the interview:** acknowledge the refusal and inform them that they can speak again to you or another team member in the future.
6 Is a clear answer difficult?	• **Acknowledge the uncertainty** faced by the person, e.g. "I can see this uncertainty is not easy for you." • **Explore** if the person can accept small chunks of certainty such as by asking the patient how quickly or slowly they feel their condition is changing. • **If the person needs to make realistic plans:** give a "best guess" response, but make it clear this is based on knowledge and experience, not certainty.
7 Is a clear answer impossible?	• **If this is because you do not have the knowledge or experience:** — acknowledge this, e.g. "I don't have the answer." — offer to refer person to someone who may be able to help.
8 Is the answer bad news?	• Go to *Breaking difficult news*, p. 23

Adapted from Faulkner, Regnard[29]

Bad news: if the answer is likely to be bad news then the decisions on *Breaking difficult news* (p. 23) can be used. Avoiding the truth is unhelpful: "The truth may hurt, but deceit hurts more."[30]

NOTES

Breaking difficult news

CLINICAL DECISION AND ACTION CHECKLIST

1 Is the setting inappropriate?
2 Three issues to check
   a. Is the person unable to understand?
   b. Does the person understand what is happening to them?
   c. Does the person want to know more?
3 Three steps to breaking difficult news
   a. Warn
   b. Pause
   c. Check
4 Three reactions a person may have
   a. Does the person want to continue?
   b. Does the person want to stop the discussion?
   c. Is the person uncertain about knowing more?

KEY POINTS

- Difficult news cannot be made easier, but telling it badly creates new difficulties.
- It is the patient who decides how much they should be told, not the professional.
- Breaking difficult news is done in stages, at the person's pace and with their permission.
- Denial is not a knowledge gap but a coping strategy that can be both necessary and effective for many patients.
- An unwillingness to openly discuss the diagnosis is not usually a barrier to informed consent to treatment.[31]

INTRODUCTION

Difficult news is any news that is unexpected and may cause distress. It is usually "bad" news, but care professionals often decide this label. There are occasions when apparently "good" news causes as much distress as "bad" news. For example, the news that radiotherapy for a frontal lobe brain tumor has resulted in a long remission may seem good news from a professional's view, but could be devastating to a relative who has now to cope with months or years of someone with an altered personality. In contrast the diagnosis of a cancer may be a relief to someone whose symptoms have been a puzzle for many months.

Many health care professionals are nervous about breaking difficult news,[32] while others believe they do it well, but observing their manner tells a different story.[28] However, following some basic principles (*see* the Key Points on the previous page) and using simple steps (*see* table opposite) can make the dialogue more helpful for the person being told and less frightening for the professional.

THREE STEPS OF THREE

Three things to check

a. *The person's understanding.* This involves making sure that the person can hear and is capable of understanding. Confusion, anxiety, and depression can all reduce concentration.
b. *The person's knowledge.* This is crucial so that you can elicit whether this news is going to be difficult for the person being told. It is unhelpful to guess what a person knows.
c. *The person's desire to know more.* This is not as difficult as it sounds, e.g. "Do you want me to explain the results of the tests?"

Three steps to breaking the news (WPC)

Most people are already worried that something might be seriously wrong. Even so they still need to be warned that this is the case.

a. **WARN:** Carer "I'm afraid the results were more serious than we thought."
b. **PAUSE:** (wait for a response) Person "What do you mean 'more serious'?"
c. **CHECK:** Carer "We found some abnormal cells. Do you want me to explain what these were?"

Many patients are clear that they want the information and only need a single Warn, Pause, and Check. However, some patients may need to go through the process several times before they give a clear answer. A few remain uncertain (*see* below).

The Warn, Pause, Check approach has another important role – that of asking the patient's consent to break the difficult news.[33] It is important to check that the person has understood the news. This WPC approach is repeated until the person has all the information they want at that time. It is equally important that the person knows that "the door is open" to return for further information or clarification. It is good practice to offer a follow-up interview.

Three reactions a person could have

a. More information is requested, e.g. "I think it's better that I know."
b. No more information is wanted, e.g. "Oh, I'll leave all that to you."
c. Uncertainty about how much information is wanted, e.g. "I'm not sure," or "You'd better speak to my wife/husband."

If the person is uncertain, the carer might ask some further questions, e.g. "Are you the sort of person who likes to know everything that is happening to them?" If the uncertainty persists this is best acknowledged and left open. The carer might say, "I can see you're not sure. That's not a problem. You can ask me sometime in the future".

DENIAL AND CONSENT FOR TREATMENT

A refusal or uncertainty about openly discussing the diagnosis does not prevent the discussion of treatment. This may seem strange, but remember this is not usually a lack of knowledge, but a struggle to cope with the knowledge they do have. Discussing treatment is a way of dealing with this knowledge. Therefore it is possible and legitimate to obtain consent for treatment in such patients. Allowing them control in this way enables them to concentrate on the benefits and burdens of the treatment

Clinical decision	If YES carry out the action below
1 Is the setting inappropriate?	• **Find somewhere confidential** and, if possible, quiet, comfortable, and free from interruptions. • **Ensure you are at the same eye level** as the person with no obstructions between you and the person. • **Ask if the person would like someone else to be present.**
2 Three things to check:	
a. Is the person unable to understand?	• **If this is reversible** (e.g. deafness responding to a hearing aid): treat the cause. • **If this is irreversible:** unless patient has previously objected, consider breaking difficult news to the relative or partner using these clinical decisions.
b. Does the person understand what is happening to them?	e.g. try asking "What have you understood about the tests?" • Go to *Helping the person with the effects of difficult news*, p. 27.
c. Does the person want to know more?	e.g. try asking "Do you want me to explain the results of the tests?" • Follow the three steps to breaking difficult news (WPC) below.
3 Three steps to breaking the news (WPC): **a. Warn:** give "warning shot" (e.g. try saying "The test results are more serious than we thought.") **b. Pause:** to give the person time to react and analyze what has been said. **c. Check:** if the person wants to continue (e.g. try asking "Do you want me to explain further?") and check if they have understood the information so far.	
4 Three reactions a person could have:	
a. Does the person want to continue?	• **Continue repeating the WPC process** above until the person has as much information as they want: — answer invitation for more information (e.g. try saying "We found some abnormal cells."). — ensure the person understands this information. — keep giving information as long as the person continues to request information. • **Consider recording** the conversation for the person or providing written material.
b. Does the person want to stop the discussion?	• **Acknowledge the refusal.** • **Offer the opportunity to discuss this further** in the future if the person wishes. • **Check if the person wants you to talk to someone else**, e.g. wife/husband, son/daughter. NB. Denial is not usually a lack of knowledge, but a way of coping with difficult news.
c. Is the person uncertain about knowing more?	• **Acknowledge the uncertainty.** • **Offer the opportunity to discuss this further** in the future if the person wishes. NB. Uncertainty is not usually a lack of knowledge, but a struggle to openly face difficult news. It is often accompanied by anxiety.

Adapted from Faulkner, Maguire, and Regnard[34]

and weigh these in the balance. In contrast, if the diagnosis is discussed against their wishes they are likely to become withdrawn, frightened, or angry and this will prevent them understanding the treatment information, making informed consent impossible.

Rarely, a patient refuses to believe the diagnosis and will also refuse treatment. These patients present quite differently, often demanding more information. Such patients will need more information and may have to be referred for second or third opinions and tests.

Helping the person with the effects of difficult news

CLINICAL DECISION AND ACTION CHECKLIST

1. Pause to check the person's reactions.
2. Acknowledge any distress.
3. Is the person accepting the difficult news?
4. Is the person overwhelmingly distressed?
5. Is the person denying or holding on to unrealistic expectations?
6. Is the person ambivalent?
7. Is collusion occurring?

KEY POINTS

- Bad news will result in emotions being expressed. Professionals can be fearful of such emotions, which in turn can hinder or prevent a patient from expressing their feelings.
- Expression of emotions is a helpful part of adjustment.
- Denial may be an effective coping mechanism for some people.
- Collusion between the patient and their partner or relative is common and is usually driven by the need to protect the other person.

INTRODUCTION

Although bad news cannot be made less bad, it can be conveyed badly. When a person perceives they have too much (or too little) information their concerns are kept hidden and unresolved. This increases the risk of clinical anxiety and depression.[35] Faced with difficult news most people respond with some acceptance or denial. Some will be firm in this reaction while many will fluctuate between the two. A few people will be ambivalent about whether they want to know more or not.

POSSIBLE REACTIONS

Distress: this indicates that the difficult news has been heard. There will be a wide range of possible reactions to difficult news such as anger, bitterness, sadness, and fear. Sometimes this is expressed openly at the time, sometimes it appears later. Professionals are often fearful of this reaction and worry that they have "upset" the person or caused psychological damage. This is often given as a reason for not exploring emotional issues.[7,10] As long as the disclosure has been at the person's pace with them in control, no damage will be caused. Open expression can be helpful to the individual and allows the professional to explore feelings further. The fact that a person has become distressed usually shows that the professional has made the person feel safe enough to express their distress.

Coping with denial or unrealistic expectations: these reactions are important and powerful protective mechanisms for anyone facing difficult news.[36] The key is deciding whether their presence is helping the individual cope. If the person is coping then no action need be taken – thoughtless intervention in such a patient shows little regard for the patient, partner, and relative.[37] Obviously, if these reactions are failing to protect the individual, gently challenging the presence of denial or unrealistic expectations may enable the person to express their distress more clearly. This expression is in itself therapeutic and may lead to some resolution of that distress.

Collusion: it takes two (or more) to collude. Both individuals know what is happening, but either deny it together, or at least in each other's company. Collusion is usually between the patient and the partner or relative. Collusion is another reaction that is seen as abnormal by professionals, and yet it is often an act of love, protecting someone they love and know well. This reaction is understandable and like denial can be left if it is working for those involved. However, collusion can cause difficulties if it is damaging the relationship through a "conspiracy of silence," in which case this cost will need to be explored and gently challenged.

Children: parents often wish to protect their dying child ("He's such a happy child . . ."), while the child may try to protect the parents ("I don't want to make her cry."). While this can work for some families, in many it hampers communication at a time when mutual trust, support. and sharing is so important. Parents are often surprised to hear that the child knows more about the situation than they admitted to the parent. Children are often relieved to hear that it is not them but the situation that is making their parents unhappy, and that crying is not always a bad thing. Carers can be in an important position to encourage such communication within the family. Since different family members may open up to different carers, team communication and support are vital.

Clinical decision	If YES carry out the action below
1 Pause to check the person's reaction.	
2 Acknowledge any distress.	
3 Is the person accepting the difficult news?	• **Acknowledge and explore any feelings and concerns.** • **Monitor regularly for feelings** of defeat, spiritual anguish, anger, and withdrawal (*see Anger*, p. 235 and *Withdrawal and depression*, p. 253).
4 Is the person overwhelmingly distressed?	• **Acknowledge the distress**, e.g. "I can see that's distressing news." NB. Although this seems a trite and obvious response from the professional, it shows the person that you have noticed. A "poker" face gives the person the impression of not caring or not wishing to deal with feelings. • **Explore the individual concerns** to work out why the reaction has been so disturbing.
5 Is the person denying or holding on to unrealistic expectations?	• **If the person is coping well with these feelings:** do not persist in challenging denial or unrealistic expectations (after all, they are coping!). • **If the person is not coping with these feelings:** — acknowledge the denial or unrealistic expectations — check for a window on the denial (e.g. "Are there times, even for a second, when you're less sure that everything is alright?") — gently challenge inconsistencies (e.g. "You say everything is fine, but you're worried about the weight loss.") — avoid being defensive about unrealistic expectations. Patients can find that holding on to such expectations helps them even although they realize they are probably unrealistic.
6 Is the person ambivalent?	• **Acknowledge the uncertainty**, e.g. "It seems that you're uncertain about this." • **Offer time for help** (e.g. "When you need more information, please ask.").
7 Is collusion occurring?	**If this is the patient wanting to withhold information from the partner or relative:** • Recognize that this is often due to a need to protect the partner. • Accept that the patient does know the partner or relative better than any professional. • Ask for permission to speak to the partner or relative to find out what they think about the situation. **If this is the partner or relative wanting to withhold information from patient:** • Accept that the carer does know the patient better than any professional. • Explore the reasons for the collusion (remember that the carer is doing what they think best at the time). • Explain that you will need to find out from the patient what they think of the situation. • Check the cost of collusion on the patient–carer relationship.

Adapted from Faulkner, Maguire, and Regnard[34]

NOTES

Identifying distress in the person with severe communication difficulty

CLINICAL DECISION AND ACTION CHECKLIST

1 Observe and document distress signs or behaviors (or ask carers).
2 Document the context.
3 Compare present signs or behaviors with previous episodes of distress, signs, and behaviors when content, and with any long-term behaviors.
4 Check through possible causes.

KEY POINTS

- Even comatose patients can show signs or behaviors of distress.
- Partners and relatives can provide valuable information and, especially in children, their perspective is essential.
- Professional carers have the skills to pick up distress, but often do so intuitively and don't necessarily have confidence in their observations.
- Distress signs and behaviors should be documented and compared with signs and behaviors in other situations.

INTRODUCTION

In some situations and conditions the ability of a patient to express their distress clearly can be severely affected. This includes adults or children with severe learning disability, people with dementia, severe dysphasia (stroke, cerebral tumor), severe depression or psychosis, and people in a comatose or semi-comatose state. There has been little research on distress in people with profound communication problems.[38,39] Carers have found it difficult to articulate their intuitive sense that the individual has an unmet need. The difficulty in identifying distress is magnified when people move between care environments or come into contact with new carers.

Although pain tools have been developed for patients with severe communication difficulties, this approach is being challenged for two reasons:

1 The recognition that pain is itself a distressing experience, so that separating pain signs and behaviors from those produced by other causes of distress may be impossible.[40–42]

2 There is no convincing published evidence that pain produces signs and behaviors that are unique to pain.[43]

Consequently, the concept of identifying distress, rather than pain, is an essential component of achieving comfort in people with severe communication difficulties. The key is to document the carers' existing skills in identifying distress, take note of the context, and then apply clinical decisions to identify the cause.[44]

WHAT ARE THE BEHAVIORS AND SIGNS OF DISTRESS?

Even in the absence of speech or the presence of severe intellectual impairment, distress can still be observed through the following:[44]

Verbal: this may be simple statements, e.g. "I'm not right" or using sounds (crying, screaming, sighing, moaning, grunting).

Facial: these may be simple expressions (grimacing, clenched teeth, shut eyes, wide open eyes, frowning, biting lower lip) or more complex.

Adaptive: rubbing or holding an area, keeping an area still, breath holding, hypersensitivity to stimuli, approaching staff, avoiding stimulation, reduced or absent function (reduced movement, lying, or sitting).

Distractive: rocking (or other rhythmic movements), pacing, biting their hand or lip, gesturing, clenched fists.

Postural: increased muscle tension (extension or flexion), altered posture, flinching, head in hands, limping, pulling cover or clothes over their head, knees drawn up.

Autonomic: this may be either sympathetic (the flight or fright response with ↑pulse rate, ↑BP, wide pupils, pallor, and sweating) or parasympathetic (in response to nausea or visceral pain with ↓BP and ↓pulse rate).

In 80% or more of distress episodes, several signs and behaviors change: facial appearance, verbal expressions, autonomic skin changes, and changes in posture, mannerisms, or the appearance of the eyes.[44] These changes may be a new sign or behavior, or the absence of signs and behavior seen during content times.

PICKING UP DISTRESS

Relatives and parents have often learnt the signs and behaviors of distress and can provide valuable information. Professional carers have the skills to observe the same signs and behaviors of distress, but often do not have confidence in their observations. Daily observation increases the number of distress signs and behaviors that are picked up and teams pick up more signs and behaviors than individuals.[44] Documenting the observations of all new signs and behaviors is a key step.

MAKING SENSE OF DISTRESS SIGNS AND BEHAVIORS

Common mistakes are to misinterpret distress as a behavior that needs treating, or to assume that distress indicates pain. There is no evidence that any single cause of distress produces distinct signs or behaviors.[43] In contrast, individuals tend to use the same signs and behaviors for different types of distress.[44] The context in which the new sign or behavior occurs is important. For example, a distress sign or behavior on moving an arm suggests arm pain, while the same behavior in a frightening situation (e.g. hospital visit) suggests fear. However, it is necessary to work through the checklist overleaf to

Clinical decision	If YES carry out the action below
1 Observe and document signs or behaviors (or ask carers) — *see* notes opposite for examples of distress signs and behaviors — establish baselines during episodes of known contentment.	
2 Document the context in which a new sign or behavior is occurring.	
3 Compare the new sign or behavior of distress with — previous episodes of distress — signs and behaviors when content — any long-term behaviors.	
4 Is the new distress sign or behavior:	
— repeated rapidly?	• **Consider these causes:** — pleuritic pain (in time with breathing): *see* cd-5e in *Emergencies*, p. 335 — colic (comes and goes every few minutes): *see* cd-4 in *Diagnosing and treating pain*, p. 49 — repetitive behavior due to boredom or fear: *see Anxiety*, p. 235, *Anger*, p. 239 or *Withdrawal and depression*, p. 253.
— associated with breathing?	• **Consider these causes:** — pleuritic pain due to infection or tumor: *see* cd-3d on p. 49. — breathlessness due to COPD, pleural effusion, tumor, mucus plugging, aspiration, bronchospasm: *see Respiratory problems*, p. 191.
— worsened or precipitated by movement?	• **Consider:** — movement-related pains: *see* cd-3 in *Diagnosing and treating pain*, p. 47 and p. 49 — a fear or dislike of an activity.
— related to eating?	• **Consider these causes:** — food refusal through illness, fear, depression, or due to swallowing problems: *see Nutrition and hydration problems*, p. 165 and *Dysphagia*, p.131 — oral problems: dental problems, mucosal infection, oromotor dysfunction: *see Oral problems*, p. 183 — upper GI problems (oral hygiene, peptic ulcer, esophageal reflux, dyspepsia) or abdominal problems: *see* cd-7 in *Diagnosing and treating pain*, p. 51.
— related to a specific situation?	• **Consider these causes:** — frightening, unfamiliar or painful situations: e.g. hospital visit, unfamiliar person — painful procedures: *see* cd-5 on p. 51.
— associated with vomiting?	• **Consider causes of nausea and vomiting:** *see Nausea and vomiting*, p. 57 and *Dyspepsia*, p. 123.
— associated with elimination (urine or fecal)?	• **Consider these causes:** — urinary problems (infection, retention): *see Urinary problems and sexual difficulties*, p. 223 — GI problems (diarrhea, constipation): *see Diarrhea*, p. 115, or *Constipation*, p. 107.
— present in a normally comfortable position or situation?	• **Consider these causes:** — pains at rest (*see Diagnosing and treating pain*, pp. 41–55) — nausea (*see Nausea and vomiting*, p. 157) — infection: check urine and chest for signs of infection — anxiety, anger or depression: *see Anxiety*, p. 235, *Anger*, p. 239 or *Withdrawal and depression*, p. 253.

Adapted from DisDAT (Disability Distress Assessment Tool)[44]
cd = clinical decision

ensure that the most likely causes have been considered.

There is now a tool available which helps to document the language of distress that a patient expresses in terms of signs and behaviors.[43] This is known as DisDAT (the Disability Distress Assessment Tool) and is available on www.disdat.co.uk.

Distress may be hidden, but it is never silent.

Discussing preferred priorities of care (advance care planning)

CLINICAL DECISION AND ACTION CHECKLIST

1 Are you uncertain if you are the right person to do this?
2 Does the patient have an impairment of mind or brain that prevents discussion of future plans?
3 Has there been a previous discussion of future plans?
4 Is the patient refusing to discuss future care?
5 Is the patient not ready to discuss end-of-life care?
6 Start discussion about future care
7 Does the patient want to refuse future treatment?
8 Does the patient want this discussion documented?

KEY POINTS

- Enabling a discussion about a patient's future care is important.
- It is a patient-controlled dialogue that evolves over time.
- It should not be a professionally driven health target.

INTRODUCTION

Enabling patients to express their wishes regarding future plans is an important part of effective communication. It is a process of discussion between an individual and their care providers irrespective of discipline, and the purpose is to convey the patient's wishes so that they can be taken into account at a future time when the patient has lost capacity. The timing, setting, and content of this discussion must be under the full control of the patient and is best completed over several meetings.[45] In Canada there is no Advance Care Planning (ACP) legislation, but at the time of writing two health authorities (Fraser in BC, Capital in Calgary, AB) have formal ACP policies, and the Canadian Hospice Palliative Care Association has recently released an information document on the topic.[46] In Canada all provinces and territories except Nunavut have Advance Health Care Directive (AHCD) legislation. In the US the Patient Self-Determination Act (1990) requires institutions to document the existence of an AHCD if the patient has completed one and to have a written policy regarding honoring them, but does not require that an AHCD be completed.[47] There are no federal documents for AHCD, and because every state is free to create its own documents AHCD legislation differs from state to state, including any surrogate decision maker's hierarchy. A Congress report recognized that an AHCD may result from informal ACP discussions,[48] but that it should not be the only result. This emphasizes that an ACP is not the same as an AHCD, which latter in Canada and the US is a legally binding document. Discussion may result in writing an advance decision to refuse treatment (*see* p. 36 and pp. 268–9) but such a result should not be the aim of the discussion and in this context must never be used as a health target.[49]

The evidence that advance care planning improves patient quality of life is weak, but communication can be improved if led by skilled caregivers.[50] However, the timing of the discussions is crucial and should be under the patient's control. Discussions held at a time of significant transition (such as admission to a residential home) can cause distress,[51] while some with advanced disease will not be ready to discuss their future care.[45,52] Patients vary over time, and from one to another, as to how much of their future care they wish to discuss.

ARE YOU THE RIGHT PERSON?

It is not possible to explore a patient's wishes and preferences about future care if you lack knowledge about their present situation and the options available in the future.

IS THERE AN IMPAIRMENT OF MIND OR BRAIN?

Capacity depends both on the complexity of the decision to be made, and the area in which the decision is being made, e.g. a patient may have capacity to make a health decision but not a financial one. If capacity is lacking for a particular decision, the decisions about future care must be made by a substitute decision maker (SDM) or health care proxy. The SDM/proxy must follow any instructions given in an AHCD, or give effect to the known wishes of the patient. If there are no instructions and the patient's wishes are not known, the SDM/proxy makes a decision in the "best interests of the patient." Health professionals should be familiar with their national and state or provincial legislation regarding AHCDs.

DISCUSSION ABOUT FUTURE CARE

If this has taken place previously it is important to check if the patient has changed their priorities. Some patients find it too difficult and distressing to discuss future care and this must be respected. Others will discuss future care, but refuse to contemplate or discuss this care in the context of the end of life. This must also be respected. In both cases the patients have the right to control the flow of information and professionals can only proceed if they have received informed consent to do so – usually this is a verbal consent to proceed.

If future care is discussed, this is best done with open questions such as:[53]

Q. In relation to your health, what has been happening to you?

Q. What are your preferences and priorities for your future care?

Q. Where would you like to be cared for in the future?

It is important to remember that any decisions a patient makes about their future care

- can only be made while they have the capacity for these decisions, and
- only become active when the patient loses that capacity.

ADVANCE REFUSAL OF FUTURE TREATMENT

A patient may demand treatment, but in Canada health professionals are under no obligation to provide non-beneficial or ineffective treatment. In the US there is no federal legislation regarding

Clinical decision	If YES carry out the action below
1 Are you uncertain if you are the right person to do this?	• **If you are uncertain or lack knowledge** of the patient's clinical condition and treatment possibilities, or their reaction to their illness, do not proceed. • **Ask a colleague** who does have this knowledge to lead the discussion.
2 Does the patient have an impairment of mind or brain?	• **If this prevents discussion of future plans:** assess the patient's capacity – *see* cd-2 in *Decisions around capacity*, p. 269. • **If the patient does not have capacity for making future plans**, then *see Decisions around capacity*, p. 267. • **If they have capacity for making future plans**, continue the discussion.
3 Has there been a previous discussion of future plans?	• **Ask the patient** if they want to change their previous priorities for care. • **Ask permission** to see any available documentation.
4 Is the patient refusing to discuss future care?	• **Review the situation regularly**, since the patient may change their mind and ask to discuss future care. • **If a patient has refused once, repeatedly checking will only cause further distress.** However, if the patient's circumstances change (e.g. acute admission to hospital) it is reasonable to check.
5 Is the patient not ready to discuss end-of-life care?	• Many patients with early or slowly progressing disease, and some with advanced disease, will not wish to discuss end-of-life care. However, they should still receive the opportunity to discuss other aspects of their future care. • Remember that the discussion and any documentation does *not have to* include questions or statements about end-of-life care.
6 Start discussion about future care: • Ask open questions, for example Q. In relation to your health, what has been happening to you? Q. What are your preferences and priorities for your future care? Q. Where would you like to be cared for in the future? • Allow the patient to control the flow of all information, i.e. if they do not want to discuss an aspect of their future care, defer that question to another time. • Check if there are any further issues, e.g. "Are there any other issues that are important to you?"	
7 Does the patient want to refuse future treatment?	• Document both the discussion and the decision. Ask if the patient has completed an AHCD, or wishes to do so. Ensure it is consistent with their stated wishes, and recommend that it be made available where likely to be needed, e.g. on the hospital chart, in the home, at their physicians' offices.
8 Does the patient want this discussion documented?	• **If they want the discussion documented:** — write the priorities for care in the patient's records. If specific documentation is used, do not use one that is restricted to end of life for a patient who does not want to discuss this aspect of their care — offer the patient a copy — ask the patient if and to whom they want copies given, e.g. care teams, family — document and date all subsequent discussions and changes. • **If they do not want the discussion documented** — document only that the discussion has taken place — review the patient's future priorities when the patient requests a review OR when their circumstances change.

Adapted from Regnard, Randall, Matthews, and Gibson[55]
cd = clinical decision

this, and most state legislation tends to be conservative and leans toward preservation of life. Health care personnel should be aware of legislation in their own state. However, some patients will wish to make specific statements to refuse future treatment, and health professionals are obliged to honor this decision if it is valid and applicable. This can be done verbally, but if the refusal concerns life-sustaining treatment, both the fact that the discussion took place and the resulting decision should be documented. A well-written AHCD is useful here, but unfortunately many patients understand poorly the term "life-sustaining therapies," so patients should be encouraged, before writing an AHCD, to discuss their wishes and how to word them, with a health care professional who knows about their case and their illness.[54] Life-sustaining treatment is any treatment that, if refused, would result in the death of the patient.

DOCUMENTATION

A patient may refuse to have any details of the discussion documented, in which case only the fact that the discussion has taken place can be documented.

There is no single format for advance care planning documentation, but if the patient agrees to documentation it should:

- be simple and contain answers to broad questions about future care
- not address end-of-life care if the patient does not wish to do so. However, these patients may well be ready to discuss other aspects of their future care. The inclusion of end-of-life care discussions in a document can encourage professionals to assume that advance care planning is only about end-of-life care.
- include advance decisions to refuse treatment or decisions on cardiopulmonary resuscitation (CPR) only if the patient wishes to discuss them.

If an (informal) ACP is decided upon, it should be documented in the chart and other appropriate places, e.g. the home, with the patient's agreement. Most patients will be happy for the document to be widely circulated or held on a central database, but patients with capacity must be given the opportunity to refuse if they wish.

REVIEWING ADVANCE CARE PLANS

These should be reviewed regularly, ideally at intervals agreed with the patient. A change in the patient's circumstances may be a trigger for a review, but this may also be a difficult time for a patient that prevents them from wanting to plan the next steps.

REFERENCES: GETTING STARTED

B = book; C = comment; Ch = chapter; CS(n) = case study (no. of cases); CT = controlled trial; E = editorial; GC = group consensus; I = interviews; LS = laboratory study; MC = multi-center; OS = open study; PhD = PhD thesis; R = review; RCT (n) = randomized controlled trial (no. of cases); RS = retrospective survey; SA = systematic or meta analysis; web = online resource.

1 Regnard C. Helping the person to share their problems. In: *CLiP (Current Learning in Palliative Care) e-learning programme*. www.helpthehospices.org.uk/clip (web)
2 Maguire P, Faulkner A, Regnard C. (1995) Eliciting the current problems. In: *Flow Diagrams in Advanced Cancer and Other Diseases*. London: Edward Arnold. pp. 1–4. (Ch)
3 Price J, Leaver L. (2002) ABC of psychological medicine: beginning treatment. *British Medical Journal*. **325**: 33–5.
4 Maguire P, Walsh S, Jeacock J, Kingston R. (1999) Physical and psychological needs of patients dying from colo-rectal cancer. *Palliative Medicine*. **13**: 45–50. (OS, I)
5 Maguire P, Parkes CM. (1998) Surgery and loss of body parts. *British Medical Journal*. **316**: 1086–8. (R)
6 Wilson KG, Chochinov HM, Skirko MG, Allard P, Chary S, Gagnon PR, Macmillan K, De Luca M, O'Shea F, Kuhl D, Fainsinger RL, Clinch

JJ. (2007) Depression and anxiety disorders in palliative cancer care. *Journal of Pain and Symptom Management*. **33**(2): 118–29. (I-381)

7 Heaven CM, Maguire P. (1996) Training hospice nurses to elicit patient concerns. *Journal of Advanced Nursing*. **23**: 280–6. (R)

8 Heaven C, Clegg J, Maguire P. (2006) Transfer of communication skills training from workshop to workplace: the impact of clinical supervision. *Patient Education and Counseling*. **60**(3): 313–25. (RCT-61)

9 Maguire P, Faulkner A, Booth K, Elliott C, Hillier V. (1996) Helping cancer patients disclose their concerns. *European Journal of Cancer*. **32A**: 78–81. (OS)

10 Maguire P. (1985) Barriers to psychological care of the dying. *British Medical Journal Clinical Research Ed*. **291**: 1711–3. (R)

11 Maguire P. (1999) Improving communication with cancer patients. *European Journal of Cancer*. **35**: 2058–65. (R)

12 Maguire P. (1999) Improving communication with cancer patients. *European Journal of Cancer*. **35**: 1415–22. (R)

13 Heaven C, Clegg J, Maguire P. (2006) Transfer of communication skills training from workshop to workplace: the impact of clinical supervision. *Patient Education and Counseling*. **60**(3): 313–25. (RCT-29)

14 Chibnall JT, Bennett ML, Videen SD, Duckro PN, Miller DK. (2004) Identifying barriers to psychosocial spiritual care at the end of life: a physician group study. *American Journal of Hospice and Palliative Medicine*. **21**(6): 419–26. (OS, I-17)

15 Hills J, Paice JA, Cameron JR, Shott S. (2005) Spirituality and distress in palliative care consultation. *Journal of Palliative Medicine*. **8**(4): 782–8. (I-31)

16 Selman L, Beynon T, Higginson IJ, Harding R. (2007) Psychological, social and spiritual distress at the end of life in heart failure patients. *Current Opinion in Supportive and Palliative Care*. **1**(4): 260–6. (R, 88 refs)

17 McSherry M, Kehoe K, Carroll JM, Kang TI, Rourke MT. (2007) Psychosocial and spiritual needs of children living with a life-limiting illness. *Pediatric Clinics of North America*. **54**(5): 609–29. (R, 48 refs)

18 Vivat B, Members of the Quality of Life Group of the European Organisation for Research and Treatment of Cancer. (2008) Measures of spiritual issues for palliative care patients: a literature review. *Palliative Medicine*. **22**(7): 859–68. (SA-29)

19 Daaleman TP, Usher BM, Williams SW, Rawlings J, Hanson LC. (2008) An exploratory study of spiritual care at the end of life. *Annals of Family Medicine*. **6**(5): 406–11. (I-12)

20 Hanson LC, Dobbs D, Usher BM, Williams S, Rawlings J, Daaleman TP. (2008) Providers and types of spiritual care during serious illness. *Journal of Palliative Medicine*. **11**(6): 907–14. (I-103)

21 Rodin G, Lo C, Mikulincer M, Donner A, Gagliese L, Zimmermann C. (2009) Pathways to distress: the multiple determinants of depression, hopelessness, and the desire for hastened death in metastatic cancer patients. *Social Science and Medicine*. **68**(3): 562–9. (I-406)

22 Fanos JH, Gelinas DF, Foster RS, Postone N, Miller RG. (2008) Hope in palliative care: from narcissism to self-transcendence in amyotrophic lateral sclerosis. *Journal of Palliative Medicine*. **11**(3): 470–5. (I-16)

23 Regnard C. Answering difficult questions. In: *CLiP (Current Learning in Palliative Care) e-learning programme*. www.helpthehospices.org.uk (click on 'e-learning'). (web)

24 Fallowfield L. (2004) Communication with the patient and family in palliative medicine. In: Doyle D, Hanks G, Cherney NI, Calman K, eds. *Oxford Textbook of Palliative Medicine, 3rd ed*. Oxford: Oxford University Press. pp. 101–7.

25 Kennedy V, Lloyd-Williams M. (2006) Maintaining hope: communication in palliative care. *Recent Results in Cancer Research*. **168**: 47–60.

26 Dein S, Thomas K. (2002) To tell or not to tell. *European Journal of Palliative Care*. **9**(5): 209–12. (R, 30 refs)

27 Fainsinger RL, Núñez-Olarte JM, Demoissac DM. (2003) The cultural differences in perceived value of disclosure and cognition: Spain and Canada. *Journal of Pain and Symptom Management*. **19**(1): 43–8. (I-200)

28 Bruera E, Palmer JL, Pace E, Zhang K, Willey J, Strasser F, Bennett MI. (2007) A randomized, controlled trial of physician postures when breaking bad news to cancer patients. *Palliative Medicine*. **21**(6): 501–5. (RCT-168)

29 Faulkner A, Regnard C. (1995) Handling difficult questions. In: *Flow Diagrams in Advanced Cancer and Other Diseases*. London: Edward Arnold. pp. 92–5. (Ch)

30 Fallowfield LJ, Jenkins VA, Beveridge HA. (2002) Truth may hurt but deceit hurts more: communication in palliative care. *Palliative Medicine*. **16**: 297–303.

31 General Medical Council. (2008) *Consent: Patients and Doctors Making Decisions Together*. London: GMC. (available at: www.gmc-uk.org/news/articles/Consent_guidance.pdf)

32 Friedrichsen M, Milberg A. (2006) Concerns about losing control when breaking bad news to terminally ill patients with cancer: physicians' perspective. *Journal of Palliative Medicine*. **9**(3): 673–82. (I-30)

33 Rudnick A. (2002) Informed consent to breaking bad news. *Nursing Ethics: an International Journal for Health Care Professionals*. **9**(1): 61–6. (R, 7 refs)

34 Faulkner A, Maguire P, Regnard C. (1995) Breaking bad news. In: *Flow Diagrams in Advanced Cancer and Other Diseases*. London: Edward Arnold; pp. 86–91. (Ch)

35 Maguire P. (1998) Breaking bad news. *European Journal of Surgical Oncology*. **24**: 188–91. (R)

36 Vos MS, de Haes JCJM. (2007) Denial in cancer patients: an explorative review. *Psycho-Oncology*. **16**: 12–25. (R)

37 Vachon MLS. (2004) The emotional problems of the patient in palliative medicine. In: Doyle D,

Hanks G, Cherney NI, Calman K, eds. *Oxford Textbook of Palliative Medicine, 3rd ed.* Oxford: Oxford University Press. pp. 961–85.
38 Hunt A. (2001) Towards an understanding of pain in the child with severe neurological impairment. Development of a behaviour rating scale for assessing pain. PhD thesis. Manchester: University of Manchester. (PhD)
39 Tuffrey-Wijne I. (2003) The palliative care needs of people with intellectual disabilities: a literature review. *Palliative Medicine.* **17**: 55–62. (R)
40 Kaasalainen S. (2007) Pain assessment in older adults with dementia: using behavioral observation methods in clinical practice. *Journal of Gerontological Nursing.* **33**(6): 6–10. (R, 40 refs)
41 Jordan AI, Regnard C, Hughes JC. (2007) Hidden pain or hidden evidence? *Journal of Pain and Symptom Management.* **33**(6): 658–60. (Let)
42 Regnard C. (2007) A pain tool for people with communication difficulties is no closer. *Clinical Medicine.* **7**(1): 89–90. (Let)
43 Regnard C, Mathews M, Gibson L, Clarke C. (2003) Difficulties in identifying distress and its causes in people with severe communication problems. *International Journal of Palliative Nursing.* **9**(3): 173–6. (R)
44 Regnard C, Reynolds J, Watson B, Matthews D, Gibson L, Clarke C. (2007) Understanding distress in people with severe communication difficulties: developing and assessing the Disability Distress Assessment Tool (DisDAT). *Journal of Intellectual Disability Research.* **51**(4): 277–92.
45 Barnes K, Jones L, Tookman A, King M. (2007) Acceptability of an advance care planning interview schedule: a focus group study. *Palliative Medicine.* **21**(1): 23–8. (I-22)
46 Available at: www.chpca.net/projects/advance_care_planning/acp_detailed_project_overview_aug_6_09.pdf
47 Galambos CM (1998) Preserving end-of-life autonomy: the Patient Self-Determination Act and the Uniform Health Care Decisions Act. *Health and Social Work.* **23**(4): 275–81.
48 Advance Directives and Advance Care Planning: Report to Congress (2008). Available at: http://aspe.hhs.gov/daltcp/reports/2008/ADCongRpt.htm#ref19
49 Parker M, Stewart C, Willmott L, Cartwright C. (2007) Two steps forward, one step back: advance care planning, Australian regulatory frameworks and the Australian Medical Association. *Internal Medicine Journal.* **37**(9): 637–43.
50 Lorenz KA, Lynn J, Dy SM, Shugarman LR, Wilkinson A, Mularski RA, Morton SC, Hughes RG, Hilton LK, Maglione M, Rhodes SL, Rolon C, Sun VC, Shekelle PG. (2008) Evidence for improving palliative care at the end of life: a systematic review. *Annals of Internal Medicine.* **148**(2): 147–59. (SA-1274)
51 White C. (2005) An exploration of decision-making factors regarding advance directives in a long-term care facility. *Journal of the American Academy of Nurse Practitioners.* **17**(1): 14–20.
52 Hofmann JC, Wenger NS, Davis RB, Teno J, Connors AF Jr., Desbiens N, *et al.* (1997) Patient preferences for communication with physicians about end-of-life decisions. SUPPORT Investigators. Study to Understand Prognoses and Preference for Outcomes and Risks of Treatment. *Annals of Internal Medicine.* **127**(1): 1–12.
53 Storey L. (2007) Preferred Priorities of Care. *Personal Communication.*
54 Thorevska N, Tilluckdarry L, Tickoo S, Havasi A, Amoateng-Adjepong Y, Manthoius CA. (2005) Patients' understanding of advance directives and cardiopulmonary resuscitation. *Journal of Critical Care.* **20**: 26–34.
55 Regnard C, Randall F, Matthews D, Gibson L. (2008) Algorithm: discussing future care with patients. In: *Advance Care Planning: a guide for health and social staff.* London: End of Life Programme.

Pain

NOTES

Diagnosing and treating pain

CLINICAL DECISION AND ACTION CHECKLIST

Do the pain descriptions, signs or behaviors suggest:

1 Severe or overwhelming pain?
2 Breakthrough pain?
3 Relation to movement?
4 Periodicity?
5 Relation to a procedure?
6 Visceral pain?
7 Relation to eating?
8 Association with skin changes?
9 Worsening by touch, or an unpleasant sensory change at rest?
10 Exacerbation when passing urine or stool?
11 It is in an area supplied by a peripheral nerve?
12 Persistence despite treatment?

KEY POINTS

- Pain treatment cannot start until an assessment has been made of the likely cause of pain.
- Work through these 12 pain clinical decisions in order – they cover most of the pains seen in advanced disease.
- Use the information provided to help you decide which pain is present.
- Finally, follow the suggestions in the tables for managing the pain.

INTRODUCTION

Most adults and older children can clearly describe pain and its nature. It is important to ask how the pain has affected feelings, daily activities, and relationships, and to ascertain the patient's expectations.[1] Information from parents and carers can be invaluable, but the basic rule is that "pain is what the patient says hurts."[2] A clinical examination is essential. Children beyond infancy, and adults with moderate learning disability, may need to use their own words for pain such as "hurt," or "feeling bad,"[3–5] However, making clear that the distress is due to pain can be difficult or impossible for a pre-verbal child, or anyone with severe anxiety, depression, confusion or cognitive impairment. There is no evidence that pain tools are of value in differentiating pain from other causes of distress, and the use of pain tools in children or adults with severe communication impairment is now being questioned.[6] However, identifying the cause of distress is still possible. *See Identifying distress in the person with severe communication difficulty*, p. 31.

CHECKLIST FOR PAIN

1 Severe or overwhelming pain

Pain of this severity needs urgent treatment (*see* cd-5 in *Emergencies*, p. 335).

2 Breakthrough pain

A brief worsening of pain can "break through" the analgesia, resulting in distress and the perception of poor pain control, despite good background analgesia with regular analgesics.[7,8] It is common, occurring in nearly two-thirds of cancer patients.[9] Since the average number of daily breakthrough episodes in cancer are four (range 1–8), with each averaging 35 minutes,[10] the main difficulty is getting an analgesic response that is quick enough to provide relief.[8]

The causes of breakthrough pain include:

- related to movement or a procedure[11]
- inadequate regular analgesia
- an unpredictable worsening of the pain, e.g. pathological fracture
- episodic pain caused by a pain less responsive to the current analgesia, e.g. colic, neuropathic pain
- reluctance of the patient to take analgesia because of misunderstanding, adverse effects or the fear of adverse effects.[12]

Since parenteral routes are impractical for long-term use, especially in the community, alternative routes are being used. The oral route is often acceptable and most opioids can start providing relief within 30 minutes. Using a lipid-soluble opioid (e.g. fentanyl, alfentanil) the buccal route can give relief within 20 minutes.[13–15] Newer routes (e.g. intranasal) and devices are becoming available, but there is no evidence that they will provide better or safer analgesia. However, such routes may have a role in the very small number of patients who need relief within 10 minutes. An alternative is to use Entonox (nitrous oxide and oxygen).[16] Severe pain that is unresponsive to systemic analgesics may need spinal analgesia or (if a single nerve is involved) a regional nerve block.

3 Pain related to movement

Fracture

Movement of the affected part by the examiner will usually result in severe pain on the slightest movement. Pathological fractures (e.g. bone metastases) are not always painful when they occur, but pain is usually a feature within minutes or hours. For severe pain, follow the advice for severe pain in cd-5 in *Emergencies*, p. 335.

Bone problems

Local tenderness over a bone suggests a local weakness. Severe skeletal instability can cause pain on minimal movement such as coughing. Osteoporosis is common in both men and women, especially those on long-term corticosteroids. In immune-compromised patients infection should be excluded, especially mycobacteria. Bone metastases are best picked up on bone scan, except for myeloma and renal carcinoma which may show up better on X-rays, CT or MRI scan.

Weak or strong opioids are first-line treatment, but such pains may be less opioid responsive.[17,18]

Radiotherapy for bone metastases: this produces complete relief after one month in 25% and partial relief in a further 40%,[19] and remains an important second-line treatment.[20,21] The pain of some patients increases after radiotherapy and can be alleviated by using dexamethasone.[22] Single fractions (e.g. 8 Gy) are as effective as, and better tolerated, than multiple fractions (e.g. 30 Gy over 10 treatments) but the need to repeat treatment is more common.[23,24] For multiple metastases radioactive compounds such as strontium isotope can be effective.[25]

Clinical decision	If YES carry out the action below
1 Is the pain severe or overwhelming?	*See* cd-5 in *Emergencies*, p. 335.
2 Is this breakthrough pain? **(i.e. pain occurring despite regular analgesia)**	NB. All breakthrough doses may need to be adjusted up or down to the individual patient: • **If already on a non-opioid analgesic:** give one dose of the regular analgesic, e.g. 1 g acetaminophen. • **If already on a regular opioid:** give 10% of the 24 hour dose e.g. 60 mg/24 hr oral morphine = approx. 5 mg dose e.g. 25 microg/hr transdermal fentanyl (i.e. 600 microg/24 hr) = approx. 50 microg buccally/SL/SC. • **If there is a response to the breakthrough dose:** Consider increasing the regular analgesic dose if the breakthrough pain tends to occur before the next regular dose or if three or more breakthrough doses are used each day. • **If there is no response after one breakthrough dose:** *For a non-opioid:* repeat in four hours. If there is no response consider changing to a weak opioid or a low dose of a strong opioid. *For an opioid:* repeat after one hour with the same dose. If there is still no response after one hour, give a third dose. • **If there is still no response after three breakthrough doses of a strong opioid:** — reconsider the cause of pain using the following pain cd-3 to cd-12. — consider Entonox (50% O_2, 50% N_2O) — *see* cd-5f in *Emergencies*, p. 335.
3 Is the pain related to movement? **(i.e. worsened or precipitated by movement)**	**a. Worsened by the slightest passive movement** • **Fracture** (deformity may be present): immobilize. *See* cd-5c in *Emergencies*, p. 335. Consider elective orthopedic surgery and radiotherapy. In osteoporosis or malignancy start bisphosphonate and calcium treatment. • **Severe soft tissue inflammation:** usually due to infection: *see* cd-8b p. 53. If the infection is deeper, movement pain may be the only sign. • **Joint problems:** (common in immobile and neurologically impaired patients) *Exclude* infection, subluxation, dislocation, metastases or a fracture involving the joint. *For inflammatory arthropathies:* ask a rheumatologist for advice. Ask the physiotherapist and occupational therapist for advice on positioning, and modifying mobility and function. *Consider:* NSAIDs, strong opioids or ketamine. • **Inflammation or irritation of muscle** (affected muscle in spasm): *see* cd-3c p. 47. • **Nerve compression:** *see* cd-11 on p. 55.

Adapted from Thompson and Regnard[26]
cd = clinical decision

NSAIDs: there is no evidence to support the routine, first-line use of NSAIDs in bone pain,[27] but they can be useful second- or third-line treatment in some patients. IV and oral ketorolac have been shown to have an opioid-sparing effect in patients with bone metastases.[28]

Bisphosphonates: these take several months before pain reduces. An exception may be intravenous ibandronic acid (not Canada) which can reduce pain within days.[29,30] When used regularly, bisphosphonates have the added advantage of reducing skeletal complications.[31,32] Adverse effects are usually mild, but care must be taken to keep patients hydrated to prevent renal failure. In patients who have had recent dental surgery, or have a poor dental state, there is a risk of osteonecrosis of the jaw.[33] If needed and practicable, the patient should receive dental attention before starting the bisphosphonate.

Gabapentin: it is not only the periosteum that contains sensory fibers, but also the marrow and mineralized bone,[34] and there is animal evidence that bone pain has a neuropathic component, making gabapentin a possible adjuvant.[35]

Stabilization: if skeletal instability is severe, operative fixation can be used followed by radiotherapy.[36] For persistent pain from vertebral metastases, vertebroplasty (injection of cement into the vertebral body metastasis) can be effective in selected patients.[37]

Chemotherapy: this can provide rapid relief in sensitive tumors such as small-cell lung carcinoma.

Joint pains

These are common in immobile patients due to muscle atrophy, weakness and poor positioning. Spasticity due to neurological impairment can be exacerbated by contractures which can be severe enough to cause subluxation or dislocation of joints. The advice of rheumatology specialists can be helpful.

Myofascial pain

This is common in advanced disease. The pain is distributed in a myotomal pattern and charts showing the typical distribution of all the main muscles are available.[38–40] A trigger point is usually present in the affected muscle and consists of a single spot, which reproduces the pain when pressed, accompanied by a palpable band of muscle in spasm beneath the trigger point.[41] They can occur in any muscle, but are particularly common in the posterior shoulder and paraspinal muscles. Acupuncture or an injection of local anesthetic into the trigger point is equally effective.[42,43] Transcutaneous electrical nerve stimulation (TENS) is effective with the frequency set low (5–10 Hz) and the electrodes positioned either side of the trigger point.[44,45]

Skeletal muscle strain

This occurs suddenly during exertion. Although a cold compress seems effective, the evidence base is poor.[46] Local warmth is more pleasant for the patient.

Spasticity and dystonia

Spasticity is characterized by an increase in muscle tone due to cerebral or spinal damage involving the upper motor neurons of the corticospinal tracts. Dystonia is a state of sustained muscle contraction producing involuntary fluctuating movements and postures, without pyramidal deficit. Pain is a common feature, often severe and can be the cause of general distress and agitation in a child.

Infection or tumor involving muscle will cause that muscle to go into painful spasm. Infection must be excluded and treated if present. The pain of tumor infiltration can be helped with dexamethasone, or possibly with a local nerve or spinal block.

Clinical decision	If YES carry out the action below
3 Is the pain related to movement? (contd.)	**b. Worsened by straining bone during examination** (e.g. percussing spine, pressing rib) • **Consider** nerve compression (*see* cd-11 on p. 55) or bone infection. • **Bone metastases** (may need to be confirmed on bone or CT/MRI scan): *If in pain at rest:* start a strong opioid. If no improvement after three dose increases, add an NSAID (e.g. diclofenac) for one week's trial. If this fails try gabapentin. *If pain is mainly on movement:* consider ketamine (*see* p. 54), and immobilization (splints, sleep positioning systems) while considering spinal analgesia (*see* p. 56). *For pain in a single site:* start dexamethasone 6 mg daily and arrange radiotherapy. *If the pain is in multiple sites:* (and patient is not hypocalcemic) use ibandronic acid (not Canada) 6 mg as 2 hour IV infusion daily for 3 days; or zoledronate 4 mg IV over 15 minutes. Ensure the patient is well hydrated and do not use if the patient has recently had dental surgery, or has bad dental hygiene. If this fails, consider referral for strontium isotope. **c. Worsened by active movement** • **Skeletal instability:** pain on any movement that strains the bone such as coughing or standing suggests there is a risk of bone fracture or collapse. Treat bone metastases as in cd-3b above. Arrange for an urgent X-ray and consider referral for orthopedic and radiotherapy opinion. • **Myofascial pain** (pain on muscle contraction, myotomal distribution, trigger point in muscle which reproduces pain when pressed): inject the trigger point with 0.25% bupivacaine, or use a TENS set at low frequency (5–10 Hz) with the electrodes either side of the trigger point. • **Skeletal muscle strain** (pain on muscle contraction, history of sudden onset during exertion): TENS, local warmth or cold. • **Spasticity:** start with baclofen 10 mg q8h and titrate the dose at weekly intervals. If the spasm persists ask for advice from a neurorehabilitation specialist about botulinum toxin injection. Other options include nerve blocks and spinal analgesia. **d. Worsened by inspiration (or breathing is more shallow)** • **Rib metastases** (local tenderness is present): refer for intercostal nerve block. For multiple sites *see* cd-3b above. • **Pleuritic pain** (local rub may be present): consider a pulmonary embolus. Treat infection if present. Consider an NSAID ± intercostal block. • **Peritoneal pain due to local metastases:** start an NSAID, e.g. diclofenac 50 mg q8h. If the pain is localized to one or two dermatomes, try an intercostal block. For peritonitis *see* cd-5d, p. 337.

Adapted from Thompson and Regnard[26]
cd = clinical decision

Spasticity is also seen in several neurological conditions such as motor neurone disease/ALS, cerebral palsy, multiple sclerosis, and spinal cord injury.[47] The advice of the physiotherapist and occupational therapist is important since correct positioning and seating can reduce the pain of the spasticity.[48] Simple measures may alleviate spasticity such as repositioning the person or gentle stretching of the muscles involved.

Multiple options are available including oral antispastic agents,[49] botulinum toxin,[50] neurolytic blocks,[51] surgical correction of deformities,[52] and intrathecal baclofen.[53,54] Antispastic drugs can be effective orally, and are more effective in younger children but are often limited by unacceptable side-effects such as weakness, sedation, and increased secretions. Diazepam can be used as a single bedtime dose, but adverse effects are common.[55] However, there is no clear evidence base to choose one treatment over another.[56] Consequently, if the spasticity does not respond to simple drug treatment, advice from a neurorehabilitation specialist may help.

Severe soft tissue inflammation

This is usually due to an acute infection. Overlying skin is usually red and swollen, and antibiotics are indicated (*see* cd-8b on p. 53). Deep infection in immunocompromised patients may have few signs and may be an abscess which needs draining and IV antibiotics. In head and neck cancer, the rapid onset of severe pain may be the only symptom of infection, but it responds rapidly to cephalexin and metronidazole.

Pleuritic pain

This is due to local pleural inflammation and persistent pain can be eased with an NSAID or an intercostal block of the affected area.

Other causes

Structures that are inflamed, infected, or distended may cause pain on movement. Recent trauma needs to be excluded, especially in frail or elderly patients.

4 Periodic pain (colic)

Smooth muscle spasm causes recurring episodes of pain lasting a few minutes. This periodic feature is characteristic of colic, although occasionally colic is continuous. Bowel is the commonest source, usually due to constipation, obstruction, diet, or mucosal irritation. The next commonest sources are the bladder (usually due to infection or irritation from a catheter) and the ureter (usually due to obstruction). Bile duct and uterus are unusual sources in advanced disease. If possible, the cause needs to be investigated to find a definitive treatment.

Opioids are only partly effective and may worsen the pain. A smooth muscle relaxant (antispasmodic) is the treatment of choice. Hyoscine butylbromide (Buscopan (Canada)) is preferred since it has fewer central effects than hyoscine hydrobromide (scopolamine) and glycopyrrolate. It must be given parenterally (e.g. SC or IV) to be effective since its oral bioavailability is less than 1%, although the oral route may have a local effect on the gut.[57] In the US use hyoscyamine (Levsin).

Renal (ureteric) colic can be severe and persistent. Strong opioids can be helpful. Rectal or parenteral NSAIDs are possibly more effective, although they can have more adverse effects.[58,59] Advice from a urology specialist is important as treatments such as stone removal and ureteric stents may be possible.

Clinical decision	If YES carry out the action below
3 (cont.) **Is the pain related to movement?** **(i.e. worsened or precipitated by movement)**	e. **Consider also:** • **Joint pain:** treat local infection if this is present. Start an NSAID, e.g. diclofenac 50 mg q8h. Check for dislocation or subluxation. Ask the physiotherapist for advice. • **Gastric distension due to gastric stasis** (fullness, early satiation, hiccups, heartburn): *see Nausea and vomiting*, p. 167. • **Local distension due to hemorrhage:** exclude bleeding disorder. Consider a strong opioid or ketamine. • **Local distension due to tumor:** Strong opioid ± high-dose dexamethasone (8–16 mg daily). A local block or spinal analgesia is sometimes needed. • **Local inflammation due to tumor, infection or trauma:** exclude and treat infection. For skin *see* cd-8 p. 53. Consider radiotherapy if this is due to tumor. • **Trauma:** do a "first aid" examination (head, neck, shoulders, limbs, back, chest, abdomen). • **Gastroesophageal reflux:** *see* cd-4 in *Dyspepsia*, p. 125.
4 **Is the pain periodic?** **(i.e. comes and goes regularly)**	a. **Occurring regularly every few seconds:** consider: —rib metastases or pleuritic pain (*see* cd-3d on p. 47) —severe skeletal instability (*see* cd-3c on p. 47) b. **Occurring regularly every few minutes:** this is likely to be smooth muscle colic. If unsure, give a single dose of hyoscine butylbromide 20 mg IV (Canada) (or 300 microg of buccal hyoscine hydrobromide) – rapid pain relief confirms this is colic. In the US use hyoscyamine 0.25 mg PO/SL • **Abdominal pain:** probably bowel colic due to constipation, bowel obstruction, diet (e.g. tube feeding, food sensitivity), or bowel irritation (drugs, radiotherapy, chemotherapy, infection): — treat the cause, but for relief use hyoscine butylbromide 10–20 mg (Canada) SC as required, or can be used as continuous SC infusion (30–180 mg/24 hr). In US use hyoscyamine 0.125–0.25 mg PO/SL tid–qid PRN. • **Suprapubic pain with urinary frequency or urgency:** this may be bladder colic due to infection, outflow obstruction, unstable bladder, or irritation by tumor or catheter. Treat the cause, but for relief use hyoscine butylbromide or hyoscyamine as for bowel colic above. *See Urinary problems and sexual difficulties*, p. 223. • **If the pain is in the loin or groin:** this may be ureteric colic due to irritation or obstruction. Treat the cause if possible. — consider starting a strong opioid (or giving a breakthrough dose of an existing opioid). An NSAID can be tried if the renal function is normal. For ureteric obstruction due to tumor, try dexamethasone 16 mg daily. *If the pain persists:* If the patient is well hydrated and renal function is normal give ketorolac 30 mg IV or SC repeated after 30 min if needed, or diclofenac100 mg PR. *For obstruction due to tumor:* try dexamethasone 6 mg once daily. Consider referral for ureteric stenting.

Adapted from Thompson and Regnard[26]
cd = clinical decision

5 Pain related to a procedure

Procedures that are painful produce increasing fear and pain with further procedures. Wounds such as pressure ulcers are often painful and pain can last an hour or more after a dressing change.[60] Using one or more of the following approaches can change an intolerable episode into one that can be tolerated repeatedly:

Change the technique: explanation together with a caring and calm approach in a warm and private setting can reduce patient anxiety. Distraction and cuddling can help a child and complementary therapies have a role.[61] Changing to non-adherent dressings reduces the pain when they are next removed.[62]

Topical drugs: for blood sample or venous cannulation, the topical application of a local anesthetic cream or gel is effective.[63,64] Preparations containing tetracaine (amethocaine) (e.g. Ametop gel) seem more effective than those with lidocaine (e.g. EMLA cream).[64] Mucosal pain can be eased by lidocaine, but the spray can cause initial stinging. Sometimes an area is highly sensitive due to inflammation. The application of topical steroids will reduce the inflammation and pain – if the area is too sensitive to apply any cream, a strong preparation of beclomethasone inhaler powder can be applied. Topical morphine[65–68] may help and appears to work through a local effect.[69] However, two trials have failed to show an effect.[70,71] The role of topical NSAIDs is even less clear with an ibuprofen-impregnated dressing showing benefit in small trials,[72,73] but locally applied benzydamine cream showing no effect.[74]

Systemic analgesia: this can be the breakthrough dose of the regular analgesic (*see* cd-2, p. 45) or a single dose of another analgesic such as gabapentin.[75] If given orally, sufficient time must be allowed for the drug to be effective, otherwise it needs to be given by the IM, IV, SC or buccal route.

Entonox (nitrous oxide and oxygen) is a quick, effective analgesia for procedure-related pain in children and adults, including the elderly.[76–80] However, it is less effective than sedation and may not control severe pain.[81,82] It should not be used in the presence of abnormal air cavities, e.g. pneumothorax or bowel distension due to obstruction.[80]

Sedation: some procedures require more than local or systemic analgesia and moderate sedation is effective in both adults and children.[83] The aim is moderate sedation that stops short of the patient losing consciousness.

Hypnosis: there is good evidence that this can reduce the pain of procedures in suitable patients.[84–88]

6 Visceral pain

This is caused by disorders of the internal organs caused by tumor, ischemia, or inflammation.[89] Cardiac pain and bowel distension are examples. Liver metastases can cause pain, but only if the liver capsule is stretched or inflamed. Damage to the celiac plexus or the lumbosacral plexus by tumor or fibrosis can cause a visceral neuropathic pain which responds to gabapentin.[90,91] Persistent celiac plexus pain may respond to a neurolytic block, but does not give a better quality of life than systemic analgesics.[92,93]

7 Pain related to eating

Pain will be caused by anything which causes inflammation of the mucosa of the mouth, pharynx, esophagus, or stomach. Related structures must also be considered such as teeth. Dyspepsia is a common cause (*see Dyspepsia*, p. 123), and gastric stasis can be a cause of epigastric discomfort (*see Nausea and vomiting*, p. 167). Although oral mucosal pain may respond to topical preparations such

Clinical decision	If YES carry out the action below
5 Is the pain related to a procedure? (e.g. a dressing change)	• **Change the technique:** e.g. calmer and more private setting, or different dressings. In children, distraction and cuddling can help. • **Topical local anesthetic:** for skin apply tetracaine (amethocaine) as Ametop gel (Canada) or Synera plaster (US) at least 30 min before the procedure. For painful mucosa try a lidocaine 10% spray (can cause stinging) or a tetracaine gel. • **If painful inflammation is present:** apply a topical steroid cream once daily. If the area is too sensitive to apply directly, use a beclomethasone inhaler (400 microg/spray) to spray steroid over the area several times daily to reduce inflammation enough to allow direct application of steroid cream and dressings. • **Consider:** *Giving a breakthrough dose* of analgesia (*see* cd-2, p. 45). *Entonox* (50% O_2, 50% N_2O) just before and during procedure. Do not use in the presence of pneumothorax or distended bowel. *Consider using topical opioid,* e.g. 0.1% solution of morphine in Intrasite gel. *Gabapentin* may have a role. *Ask for advice* from palliative care specialist. Options are ketamine 2.5–5 mg SC or buccal; fentanyl/sufentanil SL; or moderate sedation with midazolam 1–5 mg titrated IV or buccal.
6 Is this visceral pain?	• **Cardiac pain persisting despite antianginal drugs:** start regular strong opioid. Consider referral for spinal analgesia. • **Liver capsule distension:** start dexamethasone 6 mg PO daily, reducing to lowest dose that controls symptoms. Consider an opioid (*see Choosing an analgesic*, p. 57) • **Celiac plexus pain:** start gabapentin 100 mg q8h and titrate (up to 1200 mg q8h may be needed). Consider referral for a neurolytic block or spinal analgesia. • **Related to bowels or bladder:** *see* cd-4b on p. 49 and cd-7 below.
7 Is the pain related to eating?	• **Pain in the mouth:** *see* cd-5 in *Oral problems*, p. 187. • **Pain on swallowing:** *see* cd-6 in *Dysphagia*, p. 135. • **If this is dyspepsia:** *see Dyspepsia*, p. 123. • **Consider:** gastric stasis causing epigastric discomfort (start a prokinetic); tube feed rate set too high (reduce rate and start a prokinetic); sensitive gastrocolic reflex (exclude constipation, otherwise reduce size and increase frequency of meals); cholecystitis (ask for advice from gastroenterologist).

Adapted from Thompson and Regnard[26]
cd = clinical decision

as benzydamine mouthwash, systemic analgesia is often needed. Infection (e.g. candidiasis, herpes) must be treated appropriately.

8 Associated with elimination

Problems such as constipation or a urine infection can cause pain. This may be periodic (colic), due to mucosal irritation (e.g. dysuria), pressure from local tumor causing a persistent sensation of wanting to defecate (tenesmus) or rectal tumor or inflammation causing rectal pain (proctalgia).

9 Associated skin changes

Pain is common in the presence of skin damage, especially in pressure ulcers.[94] Although the damaged skin edge of an ulcer is painful, deep ulcers can be more painful than superficial ulcers (*see* cd-5, p. 207). Arterial ulcers are more likely to cause pain on lying down than venous ulcers.[95] For management *see* cd-5 on p. 51 or *Skin problems* on p. 203 and *Malignant ulcers and fistulae* on p. 149.

10 Unpleasant sensory changes at rest

Up to a third of patients with chronic pain have neuropathic pain and its presence increases the likelihood of suicidal thoughts.[96,97] It is due to persistent changes in receptor and neurotransmitter functioning in the spinal cord following nerve damage.[98] No single test can confirm the presence the basis of neuropathic pain, so it is diagnosed on the patient's descriptions, and the signs elicited on examination.[99] The features of neuropathic pain are shown in the table.

Treatment can be complex,[100] and the advice of a pain or palliative care specialist should be sought. Fortunately, the mechanisms of neuropathic pain, and the treatments, may be similar in a wide range of causes. The most effective agents are tricyclic antidepressants (TCAs), followed by opioids, then anticonvulsants,[101] but combinations of these drugs are more effective than any one used alone.[102,103]

Spontaneous symptoms:
- superficial burning pain
- deep or bruising pain
- paraesthesia, e.g. tingling
- dysesthesia, e.g. stabbing, stinging, cold, heat
- paroxysms, i.e. severe episodes.

NB. Some patients find neuropathic pain so unusual they struggle to describe the sensation.

On examination:
- reduced ability to distinguish coolness from warmth
- reduced sensation of light touch
- pain on touching (allodynia)
- increased sensitivity to touch (hyperalgesia)
- reduced vibration sensation.

Clinical features of neuropathic pain[99,104]

Opioids: pains often have multiple causes, especially in cancer, and opioids are an essential first step. In addition, neuropathic pain is opioid-responsive,[105,106] although there is no evidence that any one opioid is more effective than any other in treating neuropathic pain, including methadone.[107] However, neuropathic pain becomes less responsive after weeks or months, when an adjuvant analgesic should be added.

Antidepressants: TCAs (especially amitriptyline and imipramine) and the serotonin-norepinephrine reputake inhibitors (SNRIs) venlafaxine and duloxetine have the best evidence for efficacy in neuropathic pain.[108,109] They are equally effective but can all produce a wide range of adverse effects, especially TCAs at higher doses (dry mouth, constipation, blurred vision, hypotension, movement disorders, drowsiness, confusion).

Clinical decision	If YES carry out the action below
8 Are there associated skin changes in the area of the pain?	• **Skin ulcers:** *see Skin problems* on p. 203 and *Malignant ulcers and fistulae* on p. 159. Consider using topical preservative-free morphine injection solution in approx. 16 g Intrasite gel (approx. equivalent to a 0.1% solution). • **Red/hot skin:** *Exclude eczema or dermatitis.* *If cellulitis is suspected* start an antibiotic (amoxicillin or clindamycin in a lymphedematous limb, otherwise use cephalexin). *In head and neck soft tissue infection:* start metronidazole plus cephalexin. *Consider* if this pain is a sympathetic hypoactivity pain (*see* cd-9c below). • **Pale/cold or black skin:** *Arterial insufficiency (ischemia) (pale or black skin):* contact a vascular surgeon for advice. An opioid is only partly effective, and alternatives are ketamine as a continuous SC infusion 50–300 mg in 24 hours, a local nerve block or spinal analgesia. *Sympathetic hyperactivity pain (pale, cold skin): see* cd-9c below. • **For other skin disease:** treat the cause.
9 Is this an unpleasant sensory change at rest, or does touch make the pain worse?	**a. Pain in a dermatome** (i.e. in the distribution of a spinal nerve root): Start low-dose amitriptyline 10–25 mg once at night and titrate. If this helps but adverse effects are troublesome try imipramine 10–25 mg once at night *or* venlafaxine 37.5 mg q12h *or* duloxetine 60 mg once daily. *If the pain persists add* gabapentin 100 mg q8h and titrate (up to 1200 mg q8h may be needed). *If there is no improvement* contact the pain or palliative care specialist. Possibilities include ketamine, lidocaine, nerve blocks or spinal analgesia. **b. Pain in area supplied by a peripheral nerve:** Exclude reversible causes (e.g. B_{12} deficiency). Treat as in cd-9a above. **c. Pain in a sympathetic distribution** (i.e. the same distribution as the arterial supply since sympathetic nerves run along arteries): Start treating in the same way as in cd-9a. *If the skin is cold and pale:* this is sympathetic hyperactivity and a pain specialist may advise a chemical sympathectomy. *If the skin is warm and red or dusky:* this is sympathetic hypoactivity and this can sometimes be helped by placing TENS electrodes over the main artery supplying the area (do not use this over the carotids in the neck). **d. Hemibody (thalamic) pain:** this may be due to destructive brain lesions (metastases, CVA); it can also occur in neurologically impaired children with complex seizures. Anticonvulsants such as gabapentin may help.

Adapted from Thompson and Regnard[26]
cd = clinical decision

Anticonvulsants: carbamazepine has a strong evidence base, but has many potential interactions with drugs used in palliative care (*see Drug information*, p. 287–8) as well as the risk of red cell aplasia, requiring regular blood counts for the first few months. Gabapentin has fewer interactions and appears effective in a wide range of neuropathic pains,[110] including central (thalamic) pain.[111–113] However, increasing experience has uncovered a range of adverse effects including drowsiness and dizziness. Starting at low doses (100 mg q8h) is better tolerated in ill patients than higher starting doses. There is no evidence that pregabalin is superior to gabapentin. Topiramate and oxcarbazepine are alternatives which may be effective in neuropathic pain.[114]

Cannabinoids: these can be effective in neuropathic pain but currently available cannabinoids can have troublesome psychoactive adverse effects.[115,116]

Topical treatments: capsaicin cream is moderately effective and is useful in patients who cannot tolerate systemic drugs, but it can cause pain and stinging in the first few days of application.[117] Full benefit may take up to four weeks. Plastic food wrap can be used as a temporary measure since it protects a hypersensitive area of skin.

Other drugs: many drugs can be added to provide additional analgesia such as flecainide,[118] and ketamine,[119] have shown some benefit in small studies. Topical lidocaine may help some patients,[120] and IV lidocaine may be more effective but must be administered under ECG monitoring.[121,122] After the loading dose a SC infusion can be maintained without cardiac monitoring,[123] although clinical monitoring for lidocaine side-effects should be continued:

Early – light-headedness, perioral numbness, metallic taste, blurred vision, hypertension

Late – visual/auditory hallucinations, dissociation, twitching, hypotension

Very late – convulsions, cardio-respiratory arrest.

Lidocaine side-effects

11 Nerve compression

If the cause is a tumor, radiotherapy or chemotherapy may shrink the tumor or dexamethasone may reduce the edema around the tumor.[124] Other options are a local nerve block or spinal analgesia.

12 Persistent pain

If pain persists despite going through these clinical decisions, a complete reassessment is necessary. A new pain or poor concordance (compliance) with treatment are common reasons for persistent pain. Involving the adult or child in the management of their pain increases self-esteem and reduces pain perception. It is also important to exclude unresolved psychological and spiritual issues, since these reduce the ability to cope with pain. These will need to be addressed by an interdisciplinary team, including a chaplain and psychologist or counselor, as part of an holistic approach to enable the person to cope with their pain. However, some patients interpret psychological or spiritual approaches as implying that their pain is "all in the head," and they reject such approaches outright.

Ketamine: this may have a role in some persistent pains.[125–129] These include phantom-limb pain,[130] traumatic pain,[131] severe inflammatory bowel disease pain in children,[132] painful subcutaneous calciphylaxis,[133] neuropathic pain,[119] pain related to multiple sclerosis,[134] and arterial ischemic pain.[135] It can be given orally, subcutaneously, intranasally,[136] or by the buccal route.[119] Adverse effects are unusual at low doses, but at higher

Clinical decision	If YES carry out the action below
10 Is the pain made worse by passing urine or stool?	• **Pain on micturition:** *See* cd-4 in *Urinary problems and sexual difficulties*, p. 223. • **Pain on passing stool:** Consider these causes: hard stool (*see Constipation*, p. 107), anal fissure (use nitroglycerine (NTG) cream), hemorrhoids (use topical soothing cream), infection (treat). *Rectal pain (proctalgia) or strong sensation of a need to evacuate (tenesmus):* — exclude rectal impaction with stool. — if due to tumor, dexamethasone 6 mg PO once daily may help. — if due to inflammation of rectal mucosa (tumor, infection, radiotherapy), try local steroid (Entocort enema or Cortenema), or a compounding pharmacy can prepare, e.g. dexamethasone suppositories given q1–2 days.
11 Is the pain in an area supplied by a peripheral nerve? (e.g. sciatica)	• **If this is an unpleasant sensory change at rest:** *see* cd-9 on p. 53. • **Nerve compression:** Start an opioid. *Exclude nerve compression* caused by skeletal instability (X-rays ± bone scan, but a CT or MRI scan may be necessary). *Exclude or treat bone infection.* *If due to pressure from tumors or metastases* consider radiotherapy or dexamethasone (6–8 mg once daily – higher doses, e.g. 16 mg stat, then 16 mg/day and taper, can be used, but at higher risk of adverse effects). Occasionally a nerve block or spinal analgesia is needed.
12 Is the pain persisting?	• **Consider these as causes:** *Total pain:* unresolved fear, anger, or depression (*see Anxiety*, p. 239, *Anger*, p. 235, *Withdrawal and depression*, p. 253). *Poor concordance (compliance) with treatment:* due to fear, misunderstanding of instructions or an unacceptable form of medication. *Inappropriate analgesic dose or timing.* *Onset of a new pain:* go through previous pain clinical decisions. *Opioid-induced hyperalgesia: see* cd-12 in *Managing the adverse effects of analgesics* on p. 73. • **Consider these treatments:** multi-modal treatment (e.g. opioid/amitriptyline/gabapentin combination), lidocaine, ketamine, spinal analgesia. Because of the complexity, ask for advice from a pain or palliative care specialist.

Adapted from Thompson and Regnard[26]
cd = clinical decision

doses include drowsiness, blood pressure increase, dysphoria, hallucinations, angina, cystitis, and dizziness, and about 15% of patients have to stop ketamine because of adverse effects.[137] It is contraindicated in the presence of raised intracranial pressure, severe cardiac disease, or raised blood pressure, and caution is advised in patients with epilepsy.

Spinal analgesia: this is often needed in severe breakthrough pain that is responding poorly to systemic analgesia.[138–142] The intrathecal route has fewer complications than the epidural route when a spinal line is needed for more than three weeks.[143,144] Around two-thirds of patients benefit but there is an associated mortality due to meningitis of around 2%,[138] but the risk is reduced with implantable intrathecal pumps.[145] An important contraindication to spinal analgesia is a patient who is deteriorating on a daily basis since it can take a week or more to organize and titrate spinal analgesia. The mainstay of analgesia is a local anesthetic – usually this is bupivacaine as it has antimicrobial properties.[146] To this an opioid is usually added (usually hydromorphone or morphine), but this may be unnecessary if the patient is still on systemic opioids. Additional drugs are sometimes used, such as baclofen for spasticity or clonidine for neuropathic pain.

The drugs are usually administered through an external line connecting a programmable pump to the intrathecal line. External intrathecal lines can be kept in place for a median of three months.[138] Implantable pumps are an alternative for long-term use.[145] Full protocols for the use of intrathecal analgesia are available.[147]

Complementary therapies

Although the commonest therapies are self-administered dietary supplements,[148] a number of therapies have been shown to be effective for pain in both children and adults, and are being used increasingly often in palliative care.[149]

Acupuncture has a good evidence base, but tends to provide only short-term benefit.[150,151] It can be used safely in children.[152,153]

Hypnosis can be effective in suitable patients, including children.[154–157] It is being used in palliative care,[158] but the evidence is less convincing and more research is needed.[159]

Music therapy has a role for children,[160,161] but has also been used in adults,[162] and in palliative care.[163]

Transcutaneous electrical nerve stimulation: this can provide acupuncture-like stimulation but can do so over long periods or continuously.[164] However, the results in palliative care are unconvincing.[165]

Touch therapies: massage promotes relaxation and trust that can ease pain and anxiety.[166–168] Any discomfort following massage is mild and lasts less than 36 hours.[169]

Relaxation therapies: there are many variations of this from simple relaxation to guided visualization. It is particularly accepted by younger people, although it does not suit everyone and about two-thirds withdraw from treatment.[170]

Choosing an analgesic

CLINICAL DECISION AND ACTION CHECKLIST

1 Check through *Diagnosing and treating pain* (p. 43)
2 Is rapid control of the pain needed?
3 Is the patient vomiting or unable to swallow?
4 Is there a medical precaution or contraindication?
5 Does the patient have a preference for an opioid preparation?
6 Are adverse effects troubling the patient?
7 Is a combination of analgesics needed?

KEY POINTS

- The choice of analgesic depends on:
  - the cause of the pain
  - the route of administration
  - patient preference for a preparation
  - coexisting conditions
  - adverse effects
  - the need for combination analgesia.

INTRODUCTION

There are many analgesic types and preparations that between them will suit most patients. However, comparative trials are few. An analgesic must be chosen on the basis of the cause of the pain, its pharmacokinetics, route of administration, and suitability for the individual patient.

CHOICE BASED ON THE CAUSE OF PAIN

Pains vary in their sensitivity to opioids and some pains will only respond to other drugs (adjuvant analgesics, e.g. hyoscine butylbromide (Canada) or hyoscyamine (US) for colic) or approaches (e.g. pressure relieving devices for skin pressure pain).[171–174] Use the 12 clinical decisions in *Diagnosing and treating pain*, p. 43 to decide which drugs or approaches are needed.

CHOICE BASED ON THE ANALGESIC STAIRCASE

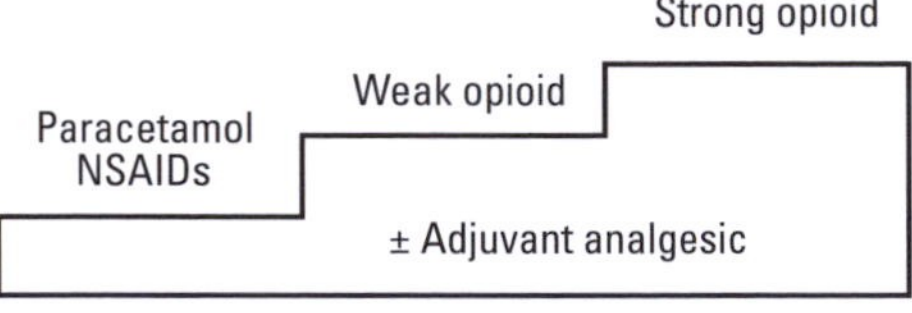

WHO analgesic staircase

This analgesic staircase uses the key principle of broad spectrum analgesia with non-opioids, opioids and adjuvant analgesics.[1] Weak opioids used to be a key step, but it is possible to switch from a non-opioid to a low dose of a strong opioid (e.g. 15 mg/24 hr oral morphine).[175,176] Morphine remains the strong opioid of choice.[177]

However, the WHO staircase is a very broad principle which fails with pain unresponsive to opioids and whose effectiveness has never been tested in a randomized controlled trial.[178] In reality, it is necessary to individualize the staircase to each patient. For example the staircase for a patient with neuropathic pain might look very different:

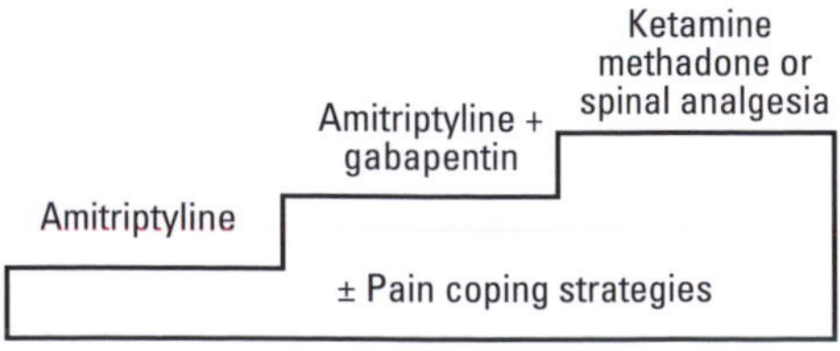

Example of analgesic staircase for neuropathic pain

CHOICE BASED ON PHARMACOKINETIC AND PHARMACEUTICAL ISSUES

The cause of the pain will often suggest the type of analgesic needed. Choosing a specific analgesic depends on the following:

Speed of response

There is a time delay before the effects of an analgesic can be assessed:

Intravenous 1–2 min
Intranasal 3–10 min
Intramuscular 3–10 min (may be faster in deltoid than gluteal muscle with some drugs, including morphine[179])
Rectal (lipid soluble drug) 5–10 min
Subcutaneous 20–30 min
Buccal (lipid soluble drug) up to 30 min
Oral 30–60 min or longer
Transdermal 24–48 hours or longer

Different routes = different speeds of response

Using a route which allows a rapid assessment is useful in severe pain,[180,181] but the rapid rise in drug levels can cause adverse effects. In addition IM injections are painful, while the need to change peripheral IV sites is distressing for patients. Consequently, the IV and IM routes are not suitable for regular, bolus doses of analgesia.[182] However, the intravenous route can be used for continuous infusions if a central line is present. In children, even the SC site can be distressing so buccal, nasogastric and gastrostomy routes are more common alternatives to the oral route.

Clinical decision	If YES carry out the action below
1 Check through clinical decisions 1–12 in *Diagnosing and treating pain*, pp. 45–56.	
2 Is a rapid control of the pain needed?	• **Use analgesic routes with a rapid action.** If pain control is needed in — less than 2 minutes: use the intravenous route — 5–10 minutes: use the intramuscular (deltoid muscle), intranasal or rectal, buccal (but some drugs can take up to 30 minutes) — 20–30 minutes: use the subcutaneous route — 30–60 minutes: use an oral instant release preparation.
3 Is the patient vomiting or unable to swallow?	• **For opioids**, use subcutaneous hydromorphone or morphine (continuous infusion or bolus). • **Alternatives for regular analgesic administration:** *Rectal:* non-opioid (acetaminophen), opioid (hydromorphone, morphine, or in the US oxycodone), NSAID (indomethacin). NB. Rectal administration of controlled release morphine (MS Contin) has been reported. *Transdermal:* fentanyl, but this route is only suitable for patients with stable pain. *Buccal:* fentanyl, but beware of adverse effects.
4 Is there a medical precaution or contra-indication?	• **Renal impairment (based on GFR):** *NSAIDs* are best avoided as they may cause further renal impairment. *Opioids in stable renal impairment:* any opioid can be used, but extra care is needed in titrating codeine, morphine, or oxycodone. *Opioids in unstable or fluctuating impairment (e.g. on dialysis):* avoid codeine, morphine and oxycodone. Alternatives are hydromorphone (in mild–moderate impairment), fentanyl, alfentanil, or methadone. • **Hepatic impairment:** *NSAIDs and acetaminophen* need to be used with care and avoided in severe impairment. *Opioids:* morphine is the preferred choice, but if severe (grade 3) hepatic encephalopathy is present, any opioid can precipitate coma and alternative methods of analgesia are needed. • **Peptic ulceration:** *Previous history of ulceration:* cover NSAIDs with a proton pump inhibitor (PPI) (e.g. omeprazole), cover corticosteroids with H_2 blocker (e.g. ranitidine) or PPI. *Current ulceration:* stop NSAIDs. Start sucralfate 1–2 g (5–10 mL) q6h. Consider using misoprostol 200 microg q6h, but be prepared to reduce or stop laxatives. If misoprostol is not tolerated, use a proton pump inhibitor. • **Children:** *see Drugs in children: starting doses*, p. 303. • **Drug interactions:** *see* pp. 283–301 for interactions of analgesics.

Ability to take oral medication

If a patient is vomiting or unable to swallow, non-oral routes are necessary. These are usually subcutaneous, transdermal, or rectal. The rectal route for controlled-release morphine (MS Contin) has been reported, and may be an alternative at home for short-term use when pumps or parenteral drugs are temporarily unavailable.[183–186]

Patient choice

Patients may prefer tablets, solutions, or transdermal patches. Controlled-release preparations are necessary for optimal pain management.[177,187]

Medical precautions and contra-indications

Analgesic choice can be influenced by:

Renal impairment: morphine and oxycodone should be used with care since the parent drug or its active metabolites will accumulate.[188–195] Hydromorphone may be safe for mild–moderate impairment.[196,197] Fentanyl and methadone may be safe in severe impairment, but caution is still required.[198]

Hepatic impairment: morphine is converted in the liver to potent, active metabolites and can be considered as being "activated" by the liver. This is in contrast to other opioids that are deactivated in the liver by being converted to inactive metabolites so that the administered opioid accumulates in hepatic impairment.[199–203] The effect of liver impairment on morphine is to produce less of the active metabolites – the overall effect is that its metabolism is affected much less than other opioids. However, once grade 3 encephalopathy develops any opioid can precipitate coma.

Peptic ulceration: with a history of previous peptic ulceration prescribe a proton pump inhibitor (PPI) (e.g. omeprazole).[204] For corticosteroids either an H_2 blocker (e.g. ranitidine) or proton pump inhibitor can be used.[205,206] With current ulceration NSAIDs need to be stopped and misoprostol or PPI started.[207]

Children: those aged 2 years and over tolerate opioids well, but infants under 1 year are very sensitive to opioids and they need to be used with caution.[208–210]

Drug interactions: these are common in palliative care.[211] *See* p. 283 for a list of interactions between drugs commonly used in palliative care.

Adverse effects

A change to a related analgesic may reduce or stop drug adverse effects (e.g. diclofenac to ibuprofen, morphine to hydromorphone).

Need for combination analgesia

Some conditions (e.g. pelvic tumors) can produce complex pains with multiple causes that need combinations of non-opioid, opioids and adjuvant analgesics.

Clinical decision	If YES carry out the action below
5 Does the patient have a preference for an opioid preparation?	• **Controlled-release opioid preparations:** *Oral tablets*, e.g. morphine (MS Contin, MOS SR), oxycodone (OxyContin), oxymorphone (US only (Opana ER)). *Capsules*, e.g. hydromorphone (Hydromorph Contin, Exalgo (US only)), morphine (M-Eslon, Kadian, Avinza (US only), Embeda (US only)) *Liquids:* no specifically formulated preparations are available but Kadian, Avinza, Hydromorph Contin, and M-Eslon capsules can be opened and sprinkled on, e.g. apple sauce. *Transdermal*, e.g. matrix fentanyl patch (Duragesic), reservoir fentanyl patch (generic). • **Instant release opioid preparations** *Oral tablets*, e.g. morphine (MS IR, MOS), hydromorphone (Dilaudid), oxycodone (Oxy-IR), oxymorphone (US only (Opana)). *Buccal/sublingual preparations*, e.g. fentanyl lozenge (US only (Actiq)), dissolvable tablet (US only (Fentora)) or injection solution. *Liquids*, e.g. morphine (MOS). *Intranasal:* fentanyl intranasal applicators are being trialed but are not generally available at this time.
6 Are adverse effects troubling the patient?	Convert to alternative analgesic, for example: — diclofenac to ibuprofen — morphine to hydromorphone, oxycodone, oxymorphone (US) or fentanyl (*see Using strong opioids*, p. 63) — hydromorphone, oxycodone, oxymorphone (US) or fentanyl to morphine — amitriptyline or carbamazepine to gabapentin.
7 Is a combination of analgesics indicated?	Review clinical decisions 1–12 in *Diagnosing and treating pain* (pp. 45–55) and list possible pain mechanisms to decide the combination of non-opioid, opioid and adjuvant analgesic needed.

cd = clinical decision

NOTES

Using strong opioids

CLINICAL DECISION AND ACTION CHECKLIST

1 Check *Diagnosing and treating pain*, p. 43, to ensure that a strong opioid is needed.
2 Check *Choosing an analgesic*, p. 57, to decide the starting strong opioid and route.
3 Are you uncertain about the starting dose, frequency, or titration rate?
4 If changing between strong opioids, check correct conversions.
5 Would advice be helpful?

KEY POINTS

- The starting dose and titration rate are tailored to the individual.
- The frequency of doses depends on the preparation used.
- Conversion ratios between strong opioids are guides only and dose adjustments may be needed.
- Final dose requirements cannot be predicted.
- Breakthrough doses may also need to be titrated to the individual.

INTRODUCTION

Advice on strong opioids can vary considerably depending on the source. This section gives basic advice on the doses of strong opioids when starting, titrating, and converting strong opioids. It assumes that the two previous sections have been read and/or are understood (*Diagnosing and treating pain* on p. 43, and *Choosing an analgesic* on p. 57).

STARTING DOSE

Because strong opioid dose requirements cannot be predicted, starting doses should be low, especially in infants under one year, or in frail or elderly adults. Starting with high doses produces adverse effects and increases the chance of the patient rejecting the analgesic. Starting doses for a frail, elderly adult previously on a non-opioid may be as low as morphine 1 mg q4h while younger adults will cope with higher doses such as morphine 2.5 mg q4h. Starting doses in children depend in part on their age (*see* p. 303). Patients on non-opioids should not be started on transdermal fentanyl. Patients already on higher doses of a regular weak opioid can start a strong opioid equivalent to their current dose.

FREQUENCY OF DOSE

This will depend on:

- the half-life of the opioid
- the duration of a controlled-release preparation.

Oral morphine is normally given q4h for an instant-release preparation, but infants and children may need it every 2–3 hours. The evidence for a double dose at bedtimes is conflicting.[212,213] Oxycodone has a longer half-life and can be given q6h. Immediate-release oxymorphone can be given q4–6h. Controlled-release (CR) morphine, oxycodone, hydromorphone, and oxymorphone are given twice daily, but some CR preparations of morphine and hydromorphone can be given once daily. Controlled-release morphine tablets are well tolerated by children,[214] but some may need to take it three times daily.

TITRATION OF ANALGESIA

It takes five half lives before a drug reaches a steady-state level. Therefore, this time must elapse before it can be evaluated and the dose adjusted. Opioids should be increased in 25–50% steps. The smaller increases are sometimes used for children.[215] Increases are usually every third day, but faster titration (e.g. twice daily) can be done under supervision if instant-release preparations are used. Faster titration is useful if urgency is an issue, but it also increases the likelihood of adverse effects and must be done under close supervision. Surveys of opioid doses show a range for the median dose for morphine of 60–120 mg/24 hr.[216–218] The variation is partly due to the use in some surveys of *oral morphine equivalents* (OME) calculated from converting doses of different opioids to the equivalent dose of oral morphine.[219]

BREAKTHROUGH MEDICATION

In recent years a simplified rule has evolved which applies to most opioids:[220]

Use 10% of the 24 hour dose

The breakthrough dose may have to be adjusted up or down to the individual patient and can vary from 5% to 20% of the 24 hour dose.[221,222]

USE OF OPIOIDS IN CHILDREN

There are important differences in using opioids in children with respect to starting doses, dosing frequency, adverse effects and useful routes. For more details *see Drugs in children: starting doses*, pp. 303–4.

Clinical decision	If YES carry out the action below
1 Check through clinical decisions 1–12 in *Diagnosing and Treating Pain*, p. 43.	
2 Check *Choosing an Analgesic*, p. 57 to decide the starting strong opioid and route.	
3 Are you uncertain about starting dose, frequency, or titration rate?	• **What is the starting dose for oral morphine?** *If opioid-naïve* (e.g. on only acetaminophen): 2.5 mg instant-release q4h or 10 mg controlled-release q12h. These doses should be halved in frail elderly patients. *See* p. 303 for starting doses in children. *If on previous opioids* (e.g. codeine, etc.): add up total daily dose and convert to equivalent oral morphine dose then give in divided doses (q4h for instant-release, q12h for controlled-release). • **How often should doses of strong opioids be given?** Strong opioids must be given regularly to control continuous or frequent pain. The actual frequency depends on the length of action of the preparation, e.g. — normal-release morphine, hydromorphone = q4h — normal-release oxycodone = q6h — normal-release oxymorphone = q4-6h — controlled-release morphine, hydromorphone, oxycodone, oxymorphone = q12h (some preparations are approved for q12h or q24h dosing) — transdermal fentanyl = patch change q72 hours. • **What about pain between regular doses?** *Give 10% of the total 24 hour dose q1h as required.* *See* cd-2 on breakthrough pain in *Diagnosing and treating pain*, p. 45. • **How should strong opioids be titrated?** *Wait 5 times the half-life of the drug and then increase in 25–50% steps.* For normal-release morphine this is every 24 hours, for controlled-release this is every 2–3 days. The amount of dose increase is often estimated by adding the total amount of opioid taken in the previous 24 hours (regular doses and extra doses) and using that to guide the next increment of regular dose. More frequent dose increases are possible for severe pain, when normal release preparations should be used to get on top of the pain, but the patient must be reviewed before and after each dose increase. When titrating rapidly, it is wise to monitor the respiratory rate; rates below 8 per minute suggest toxicity. NB. More frequent dose increases should not be used with transdermal opioids since these are unsuitable for unstable pain. • **What is the median dose of opioid that is usually needed?** The median daily dose of oral morphine is 90 mg/24 hours, or 15 mg q4h. • **When should I convert to a different opioid?** Only convert to a different opioid if — the reason is to reduce or avoid opioid adverse effects — a parenteral preparation for that opioid is not available — you are familiar with the other opioid and its conversion ratio — you will review the patient within 24 hours after conversion and adjust the dose to the patient's response.

cd = clinical decision

CONVERSIONS

The table opposite is a guide to conversions. However, conversion values are approximations and caution is needed.[177,223–228] When changing opioids it is often safest to convert to the equivalent dose of the current opioid, and then observe the patient. In particular look out for opioid toxicity or opioid withdrawal. Some recommend reducing the dose of the new opioid by 25–50% due to incomplete cross-tolerance.[227–230]

Rules of opioid conversion:

1. Know your opioid.
2. Use a conversion factor with which you are familiar.
3. Be prepared to re-titrate the dose.
4. If in doubt, ask for advice.

More potent opioids or routes *do not* provide greater efficacy, e.g. a pain that is not responsive to titrated oral morphine will not respond to injectable morphine either, even though this route is twice as potent. However, an alternative route may be needed to ensure adequate absorption.

Example of conversion

Oral morphine to hydromorphone infusion:

- conversion factor is ÷ 10
- so 60 mg/24 hours oral morphine ≡ 6 mg/24 hours SC hydromorphone.

Transdermal fentanyl

This is approximately 100 times more potent than oral morphine, and because it is prescribed in microg/hr rather than mg/24 hours, errors are easy to make. The manufacturer's conversion tables give suggested dose ranges.

A useful check is the following:

Divide the oral morphine dose in mg/24 hr by 3 = TD fentanyl in microg/hr

(e.g. 75 mg oral morphine/day ≈ 25 microg/hr TD fentanyl

As with all conversions this is an approximation and doses may then have to be adjusted up or down.

Transdermal opioids are less flexible than other opioid preparations and should be reserved for patients with stable pain.[177] Fentanyl TD can be used in children.[231]

Methadone

Conversion to methadone should be done cautiously and under specialist advice since, a) cross-tolerance between methadone and other opioids is often incomplete, b) it has a long and variable half-life (12–100 hours), and c) its pharmacokinetics are non-linear. There are several conversion methods, but the method on p. 68 is widely used.

Clinical decision	If YES carry out the action below
4 Are you uncertain about dose conversions?	• Check the dose conversion chart below. Important: conversions are approximations and doses may have to be adjusted up or down after conversion.
5 Would advice be helpful?	• **Ask for help if** — you need to convert to an unfamiliar opioid — there have been four dose increases with no pain relief (this suggests this pain is poorly opioid-responsive) — the patient has reached doses equivalent to 500 mg/24 hours or more of oral morphine — the pain is still 50% of its starting severity after 1 week — there are severe or persistent adverse effects — the patient has episodes of severe pain (breakthrough pain).

OPIOID DOSE CONVERSIONS[220]

1 These are conservative approximations and doses may have to be adjusted up or down after conversion.
2 If converting because of opioid toxicity, *reduce* the conversion dose of the new opioid by at least one-third.

	Approx. conversion ratio from oral morphine	Approx. 24 hr dose equivalent	Approx. 12 hourly dose equivalent	Approx. breakthrough equivalent*	Approx. hourly dose equivalent
PO codeine	× 10	600 mg	300 mg	60 mg	n/a
PO tramadol	× 10	600 mg	300 mg	60 mg	n/a
PO morphine	**× 1**	**60 mg**	**30 mg**	**6 mg**	**2.5 mg**
PO oxycodone	÷ 1.5	40 mg	20 mg	4 mg	n/a
SC or continuous IV morphine**	÷ 2	30 mg	15 mg	3 mg	n/a
PO oxymorphone†	÷ 3	20 mg	10 mg	2 mg	n/a
PO hydromorphone	÷ 5	12 mg	6 mg	1.2 mg	n/a
SC or continuous IV hydromorphone**	÷ 10	6 mg	3 mg	0.6 mg	n/a
SC or continuous IV oxymorphone **†**	÷ 20	3 mg	1.5 mg	0.3 mg	n/a
TD fentanyl	÷ 100	n/a	n/a	50 microg	25 microg

*Breakthrough doses are based on 10% of the 24 hr opioid dose; these may also have to be adjusted up or down.

**Bolus IV administration has very different pharmacokinetics compared to SC or continuous IV administration and potencies cannot be directly compared.

†Oxymorphone data from: product monograph; Houde RW, Wallenstein SL, Beaver WT. (1965) Clinical measurement of pain. In: de Stevens G, ed. *Analgetics.* New York: Academic Press, pp. 75–122; and Eddy NB, Lee LE. (1959) The analgesic equivalence to morphine and relative side action liability of oxymorphone (4-hydroxydihydromorphinone). *Journal of Pharmacology and Experimental Therapeutics.* **125**: 116–21.

1. Stop strong opioid.

2. Calculate loading methadone dose:

(NB. Skip this step, i.e. do not give a loading dose, if the patient is on transdermal fentanyl since this drug continues to be active for 24 hr or more).[232]

Loading dose = 10% of previous total 24 hour PO morphine dose (up to a maximum of 30 mg).

3. Start methadone.

If on instant-release morphine:

– if pain is present wait 2 hours to give first dose
– if pain-free wait 4 hours to give first dose.

If on q12h controlled-release morphine:

– if pain is present wait 6 hours to give first dose
– if pain-free wait 12 hours to give first dose.

If on once daily controlled-release morphine:

– if pain is present wait 12 hours to give first dose
– if pain-free wait 24 hours to give first dose.

4. For subsequent doses:

– give one-third of the loading dose (i.e. one-thirtieth of the previous 24-hour PO morphine dose)
– give this q3h PRN, unless the pain is severe in which case it can be given q1h PRN.

5. On day 6:

– add up the total amount of methadone given in the previous 48 hours
– give 25% of this amount q12h
– use 10% of the new daily dose q3h PRN for breakthrough pain.

Methadone titration (adapted from[220])

Managing the adverse effects of analgesics

CLINICAL DECISION AND ACTION CHECKLIST

1 Is coma or respiratory depression present?
2 Is there nausea and vomiting?
3 Has the stool consistency changed?
4 Are CNS symptoms present (drowsiness, confusion, nightmares, or hallucinations)?
5 Are antimuscarinic symptoms present?
6 Is movement affected?
7 Is the patient fearful of the opioid?
8 Is there evidence of recent liver or renal impairment?
9 Has blood pressure changed recently?
10 Is the problem due to a drug interaction?
11 Is itching present?
12 Has analgesia reduced or been lost?

KEY POINTS

- NSAID adverse effects are common.
- Tolerance develops to some opioid effects (e.g. nausea) but not to others (e.g. constipation).
- Adjuvant analgesics (co-analgesics) are often forgotten as a cause of troublesome adverse effects.

INTRODUCTION

Although there is no evidence that death is a consequence of the correct use of oral morphine in palliative care,[2,233–235] analgesics are not free of adverse effects and minimizing their impact on patients is part of effective symptom control.

NON-OPIOID ANALGESICS

Acetaminophen

This is usually well tolerated in doses of 1 g 4–6 hourly,[236] but hepatotoxicity can occur.[237]

Non-steroidal anti-inflammatory drugs (NSAIDs)

These can be effective in some cancer pains[238] and may have a role in cachexia,[239] but adverse effects are common,[240] with a similar frequency in adults and children.[241,242]

Gastrointestinal bleeding: mucosal damage is the commonest problem, risking dyspepsia, ulceration, and bleeding.[243] This damage can occur anywhere in the gut.[244] The risk is higher for patients also on dexamethasone (×15 higher risk), acetaminophen,[245] warfarin, selective serotonin reuptake inhibitor (SSRI) antidepressants, for older patients (especially over 80), those with liver disease, a past history of peptic ulceration, current peptic ulceration, or current *H. pylori* infection. COX-2 specific NSAIDs only reduce peptic ulceration by half,[246] and bleeding from the gut can still occur.[243,247,248] Ibuprofen has the lowest risk.

Renal impairment is a risk, especially with longer acting NSAIDs (e.g. piroxicam)[249] and is not reduced by using COX-2 NSAIDs.[250] Dehydration increases the risk. Over one-third of acute interstitial nephritis is due to NSAIDs.[251]

Cerebrovascular toxicity: there is an increased risk of stroke with all NSAIDs, especially COX-2 NSAIDs.[252,253]

Cardiovascular toxicity: there is an increased risk of thrombotic events, hypertension, and heart failure with all NSAIDs.[254]

NSAID protection: proton pump inhibitors (PPIs) (e.g. lansoprazole, omeprazole) reduce the risk of gastrointestinal events by 70%.[255] Misoprostol is as effective as a PPI, but is more effective if gastric ulceration is already present.[207] Misoprostol causes diarrhea but this can be useful if the patient needs laxatives for other reasons. H_2-receptor antagonists (e.g. ranitidine, cimetidine) prevent NSAID-related duodenal ulceration, but they do not prevent NSAID-related gastric ulceration.[256]

OPIOID ANALGESICS

The frequency of adverse effects from opioids is similar in neonates, children, and adults.[257] A few are common but treatable, while tolerance to others develops within days. Serious adverse effects are unusual.

Respiratory depression is rarely a problem in patients on opioids prescribed in the way described in *Using strong opioids*, p. 63. Over the last 25 years published evidence shows that respiratory function is unaffected if morphine is given to patients as a treatment for breathlessness,[258] even if they are elderly,[259] are opioid-naïve,[260] have poor respiratory function,[261] have restrictive respiratory failure,[262] or have motor neurone disease/ALS.[263] Morphine does not cause an acute chest syndrome in children with sickle-cell disease crises.[264] In addition, opioids do not hasten death or shorten survival even when given as a double dose at bedtime,[226] or used after ventilator withdrawal.[265]

However, there is a risk of respiratory depression if:

- the starting dose is too high
- titration is rapid and poorly monitored
- opioid conversions are incorrect
- pain is suddenly relieved without prior dose reduction, e.g. after a nerve block.

Clinical decision	If YES carry out the action below
1 Is coma or respiratory depression present?	*See* cd-3b in *Emergencies*, p. 333.
2 Is there nausea or vomiting?	• **Gastric irritation** (NSAID any type, corticosteroids): start a proton pump inhibitor (PPI), e.g. lansoprazole 30 mg daily or omeprazole 20 mg daily (a PPI is preferable to misoprostol). If vomit or stool are positive for blood, stop the NSAID and start sucralfate 2 g q6h. • **Central effects** (*opioid, carbamazepine, dantrolene*): when the pattern is a non-specific pattern of nausea and vomiting start haloperidol 1.5–3 mg once at night. Consider switching to a different opioid. If constipation is present: *see Constipation* on p. 107. • **Gastric stasis** (*opioid, amitriptyline*): if large volume vomiting is the main problem this suggests gastric stasis. *See* cd-2a in *Nausea and vomiting*, p. 169.
3 Has the stool consistency changed?	• **Consider these drugs as causes:** amitriptyline, carbamazepine, dantrolene, NSAIDs, opioids. • *See Constipation*, p.107; *see Diarrhea*, p. 115.
4 Are CNS symptoms present?	(e.g. drowsiness, confusion, nightmares, or hallucinations) • **Consider these drugs as causes:** amitriptyline, carbamazepine, dantrolene, baclofen, gabapentin, ketamine, NSAIDs, opioids. Reduce the dose or change to an alternative drug. *See Confusional states*, p. 245. • **If drowsiness persists:** check for other causes (*see Fatigue, drowsiness, lethargy and weakness*, p. 149). Consider using methylphenidate 2.5–5 mg in the morning, increasing if necessary to 10–15 mg. A second dose can be given, but no later than lunchtime to avoid insomnia.
5 Are antimuscarinic symptoms present?	(i.e. blurred vision, constipation, drowsiness, dry mouth, hypotension, urinary retention) • **Consider these drugs as causes:** amitriptyline, hyoscine hydrobromide (scopolamine), hyoscyamine, or opioids. Reduce dose or change to an alternative analgesic.
6 Is movement affected?	• **Myoclonus (opioids):** if on a strong opioid, myoclonus suggests toxicity – reduce dose or change opioid. Consider adding dantrolene or SC midazolam. • **Dyskinesia, Parkinson's:** consider amitriptyline, carbamazepine, gabapentin, haloperidol, metoclopramide, or phenothiazines as possible causes. Reduce the dose or change to a different drug. Alternatively, give benztropine 1–2 mg od or bid, or try procyclidine (Canada only) 2.5 mg q8h and titrate dose. • **Muscle weakness** (baclofen, corticosteroids): reduce the dose.
7 Is the patient fearful of the opioid?	Usually, this is due to a fear of opioid adverse effects or addiction. • Explain the facts about opioids (*see* text). Offer written information.[266]
8 Is there evidence of recent liver or renal impairment?	• **Liver impairment:** consider accumulation of carbamazepine, gabapentin, NSAIDs, acetaminophen, oxycodone, fentanyl, or alfentanil. • **Renal impairment:** consider accumulation of carbamazepine, or the accumulation of metabolites of hydromorphone or morphine. Consider NSAIDs as a cause of renal impairment.

cd = clinical decision

Transdermal fentanyl has long been known to cause unexpected respiratory depression,[267] and safety alerts have been issued in Canada, the US and UK.[268] Very little is known about the pharmacokinetics of lipid soluble strong opioids, but there is now evidence that cachectic patients handle fentanyl differently.[269]

If reversal with naloxone is necessary, this must be done in a titrated way to reverse respiratory effects without reversing analgesia (*see* cd-3b in *Emergencies*, p. 333.

Constipation occurs in over 90% of patients on opiods and concurrent laxatives are essential for these patients.[270] Patients taking fentanyl are as likely to need laxatives as patients on other opioids, but pass stool less frequently.[271] Treatment is a combination of a stimulant and softening laxative (*see Constipation*, p. 107), and it is unusual to fail to prevent opioid-induced constipation.

Nausea and vomiting: *see Nausea and vomiting*, p. 167. Although nausea is reported in nearly half of patients on opioids,[272] this is usually due to other causes.[273] However, opioids can cause nausea and vomiting in several ways. Stimulation of dopamine receptors in the chemoreceptor trigger zone (CTZ) in the floor of the fourth ventricle results in a non-specific pattern of nausea and vomiting, which responds to haloperidol.[274] Opioids also reduce gastric emptying which produces the typical pattern of gastric stasis and responds to prokinetics. Finally, constipation due to opioids can cause nausea and vomiting.

Tolerance: opioids show "selective tolerance"[275] so that tolerance to euphoria takes 1–2 days, to drowsiness 5–7 days, and to nausea within a few days or weeks (although it can become more chronic).[276] In contrast, no tolerance develops to constipation and tolerance to analgesia is not usually a clinical problem.[277]

Addiction (a craving for a chemical or situation)[278] is rare in patients with advanced disease taking opioids for pain.[279,280] Physical dependence does occur but withdrawal symptoms are unusual (usually colic, diarrhea) and do not prevent gradual reductions over 5 days.[281]

Drowsiness: this usually wears off over a few days, but persistent drowsiness may need a switch to a different opioid. If this is not possible an alternative is to use a psychostimulant such as methylphenidate.[282]

Dry mouth is common, occurring in up to 40% of patients.[283]

Myoclonus (intermittent jerks of the limbs or body) is seen with morphine,[284] but has also been reported with hydromorphone,[275] methadone,[285] and fentanyl.[286–288] It is a useful sign of opioid toxicity[289] and an indication to reduce the dose or change opioid. A few patients develop myoclonus without other signs of toxicity and dantrolene or midazolam can reduce the myoclonus.[290,291]

Other adverse effects

Delirium and hallucinations: opioids are an unusual cause and other causes should be considered.[292]

Itching: opioids can cause histamine release. Although opioids can cause histamine release from peripheral mast cells,[293] this release is also centrally mediated and responds to low-dose naloxone.[294–296] It is uncommon in palliative care practice, but if persistent low-dose naloxone is effective.[297]

Clinical decision	If YES carry out the action below
9 Has blood pressure changed recently?	• **Increased:** consider dantrolene, dexamethasone, ketamine, prednisolone, or tramadol as causes • **Decreased:** consider amitriptyline, baclofen, dantrolene, or tramadol as causes.
10 Is the problem due to a drug interaction?	• **Check interactions** of analgesic drugs with other drugs used in palliative care, p. 283.
11 Is itching present?	• **If recently started on a strong opioid:** consider centrally mediated histamine release (this is not an allergic response). Consider changing to an alternative opioid, or using low-dose naloxone continuous subcutaneous infusion (CSCI) (5 microg/kg/24 hr) • **If not on a strong opioid:** look for allergic causes.
12 Has analgesia reduced or been lost?	• **Consider:** a new non-opioid-responsive pain (*see* cd3-12 in *Diagnosing and treating pain*, pp. 45–55); vomiting (*see Nausea and vomiting*); incorrect dose conversion; or altered metabolism. • **Opioid-hyperalgesia:** start acetaminophen 1 g every 4–6 hours. Consider switching to methadone. Ultra-low-dose naloxone CSCI may help (1.5 microg/kg/24 hr). Alternatively, consider spinal analgesia and reduce opioid.

cd = clinical decision

Loss of analgesia: this may be due to inaccurate dose conversion, inadequate absorption (e.g. vomiting), or altered metabolism. For example, some patients on oxycodone require high doses and this may be due to these patients metabolizing oxycodone rapidly to non-analgesic metabolites.[298]

Opioid-induced hyperalgesia is a paradoxical effect of opioids that increases the sensitivity to pain. It produces pain that may be different to the original pain, often with hypersensitivity and allodynia.[299,300] Opioid-induced hyperalgesia should be suspected in patients who experience worsening pain after receiving rapidly escalating doses of opioids. It can be managed by decreasing the opioid dose or rotating to a different opioid, as these strategies reduce the levels of the opioid and its metabolites.[274] Some drugs may reduce hyperalgesia (e.g. acetaminophen, clonidine, ketamine, lidocaine), while some opioids are less likely to cause hyperalgesia or even counteract this effect (e.g. methadone).[301,302] In humans ultra low doses have been used without reversing analgesia or precipitating withdrawal symptoms,[303] and they can reduce opioid requirements.[304] Higher rates of infusion have been used,[305] but there is a risk that non-pain-related opioid withdrawal symptoms can develop (e.g. diarrhea). A CSCI of 1.5 microg/kg/24 hr is suggested as a starting dose.

ADJUVANT ANALGESICS

These drugs have a wide range of adverse effects and the manufacturers' product information monographs should be consulted.

Antidepressants: switch to an alternative drug (e.g. amitriptyline to imipramine).

Anticonvulsants: carbamazepine has a high rate of adverse effects and interactions and gabapentin is a safer alternative in advanced disease.[108]

Corticosteroids: although often beneficial in the short term, the adverse effects may come to outweigh the benefits. Troublesome adverse effects can occur within days of starting higher doses (e.g. above 12 mg daily), such as diabetes, insomnia, or a hyperactive delirium (steroid-induced psychosis). Patients on long-term treatment can develop adverse effects that develop over weeks or months, such as edema, proximal weakness (due to an irreversible myopathy), and osteoporosis.[306] Steroid withdrawal is a risk in any patient who has been on steroids for more than three weeks and abruptly stops taking the drug. Symptoms include fever, anorexia, nausea, lethargy, arthralgia, and, less commonly, hypotension, vomiting, and abdominal pain.[307]

Smooth muscle relaxants (anti-spasmodics): hyoscine butylbromide (Canada only) usually has few adverse effects, but hyoscine hydrobromide (scopolamine) and hyoscyamine can cause marked central antimuscarinic effects.

Skeletal muscle relaxants (anti-spasmodics): these can cause a wide range of effects from confusion to weakness, but can be beneficial in carefully selected patients.

REFERENCES: PAIN

B = book; C = comment; Ch = chapter; CS-n = case study-no. of cases; CT-n = controlled trial-no. of cases; E = editorial; GC = group consensus; I = interviews; LS = laboratory study; MC = multi-center; OS-n = open study-no. of cases; QS = questionnaire based study-no of cases; R = review; Rep = report; RCT-n = randomized controlled trial-no. of cases; RS-n = retrospective survey-no. of cases; SA = systematic or meta analysis.

1 Vachon M. (2009). The emotional problems of the patient in palliative medicine. In: Hanks G, Cherney NI, Christakis NA, Fallon M, Kaasa S, Portenoy RK. *The Oxford Textbook of Palliative Medicine, 4th ed.* Oxford/New York: Oxford University Press.

2 Pain relief. In: Twycross R, Wilcock A, Stark Toller C. (2009) *Symptom Management in Advanced Cancer, 4th ed.* Nottingham: palliativedrugs.com. pp. 13–59. (Ch)

3 Eland JM. (1985) Paediatrics. In: *Pain.* Springhouse, PA: Springhouse Corporation. (Ch)

4 McGrath PJ, McAlpine L. (1993) Psychologic aspects on paediatric pain. *Journal of Paediatrics.* **5**(2): S2–8.

5 Kaasalainen S. (2007) Pain assessment in older adults with dementia: using behavioral observation methods in clinical practice. *Journal of Gerontological Nursing.* **33**(6): 6–10. (R, 40 refs)

6 Regnard C, Mathews M, Gibson L, Clarke C. (2003) Difficulties in identifying distress and its causes in people with severe communication problems. *International Journal of Palliative Nursing.* **9**(3): 173–6.

7 Portenoy RK, Payne D, Jacobsen P. (1999) Breakthrough pain: characteristics and impact in patients with cancer pain. *Pain.* **81**(1–2): 129–34. (OS-164)

8 William L, Macleod R. (2008) Management of breakthrough pain in patients with cancer. *Drugs.* **68**(7): 913–24. (R, 121 refs)

9 Caraceni A, Martini C, Zecca E, Portenoy RK, Ashby MA, *et al.* (2004) Working Group of an IASP Task Force on Cancer Pain. Breakthrough pain characteristics and syndromes in patients with cancer pain. An international survey. *Palliative Medicine.* **18**(3): 177–83. (RS-1095)

10 Zeppetella G. (2008) Opioids for cancer breakthrough pain: a pilot study reporting patient assessment of time to meaningful pain relief. *Journal of Pain and Symptom Management.* **35**(5): 563–7. (OS)

11 Swanwick M, Haworth M, Lennard RF. (2001) The prevalence of episodic pain in cancer: a survey of hospice patients on admission. *Palliative Medicine.* **15**(1): 9–18. (OS-245)

12 Davies AN, Vriens J, Kennett A, McTaggart M. (2008) An observational study of oncology patients' utilization of breakthrough pain medication. *Journal of Pain and Symptom Management.* **35**(4): 406–11. (OS-87)

13 Portenoy RK, Taylor D, Messina J, Tremmel L. (2006) A randomized, placebo-controlled study of fentanyl buccal tablet for breakthrough pain in opioid-treated patients with cancer. *Clinical Journal of Pain.* **22**(9): 805–11. (RCT-77)

14 Zeppetella G, Ribeiro MD. (2006) Opioids for the management of breakthrough (episodic) pain in cancer patients. *Cochrane Database of Systematic Reviews.* **1**: CD004311. (SA-4, 26 refs)

15 Hanks GW, Nugent M, Higgs CM, Busch MA. (2004) OTFC Multicentre Study Group. Oral transmucosal fentanyl citrate in the management of breakthrough pain in cancer: an open, multicentre, dose-titration and long-term use study. *Palliative Medicine.* **18**(8): 698–704. (OS-58)

16 Parlow JL, Milne B, Tod DA, Stewart GI, Griffiths JM, Dudgeon DJ. (2005) Self-administered nitrous oxide for the management of incident pain in terminally ill patients: a blinded case series. *Palliative Medicine.* **19**(1): 3–8. (RCT-7)

17 Luger NM, Sabino MAC, Schwei MJ, Mach DB, *et al.* (2002) Efficacy of systemic morphine suggests a fundamental difference in the mechanisms that generate bone cancer vs. inflammatory pain. *Pain.* **99**: 397–406. (LS)

18 Mercadante S, Villari P, Ferrera P, Casuccio A. (2004) Optimization of opioid therapy for preventing incident pain associated with bone metastases. *Journal of Pain and Symptom Management*. **28**(5): 505–10. (OS-25)
19 McQuay HJ, Collins SL, Carroll D, Moore RA. (2000) Radiotherapy for the palliation of painful bone metastases. *Cochrane Database of Systematic Reviews*. **2**: CD001793. (SA, 27 refs)
20 Agarawal JP, Swangsilpa T, van der Linden Y, Rades D, Jeremic B, Hoskin PJ. (2006) The role of external beam radiotherapy in the management of bone metastases. *Clinical Oncology (Royal College of Radiologists)*. **18**(10): 747–60. (R, 86 refs)
21 Wu JS, Monk G, Clark T, Robinson J, Eigl BJ, Hagen N. (2006) Palliative radiotherapy improves pain and reduces functional interference in patients with painful bone metastases: a quality assurance study. *Clinical Oncology (Royal College of Radiologists)*. **18**(7): 539–44. (OS-84)
22 Chow E, Loblaw A, Harris K, Doyle M, *et al.* (2007) Dexamethasone for the prophylaxis of radiation-induced pain flare after palliative radiotherapy for bone metastases: a pilot study. *Supportive Care in Cancer.* **15**(6): 643–7. (OS-33)
23 Hartsell WF, Scott CB, Bruner DW, Scarantino CW, *et al.* (2005) Randomized trial of short- versus long-course radiotherapy for palliation of painful bone metastases. *Journal of the National Cancer Institute*. **97**(11): 798–804. (RCT-898)
24 van der Linden YM, Lok JJ, Steenland E, Martijn H, van Houwelingen H, Marijnen CA, Leer JW. (2004) Dutch Bone Metastasis Study Group. Single fraction radiotherapy is efficacious: a further analysis of the Dutch Bone Metastasis Study controlling for the influence of retreatment. *International Journal of Radiation Oncology, Biology, Physics*. **59**(2): 528–37. (RCT)
25 Nilsson S, Strang P, Ginman C, Zimmermann R, *et al.* (2005) Palliation of bone pain in prostate cancer using chemotherapy and strontium-89. A randomized phase II study. *Journal of Pain and Symptom Management*. **29**(4): 352–7. (RCT-35)
26 Thompson JW, Regnard C. (1995) Pain. In: *Flow Diagrams in Advanced Cancer and Other Diseases*. London: Edward Arnold. pp. 5–10. (Ch)
27 Eisenberg E, Berkey CS, Carr DB, Mosteller F, Chalmers TC. (1994) Efficacy and safety of nonsteroidal antiinflammatory drugs for cancer pain: a meta-analysis. *Journal of Clinical Oncology*. **12**(12): 2756–65. (SA)
28 Joishy SK, Walsh D. (1998) The opioid-sparing effects of intravenous ketorolac as an adjuvant analgesic in cancer pain: application in bone metastases and the opioids bowel syndrome. *Journal of Pain and Symptom Management*. **16**: 334–9. (CS-10)
29 Clemons M, Dranitsaris G, Ooi W, Cole DE. (2008) A Phase II trial evaluating the palliative benefit of second-line oral ibandronate in breast cancer patients with either a skeletal related event (SRE) or progressive bone metastases (BM) despite standard bisphosphonate (BP) therapy. *Breast Cancer Research and Treatment*. **108**(1): 79–85. (OS-30)
30 Cameron D, Fallon M, Diel I. (2006) Ibandronate: its role in metastatic breast cancer. *Oncologist*. **11**(Suppl. 1): S27–33. (R, 43 refs)
31 Pavlakis N, Schmidt R, Stockler M. (2005) Bisphosphonates for breast cancer. *Cochrane Database of Systematic Reviews*. **3**: CD003474. (SA, R, 54 refs)
32 Saad F, Chen YM, Gleason DM, Chin J. (2007) Continuing benefit of zoledronic acid in preventing skeletal complications in patients with bone metastases. *Clinical Genitourinary Cancer.* **5**(6): 390–6. (RCT-422)
33 Coleman RE. (2008) Risks and benefits of bisphosphonates. *British Journal of Cancer*. **98**(11): 1736–40. (R, 36 refs)
34 Peters CM, Ghilardi JR, Keyser CP, Kubota K, Lindsay TH, Luger NM, Mach DB, Schwei MJ, Sevcik MA, Mantyh PW. (2005) Tumor-induced injury of primary afferent sensory nerve fibers in bone cancer pain. *Experimental Neurology*. **193**(1): 85–100. (LS)
35 Donovan-Rodriguez T, Dickenson AH, Urch CE. (2005) Gabapentin normalizes spinal neuronal responses that correlate with behavior in a rat model of cancer-induced bone pain. *Anesthesiology*. **102**(1): 132–40. (LS)
36 Townsend PW, Smalley SR, Cozad SC, Rosenthal HG, Hassanein RE. (1995) Role of postoperative radiation therapy after stabilization of fractures caused by metastatic disease. *International Journal of Radiation Oncology, Biology, Physics*. **31**: 43–9. (OS-60)
37 Bartels RH, van der Linden YM, van der Graaf WT. (2008) Spinal extradural metastasis: review of current treatment options. *CA: a Cancer Journal for Clinicians*. **58**(4): 245–59. (R, 115 refs)
38 Borg-Stein J, Simons DG. (2002) Focused review: myofascial pain. *Archives of Physical Medicine and Rehabilitation*. **83**(Suppl. 2): S40–7. (R, 99refs)
39 Travell JG, Simons DG. (1989) Myofascial pain. In: Wall PD, Melzack R, eds. *Textbook of Pain, 2nd ed.* Edinburgh: Churchill Livingstone. (Ch)
40 Bennett R. (2007) Myofascial pain syndromes and their evaluation. *Best Practice and Research in Clinical Rheumatology*. **21**(3): 427–45. (R, 81 refs)
41 Chen Q, Bensamoun S, Basford JR, Thompson JM, An KN. (2007) Identification and quantification of myofascial taut bands with magnetic resonance elastography. *Archives of Physical Medicine and Rehabilitation*. **88**(12): 1658–61. (OS-3)
42 Ga H, Choi JH, Park CH, Yoon HJ. (2007) Acupuncture needling versus lidocaine injection of trigger points in myofascial pain syndrome in elderly patients – a randomised trial. *Acupuncture in Medicine*. **25**(4): 130–6. (RCT-39)
43 Iwama H, Ohmori S, Kaneko T, Watanabe K. (2001) Water-diluted local anesthetic for trigger-point injection in chronic myofascial pain syndrome: evaluation of types of local anesthetic and concentrations in water. *Regional Anesthesia and Pain Medicine*. **26**(4): 333–6. (OS-40)
44 Offenbacher M, Stucki G. (2000) Physical therapy

in the treatment of fibromyalgia. *Scandinavian Journal of Rheumatology*. Supplement. **113**: 78–85. (R, 58 refs)

45 Graff-Radford SB, Reeves JL, Baker RL, Chiu D. (1989) Effects of transcutaneous electrical nerve stimulation on myofascial pain and trigger point sensitivity. *Pain*. **37**(1): 1–5. (CT-60)

46 Sauls J. (1999) Efficacy of cold for pain: fact or fallacy? *Online Journal of Knowledge Synthesis for Nursing*. **6**(7): 101–11.

47 Barnes M. (2001) An overview of the clinical management of spasticity. In: Barnes MP, Garth RJ, eds. *Upper Motor Neurone Syndrome and Spasticity: clinical management and neurophysiology*. Cambridge: Cambridge University Press. (Ch)

48 Gracies JM. (2001) Physical modalities other than stretch in spastic hypertonia. *Physical Medicine and Rehabilitation Clinics of North America*. **12**(4): 769–92. (R, 222 refs)

49 Meleger AL. (2006) Muscle relaxants and antispasticity agents. *Physical Medicine and Rehabilitation Clinics of North America*. **17**(2): 401–13. (R, 25 refs)

50 Bergfeldt U, Borg K, Kullander K, Julin P. (2006) Focal spasticity therapy with botulinum toxin: effects on function, activities of daily living and pain in 100 adult patients. *Journal of Rehabilitation Medicine*. **38**(3): 166–71. (CT-100)

51 Zafonte RD, Munin MC. (2001) Phenol and alcohol blocks for the treatment of spasticity. *Physical Medicine and Rehabilitation Clinics of North America*. **12**(4): 817–32. (R, 53 refs)

52 Grabb PA, Doyle JS. (2001) The contemporary surgical management of spasticity in children. *Physical Medicine and Rehabilitation Clinics of North America*. **12**(4): 907–22. (R, 53 refs)

53 Guillaume D, Van Havenbergh A, Vloeberghs M, Vidal J, Roeste G. (2005) A clinical study of intrathecal baclofen using a programmable pump for intractable spasticity. *Archives of Physical Medicine and Rehabilitation*. **86**(11): 2165–71. (CT, MC-133)

54 Bhimani R. (2008) Intrathecal baclofen therapy in adults and guideline for clinical nursing care. *Rehabilitation Nursing*. **33**(3): 110–16. (R, 14 refs)

55 Abbruzzese G. (2002) The medical management of spasticity. *European Journal of Neurology*. **9**(Suppl. 1): 30–4; discussion 53–61. (R, 27 refs)

56 Shakespeare DT, Young CA, Boggild M. (2000) Anti-spasticity agents for multiple sclerosis. *Cochrane Database of Systematic Reviews*. **4**: CD001332. (SA, 172 refs)

57 Tytgat GN. (2007) Hyoscine butylbromide: a review of its use in the treatment of abdominal cramping and pain. *Drugs*. **67**(9): 1343–57. (R, 38 refs)

58 Holdgate A, Pollock T. (2005) Nonsteroidal anti-inflammatory drugs (NSAIDs) versus opioids for acute renal colic. *Cochrane Database of Systematic Reviews*. **2**: CD004137. (R, 63 refs)

59 Holdgate A, Pollock T. (2004) Systematic review of the relative efficacy of non-steroidal anti-inflammatory drugs and opioids in the treatment of acute renal colic. *British Medical Journal*. **328**: 1401. (R, 35 refs)

60 Price PE, Fagervik-Morton H, Mudge EJ, Beele H, *et al.* (2008) Dressing-related pain in patients with chronic wounds: an international patient perspective. *International Wound Journal*. **5**(2): 159–71. (RS-2018)

61 Kane FM, Brodie EE, Coull A, Coyne L, *et al.* (2004) The analgesic effect of odour and music upon dressing change. *British Journal of Nursing*. **13**(19): S4–12. (CT-8)

62 Franks PJ, Moody M, Moffatt CJ, Hiskett G, *et al.* (2007) Wound Healing Nursing Research Group. Randomized trial of two foam dressings in the management of chronic venous ulceration. *Wound Repair and Regeneration*. **15**(2): 197–202. (RCT-156)

63 Nahum Y, Tenenbaum A, Isaiah W, Levy-Khademi F. (2007) Effect of eutectic mixture of local anesthetics (EMLA) for pain relief during suprapubic aspiration in young infants: a randomized, controlled trial. *Clinical Journal of Pain*. **23**(9): 756–9. (RCT-52)

64 Lander JA, Weltman BJ, So SS. (2006) EMLA and amethocaine for reduction of children's pain associated with needle insertion. *Cochrane Database of Systematic Reviews*. **3**: CD004236. (SA-23 refs)

65 Back IN, Finlay I. (1995) Analgesic effect of topical opioids on painful skin ulcers. *Journal of Pain and Symptom Management* **10**: 493. (Let)

66 Krajnik M, Zylicz Z. (1997) Topical morphine for cutaneous cancer pain. *Palliative Medicine*. **11**: 325–6. (CS-6)

67 Twillman RK, Long TD, Cathers TA, Mueller DW. (1999) Treatment of painful skin ulcers with topical opioids. *Journal of Pain and Symptom Management*. **17**(4): 288–92. (CS-9)

68 Ashfield T. (2005) The use of topical opioids to relieve pressure ulcer pain. *Nursing Standard*. **19**(45): 90–2. (R, 17 refs)

69 Ribeiro MD, Joel SP, Zeppetella G. (2004) The bioavailability of morphine applied topically to cutaneous ulcers. *Journal of Pain and Symptom Management*. **27**(5): 434–9. (OS, LS-6)

70 Vernassiere C, Cornet C, Trechot P, Alla F, *et al.* (2005) Study to determine the efficacy of topical morphine on painful chronic skin ulcers. *Journal of Wound Care*. **14**(6): 289–93. (RCT-24)

71 Welling A. (2007) A randomised controlled trial to test the analgesic efficacy of topical morphine on minor superficial and partial thickness burns in accident and emergency departments. *Emergency Medicine Journal*. **24**(6): 408–12. (RCT-59)

72 Sibbald RG, Coutts P, Fierheller M, Woo K. (2007) A pilot (real-life) randomised clinical evaluation of a pain-relieving foam dressing: (ibuprofen-foam versus local best practice). *International Wound Journal*. **4**(Suppl. 1): 16–23. (RCT-24)

73 Gottrup F, Jorgensen B, Karlsmark T, Sibbald RG, *et al.* (2007) Less pain with Biatain-Ibu: initial findings from a randomised, controlled, double-blind clinical investigation on painful venous leg ulcers. *International Wound Journal*. **4**(Suppl. 1): 24–34. (RCT-12)

74 Prentice WM, Roth LJ, Kelly P. (2004) Topical benzydamine cream and the relief of pressure pain. *Palliative Medicine*. **18**(6): 520–4. (RCT-31)

75 Devulder J, Lambert J, Naeyaert JM. (2001) Gabapentin for pain control in cancer patients' wound dressing care. *Journal of Pain and Symptom Management.* **22**(1): 622–6. (CS-1)
76 Masood J, Shah N, Lane T, Andrews H, Simpson P, Barua JM. (2002) Nitrous oxide (Entonox) inhalation and tolerance of transrectal ultrasound guided prostate biopsy: a double-blind randomized controlled study. *Journal of Urology.* **168**(1): 116–20. (RCT-110)
77 Cleary AG, Ramanan AV, Baildam E, Birch A, Sills JA, Davidson JE. (2002) Nitrous oxide analgesia during intra-articular injection for juvenile idiopathic arthritis. *Archives of Disease in Childhood.* **86**(6): 416–8. (OS-55)
78 Carbajal R, Biran V, Lenclen R, Epaud R, *et al.* (2008) EMLA cream and nitrous oxide to alleviate pain induced by palivizumab (Synagis) intramuscular injections in infants and young children. *Pediatrics.* **121**(6): e1591–8. (RCT, MC-55)
79 Paris A, Horvath R, Basset P, Thiery S, *et al.* (2008) Nitrous oxide-oxygen mixture during care of bedsores and painful ulcers in the elderly: a randomized, crossover, open-label pilot study. *Journal of Pain and Symptom Management.* **35**(2): 171–6. (RCT, MC-34)
80 Sealey L. (2002) Nurse administration of Entonox to manage pain in ward settings. *Nursing Times.* **98**(46): 28–9. (R, 9 refs)
81 Forbes GM, Collins BJ. (2000) Nitrous oxide for colonoscopy: a randomized controlled study. *Gastrointestinal Endoscopy.* **51**(3): 271–7. (RCT-102)
82 Enting RH, Oldenmenger WH, van der Rijt CCD, Koper P, Smith PAE. (2002) Nitrous oxide is not beneficial for breakthrough cancer pain. *Palliative Medicine.* **16**: 257–9. (CS-2)
83 Iannalfi A, Bernini G, Caprilli S, Lippi A, Tucci F, Messeri A. (2005) Painful procedures in children with cancer: comparison of moderate sedation and general anesthesia for lumbar puncture and bone marrow aspiration. *Pediatric Blood and Cancer.* **45**(7): 933–8. (OS-14)
84 Shakibaei F, Harandi AA, Gholamrezaei A, Samoei R, Salehi P. (2008) Hypnotherapy in management of pain and reexperiencing of trauma in burn patients. *International Journal of Clinical and Experimental Hypnosis.* **56**(2): 185–97. (CT-44)
85 Thornberry T, Schaeffer J, Wright PD, Haley MC, Kirsh KL. (2007) An exploration of the utility of hypnosis in pain management among rural pain patients. *Palliative and Supportive Care.* **5**(2): 147–52. (RS-300)
86 Lutgendorf SK, Lang EV, Berbaum KS, Russell D, *et al.* (2007) Effects of age on responsiveness to adjunct hypnotic analgesia during invasive medical procedures. *Psychosomatic Medicine.* **69**(2): 191–9. (CT-241)
87 Lang EV, Berbaum KS, Faintuch S, Hatsiopoulou O. (2006) Adjunctive self-hypnotic relaxation for outpatient medical procedures: a prospective randomized trial with women undergoing large core breast biopsy. *Pain.* **126**(1–3): 155–64. (CT-236)
88 Uman LS, Chambers CT, McGrath PJ, Kisely S. (2006) Psychological interventions for needle-related procedural pain and distress in children and adolescents. *Cochrane Database of Systematic Reviews.* **4**: CD005179. (SA, 122 refs)
89 Al-Chaer ED, Traub RJ. (2002) Biological basis of visceral pain: recent developments. *Pain.* **96**: 221–5. (R, 39 refs)
90 Pelham A, Lee MA, Regnard CBF. (2002) Gabapentin for coeliac plexus pain. *Palliative Medicine.* **16**: 355–6. (CS-3)
91 Ceyhan GO, Michalski CW, Demir IE, Muller MW, Friess H. (2008) Pancreatic pain. *Best Practice and Research in Clinical Gastroenterology.* **22**(1): 31–44. (R, 89 refs)
92 Zhang CL, Zhang TJ, Guo YN, Yang LQ, *et al.* (2008) Effect of neurolytic celiac plexus block guided by computerized tomography on pancreatic cancer pain. *Digestive Diseases and Sciences.* **53**(3): 856–60. (RCT–56)
93 Wong GY, Schroeder DR, Carns PE, Wilson JL, *et al.* (2004) Effect of neurolytic celiac plexus block on pain relief, quality of life, and survival in patients with unresectable pancreatic cancer: a randomized controlled trial. *Journal of the American Medical Association.* **291**(9): 1092–9. (RCT-100)
94 Girouard K, Harrison MB, VanDenKerkof E. (2008) The symptom of pain with pressure ulcers: a review of the literature. *Ostomy Wound Management.* **54**(5): 30–42. (R, 52 refs)
95 Closs SJ, Nelson EA, Briggs M. (2008) Can venous and arterial leg ulcers be differentiated by the characteristics of the pain they produce? *Journal of Clinical Nursing.* **17**(5): 637–45. (I-52)
96 Bouhassira D, Lanteri-Minet M, Attal N, Laurent B, Touboul C. (2008) Prevalence of chronic pain with neuropathic characteristics in the general population. *Pain.* **136**(3): 380–7. (QS-24,497)
97 Smith MT, Edwards RR, Robinson RC, Dworkin RH. (2004) Suicidal ideation, plans, and attempts in chronic pain patients: factors associated with increased risk. *Pain.* **111**(1–2): 201–8. (I-153)
98 Portenoy RK. (1992) Cancer pain: pathophysiology and syndromes. *Lancet.* **339**: 1026–31. (R, 34 refs)
99 Jensen TS, Baron R. (2003) Translation of symptoms and signs into mechanisms in neuropathic pain. *Pain.* **102**: 1–8. (R, 40 refs)
100 Hanks GW, Justins DM. (1992) Cancer pain: management. *Lancet.* **339**: 1031–6. (R, 34 refs)
101 Finnerup NB, Otto M, McQuay HJ, Jensen TS, Sindrup SH. (2005) Algorithm for neuropathic pain treatment: an evidence based proposal. *Pain.* **118**(3): 289–305. (R, 119 refs)
102 Keskinbora K, Pekel AF, Aydinli I. (2007) Gabapentin and an opioid combination versus opioid alone for the management of neuropathic cancer pain: a randomized open trial. *Journal of Pain and Symptom Management.* **34**(2): 183–9. (CT-75)
103 Gilron I, Bailey JM, Tu D, Holden RR, Weaver DF, Houlden RL. (2005) Morphine, gabapentin, or their combination for neuropathic pain. *New England Journal of Medicine.* **352**(13): 1324–34. (RCT–57)

104 Lefaucheur JP, Drouot X, Menard-Lefaucheur I, Keravel Y, Nguyen JP. (2008) Motor cortex rTMS in chronic neuropathic pain: pain relief is associated with thermal sensory perception improvement. *Journal of Neurology, Neurosurgery and Psychiatry*. **79**(9): 1044–9. (OS-46)

105 Eisenberg E, McNicol ED, Carr DB. (2006) Efficacy of mu-opioid agonists in the treatment of evoked neuropathic pain: systematic review of randomized controlled trials. *European Journal of Pain*. **10**(8): 667–76. (R, 30 refs)

106 Eisenberg E, McNicol E, Carr DB. (2006) Opioids for neuropathic pain. *Cochrane Database of Systematic Reviews*. **3**: CD006146. (SA, 80 refs)

107 Nicholson AB. (2007) Methadone for cancer pain. *Cochrane Database of Systematic Reviews*. **4**: CD003971. (SA, 62 refs)

108 Quilici S, Chancellor J, Lothgren M, Simon D, *et al.* (2009) Meta-analysis of duloxetine vs. pregabalin and gabapentin in the treatment of diabetic peripheral neuropathic pain. *BMC Neurology*. **9**: 6. (SA)

109 Saarto T, Wiffen PJ. (2007) Antidepressants for neuropathic pain. *Cochrane Database of Systematic Reviews*. **4**: CD005454. (SA, 134 refs)

110 Serpell MG. (2002) Neuropathic Pain Study Group. Gabapentin in neuropathic pain syndromes: a randomised, double-blind, placebo-controlled trial. *Pain*. **99**: 557–66. (RCT-305)

111 Holtom N. (2000) Gabapentin for treatment of thalamic pain syndrome. *Palliative Medicine*. **14**(2): 167. (Let, CS-1)

112 Nasreddine ZS, Saver JL. (1997) Pain after thalamic stroke: right diencephalic predominance and clinical features in 180 patients. *Neurology*. **48**(5): 1196–9. (SA)

113 Segatore M. (1996) Understanding central post-stroke pain. *Journal of Neuroscience Nursing*. **28**(1): 28–35. (R, 74 refs)

114 Zin CS, Nissen LM, Smith MT, O'Callaghan JP, Moore BJ. (2008) An update on the pharmacological management of post-herpetic neuralgia and painful diabetic neuropathy. *CNS Drugs*. **22**(5): 417–42. (R, 117 refs)

115 Hosking RD, Zajicek JP. (2008) Therapeutic potential of cannabis in pain medicine. *British Journal of Anaesthesia*. **101**(1): 59–68. (R, 64 refs)

116 Ashton JC, Milligan ED. (2008) Cannabinoids for the treatment of neuropathic pain: clinical evidence. *Current Opinion in Investigational Drugs*. **9**(1): 65–75. (R, 79 refs)

117 Mason L, Moore RA, Derry S, Edwards JE, McQuay HJ. (2004) Systematic review of topical capsaicin for the treatment of chronic pain. *British Medical Journal*. **328**: 991. (SA, 33 refs)

118 von Gunten CF, Eappen S, Cleary JF, Taylor SG 4th, *et al.* (2007) Flecainide for the treatment of chronic neuropathic pain: a Phase II trial. *Palliative Medicine*. **21**(8): 667–72. (CT, MC-19)

119 Webster LR, Walker MJ. (2006) Safety and efficacy of prolonged outpatient ketamine infusions for neuropathic pain. *American Journal of Therapeutics*. **13**(4): 300–5. (OS-13)

120 Dworkin RH, O'Connor AB, Backonja M, Farrar JT, *et al.* (2007) Pharmacologic management of neuropathic pain: evidence-based recommendations. *Pain*. **132**(3): 237–51. (R, 135 refs)

121 Tremont-Lukats IW, Hutson PR, Backonja MM. (2006) A randomized, double-masked, placebo-controlled pilot trial of extended IV lidocaine infusion for relief of ongoing neuropathic pain. *Clinical Journal of Pain*. **22**(3): 266–71. (RCT)

122 Tremont-Lukats IW, Challapalli V, McNicol ED, Lau J, Carr DB. (2005) Systemic administration of local anesthetics to relieve neuropathic pain: a systematic review and meta-analysis. *Anesthesia and Analgesia*. **101**(6): 1738–49. (SA, 86 refs)

123 Ferrini R. (2000) Parenteral lidocaine for severe intractable pain in six hospice patients continued at home. *Journal of Palliative Medicine*. **3**(2): 193–200. (CS-6)

124 Twycross R. (1994) The risks and benefits of corticosteroids in advanced cancer. *Drug Safety*. **11**(3): 163–78. (R)

125 Campbell-Fleming JM, Williams A. (2008) The use of ketamine as adjuvant therapy to control severe pain. *Clinical Journal of Oncology Nursing*. **12**(1): 102–7. (R, 24 refs)

126 Legge J, Ball N, Elliott DP. (2006) The potential role of ketamine in hospice analgesia: a literature review. *Consultant Pharmacist*. **21**(1): 51–7. (SA, 24 refs)

127 Mercadante S, Arcuri E, Ferrera P, Villari P, Mangione S. (2005) Alternative treatments of breakthrough pain in patients receiving spinal analgesics for cancer pain. *Journal of Pain and Symptom Management*. **30**(5): 485–91. (OS-20)

128 Bell RF, Eccleston C, Kalso E. (2003) Ketamine as adjuvant to opioids for cancer pain: a qualitative systematic review. *Journal of Pain and Symptom Management*. **26**(3): 867–75. (SA, 50 refs)

129 Finkel JC, Pestieau SR, Quezado ZM. (2007) Ketamine as an adjuvant for treatment of cancer pain in children and adolescents. *Journal of Pain*. **8**(6): 515–21. (OS-11)

130 Eichenberger U, Neff F, Sveticic G, Bjorgo S, *et al.* (2008) Chronic phantom limb pain: the effects of calcitonin, ketamine, and their combination on pain and sensory thresholds. *Anesthesia and Analgesia*. **106**(4): 1265–73. (RCT-20)

131 Galinski M, Dolveck F, Combes X, Limoges V, *et al.* (2007) Management of severe acute pain in emergency settings: ketamine reduces morphine consumption. *American Journal of Emergency Medicine*. **25**(4): 385–90. (RCT, MC-73)

132 White M, Shah N, Lindley K, Lloyd-Thomas A, Thomas M. (2006) Pain management in fulminating ulcerative colitis. *Paediatric Anaesthesia*. **16**(11): 1148–52. (CS-3)

133 Polizzotto MN, Bryan T, Ashby MA, Martin P. (2006) Symptomatic management of calciphylaxis: a case series and review of the literature. *Journal of Pain and Symptom Management*. **32**(2): 186–90. (R, 20 refs)

134 Sakai T, Tomiyasu S, Ono T, Yamada H, Sumikawa K. (2004) Multiple sclerosis with severe pain and

allodynia alleviated by oral ketamine. *Clinical Journal of Pain*. **20**(5): 375–6. (CS-1)
135 Persson J, Hasselstrom J, Wiklund B, Heller A, Svensson JO, Gustafsson LL. (1998) The analgesic effect of racemic ketamine in patients with chronic ischemic pain due to lower extremity arteriosclerosis obliterans. *Acta Anaesthesiologica Scandinavica*. **42**(7): 750–8. (RCT-8)
136 Carr DB, Goudas LC, Denman WT, Brookoff D, *et al.* (2004) Safety and efficacy of intranasal ketamine for the treatment of breakthrough pain in patients with chronic pain: a randomized, double-blind, placebo-controlled, crossover study. *Pain*. **108**(1–2): 17–27. (RCT-20)
137 Cvrcek P. (2008) Side effects of ketamine in the long-term treatment of neuropathic pain. *Pain Medicine*. **9**(2): 253–7. (OS-32)
138 Baker L, Lee M, Regnard C, Crack L, Cullin S. (2004) Evolving spinal analgesia practice in palliative care. *Palliative Medicine*. **18**(6): 507–15. (OS-76)
139 Mercadante S, Arcuri E, Ferrera P, Villari P, Mangione S. (2005) Alternative treatments of breakthrough pain in patients receiving spinal analgesics for cancer pain. *Journal of Pain and Symptom Management*. **30**(5): 485–91. (OS-12)
140 Koulousakis A, Kuchta J, Bayarassou A, Sturm V. (2007) Intrathecal opioids for intractable pain syndromes. *Acta Neurochirurgica* – Supplement. **97**(Pt. 1): 43–8. (OS-165)
141 Smith HS, Deer TR, Staats PS, Singh V, Sehgal N, Cordner H. (2008) Intrathecal drug delivery. *Pain Physician*. **11**(2 Suppl.): S89–104. (R, 89 refs)
142 Shaladi A, Saltari MR, Piva B, Crestani F, *et al.* (2007) Continuous intrathecal morphine infusion in patients with vertebral fractures due to osteoporosis. *Clinical Journal of Pain*. **23**(6): 511–7. (OS-24)
143 Dahm P, Nitescu P, Appelgren L, Curelaru I. (1998) Efficacy and technical complications of long-term continuous intraspinal infusions of opioid and/or bupivacaine in refractory nonmalignant pain: a comparison between the epidural and the intrathecal approach with externalized or implanted catheters and infusion pumps. *Clinical Journal of Pain*. **14**(1): 4–16.
144 Nitescu P, Applegren L, Lindler L. (1990) Epidural versus intrathecal morphine-bupivacaine: assessment of consecutive treatments in advanced cancer pain. *Journal of Pain and Symptom Management*. **5**: 18–26.
145 Williams JE, Louw G, Towlerton G. (2000) Intrathecal pumps for giving opioids in chronic pain: a systematic review. *Health Technology Assessment*. 4(32): 1–65.
146 Tamanai-Shacoori Z, Shacoori V, Vo Van JM, Robert JC, Bonnaure-Mallet M. (2004) Sufentanil modifies the antibacterial activity of bupivacaine and ropivacaine. *Canadian Journal of Anaesthesia*. **51**(9): 911–14. (LS)
147 North East Spinals Group. Spinal line guidelines, September 2008. Available from claudregnard@stoswaldsuk.org
148 Wilkinson S, Farrelly S, Low J, Chakraborty A, *et al.* (2008) The use of complementary therapy by men with prostate cancer in the UK. *European Journal of Cancer Care*. **17**: 492–9. (QS-405)
149 Pan CX, Morrison RS, Ness J, Fugh-Berman A, Leipzig RM. (2000) Complementary and alternative medicine in the management of pain, dyspnea, and nausea and vomiting near the end of life: a systematic review. *Journal of Pain and Symptom Management*. **20**(5): 374–87. (SA)
150 Wang SM, Kain ZN, White P. (2008) Acupuncture analgesia: I. The scientific basis. *Anesthesia and Analgesia*. **106**(2): 602–10. (SA, 67 refs)
151 Wang SM, Kain ZN, White P. (2008) Acupuncture analgesia: II. Clinical considerations. *Anesthesia and Analgesia*. **106**(2): 611–21. (SA, 66 refs)
152 Kundu A, Berman B. (2007) Acupuncture for pediatric pain and symptom management. *Pediatric Clinics of North America*. **54**(6): 885–9. (R, 95 refs)
153 Jindal V, Ge A, Mansky PJ. (2008) Safety and efficacy of acupuncture in children: a review of the evidence. *Journal of Pediatric Hematology/Oncology*. **30**(6): 431–42. (SA)
154 Rogovik AL, Goldman RD. (2007) Hypnosis for treatment of pain in children. *Canadian Family Physician*. **53**(5): 823–5. (R, 20 refs)
155 Wood C, Bioy A. (2008) Hypnosis and pain in children. *Journal of Pain and Symptom Management*. **35**(4): 437–46. (R, 52 refs)
156 Shakibaei F, Harandi AA, Gholamrezaei A, Samoei R, Salehi P. (2008) Hypnotherapy in management of pain and reexperiencing of trauma in burn patients. *International Journal of Clinical and Experimental Hypnosis*. **56**(2): 185–97. (CT-40)
157 Uman LS, Chambers CT, McGrath PJ, Kisely S. (2006) Psychological interventions for needle-related procedural pain and distress in children and adolescents. *Cochrane Database of Systematic Reviews*. **4**: CD005179. (SA, 122 refs)
158 Finlay IG, Jones OL. (1996) Hypnotherapy in palliative care. *Journal of the Royal Society of Medicine*. **89**(9): 493–6. (OS-256)
159 Rajasekaran M, Edmonds PM, Higginson IL. (2005) Systematic review of hypnotherapy for treating symptoms in terminally ill adult cancer patients. *Palliative Medicine*. **19**(5): 418–26. (SA, 43 refs)
160 Whitehead-Pleaux AM, Zebrowski N, Baryza MJ, Sheridan RL. (2007) Exploring the effects of music therapy on pediatric pain: phase 1. *Journal of Music Therapy*. **44**(3): 217–41. (CT-9)
161 Klassen JA, Liang Y, Tjosvold L, Klassen TP, Hartling L. (2008) Music for pain and anxiety in children undergoing medical procedures: a systematic review of randomized controlled trials. *Ambulatory Pediatrics*. **8**(2): 117–28. (SA, 38 refs)
162 Nilsson U. (2008) The anxiety- and pain-reducing effects of music interventions: a systematic review. *AORN Journal*. **87**(4): 780–807. (R, 70 refs)
163 Freeman L, Caserta M, Lund D, Rossa S, Dowdy A, Partenheimer A. (2006) Music thanatology: prescriptive harp music as palliative care for the dying patient. *American Journal of Hospice and Palliative Care*. **23**(2): 100–4. (OS)

164 Johnson M, Martinson M. (2007) Efficacy of electrical nerve stimulation for chronic musculoskeletal pain: a meta-analysis of randomized controlled trials. *Pain.* **130**(1–2): 157–65. (SA-38)

165 Robb KA, Newham DJ, Williams JE. (2007) Transcutaneous electrical nerve stimulation vs. transcutaneous spinal electroanalgesia for chronic pain associated with breast cancer treatments. *Journal of Pain and Symptom Management.* **33**(4): 410–19. (RCT-40)

166 Russell NC, Sumler SS, Beinhorn CM, Frenkel MA. (2008) Role of massage therapy in cancer care. *Journal of Alternative and Complementary Medicine.* **14**(2): 209–14. (R, 33 refs)

167 Hughes D, Ladas E, Rooney D, Kelly K. (2008) Massage therapy as a supportive care intervention for children with cancer. *Oncology Nursing Forum Online.* **35**(3): 431–42. (R, 81 refs)

168 Liu Y, Fawcett TN. (2008) The role of massage therapy in the relief of cancer pain. *Nursing Standard.* **22**(21): 35–40. (R)

169 Cambron JA, Dexheimer J, Coe P, Swenson R. (2007) Side-effects of massage therapy: a cross-sectional study of 100 clients. *Journal of Alternative and Complementary Medicine.* **13**(8): 793–6. (OS-100)

170 Miller J, Hopkinson C. (2008) A retrospective audit exploring the use of relaxation as an intervention in oncology and palliative care. *European Journal of Cancer Care.* **17**: 488–91. (RS-327)

171 Hanks GW, Forbes K. (1997) Opioid responsiveness. *Acta Anaesthesiologica Scandinavica.* **41**(1 Pt. 2): 154–8. (R)

172 Mercadante S, Portenoy RK. (2001) Opioid poorly-responsive cancer pain. Part 3: clinical strategies to improve opioid responsiveness. *Journal of Pain and Symptom Management.* **21**(4): 338–54. (R, 189 refs)

173 Mercadante S, Portenoy RK. (2001) Opioid poorly-responsive cancer pain. Part 2: basic mechanisms that could shift dose response for analgesia. *Journal of Pain and Symptom Management.* **21**(3): 255–64. (R, 86 refs)

174 Mercadante S, Portenoy RK. (2001) Opioid poorly-responsive cancer pain. Part 1: clinical considerations. *Journal of Pain and Symptom Management.* **21**(2): 144–50. (R, 56 refs)

175 Mercadante S, Porzio G, Ferrera P, Fulfaro F, *et al.* (2006) Low morphine doses in opioid-naive cancer patients with pain. *Journal of Pain and Symptom Management.* **31**(3): 242–7. (CT, MC-110)

176 Maltoni M, Scarpi E, Modonesi C, Passardi A, *et al.* (2005) A validation study of the WHO analgesic ladder: a two-step vs. three-step strategy. *Supportive Care in Cancer.* **13**(11): 888–94. (RCT-54)

177 Hanks GW, Conno F, Cherny N, Hanna M, *et al.* (2001) Expert Working Group of the Research Network of the European Association for Palliative Care. Morphine and alternative opioids in cancer pain: the EAPC recommendations. *British Journal of Cancer.* **84**(5): 587–93. (GC)

178 Azevedo Sao Leao Ferreira K, Kimura M, Jacobsen Teixeira M. (2006) The WHO analgesic ladder for cancer pain control, twenty years of use: how much pain relief does one get from using it? *Supportive Care in Cancer.* **14**(11): 1086–93. (R, 59 refs)

179 Kirkpatrick T, Henderson PD, Nimmo WS. (1988) Plasma morphine concentrations after intramuscular injection into the deltoid or gluteal muscles. *Anaesthesia.* **43**(4): 293–5. (OS-10)

180 Mercadante S, Intravaia G, Villari P, Ferrera P, Riina S, Mangione S. (2008) Intravenous morphine for breakthrough (episodic-) pain in an acute palliative care unit: a confirmatory study. *Journal of Pain and Symptom Management.* **35**(3): 307–13. (CT-99)

181 Mercadante S, Villari P, Ferrera P, Casuccio A, Fulfaro F. (2002) Rapid titration with intravenous morphine for severe cancer pain and immediate oral conversion. *Cancer.* **95**(1): 203–8. (OS-49)

182 Hanks GW, Thomas EA. (1985) Intravenous opioids in chronic cancer pain. *British Medical Journal Clinical Research Ed.* **291**(6502): 1124–5. (C)

183 Kaiko RF, Fitzmartin RD, Thomas GB, Goldenheim PD. (1992) The bioavailability of morphine in controlled-release 30-mg tablets per rectum compared with immediate-release 30-mg rectal suppositories and controlled-release 30-mg oral tablets. *Pharmacotherapy.* **12**: 107–13. (RCT-14)

184 Wilkinson TJ, Robinson BA, Begg EJ, Duffull SB, Ravenscroft PJ. (1992) Pharmacokinetics and efficacy of rectal versus oral sustained-release morphine in cancer patients. *Cancer Chemotherapy and Pharmacology.* **31**: 251–4. (RCT-10)

185 Campbell WI. (1996) Rectal controlled-release morphine: plasma levels of morphine and its metabolites following the rectal administration of MST Continus 100 mg. *Journal of Clinical Pharmacology and Therapeutics.* **21**: 65–71. (OS-8)

186 Maloney CM, Kesner RK, Klein G, Bockenstette J. (1989) The rectal administration of MS Contin®: clinical implications of use in end stage cancer. *American Journal of Hospice Care.* **6**: 34–5. (OS-39)

187 Davis M, Wilcock A. (2001) Modified-release opioids. *European Journal of Palliative Care.* **8**: 142–6. (R)

188 Portenoy RK, Thaler HT, Inturrisi CE, Friedlander-Klar H, Foley KM. (1992) The metabolite morphine-6-glucuronide contributes to the analgesia produced by morphine infusion in patients with pain and normal renal function. *Clinical Pharmacology and Therapeutics.* **51**: 422–31. (OS-14)

189 Faura CC, Moore A, Horga JF, Hand CW, McQuay HJ. (1996) Morphine and morphine-6-glucuronide plasma concentrations and effect in cancer pain. *Journal of Pain and Symptom Management.* **11**: 95–102. (OS-39)

190 Mazoit JX, Sardouk P, Zetlaoui P, Scherrmann JM. (1987) Pharmacokinetics of unchanged morphine in normal and cirrhotic patients. *Anaesthesia and Analgesia.* **66**: 293–8. (CT-14)

191 Portenoy RK, Foley KM, Stulman J, *et al.* (1991) Plasma morphine and morphine-6-glucuronide during chronic morphine therapy for cancer pain: plasma profiles, steady state concentrations and

the consequences of renal failure. *Pain*. **47**: 13–19. (CS-2)

192 Ashby M, Fleming B, Wood M, Somogyi A. (1997) Plasma morphine and glucuronide (M3G and M6G) concentrations in hospice patients. *Journal of Pain and Symptom Management*. **14**: 157–67. (OS-36)

193 Kirvela M, Lindgren L, Seppala T, Olkkola KT. (1996) The pharmacokinetics of oxycodone in uremic patients undergoing renal transplantation. *Journal of Clinical Anesthesia*. **8**(1): 13–18. (CT-20)

194 Foral PA, Ineck JR, Nystrom KK. (2007) Oxycodone accumulation in a haemodialysis patient. *Southern Medical Journal*. **100**(2): 212–14. (CS–1)

195 Dean M. (2004) Opioids in renal failure and dialysis patients. *Journal of Pain and Symptom Management*. **28**(5): 497–504. (R, 56 refs)

196 Lee MA, Leng ME, Tiernan EJ. (2001) Retrospective study of the use of hydromorphone in palliative care patients with normal and abnormal urea and creatinine. *Palliative Medicine*. **15**(1): 26–34. (RS-55)

197 Babul N, Darke AC, Hagen N. (1995) Hydromorphone metabolite accumulation in renal failure. *Journal of Pain and Symptom Management*. **10**(3): 184–6. (C)

198 Davies G, Kingswood C, Street M. (1996) Pharmacokinetics of opioids in renal dysfunction. *Clinical Pharmacokinetics*. **31**(6): 410–22. (R, 93 refs)

199 Tegeder I, Lotsch J, Geisslinger G. (1999) Pharmacokinetics of opioids in liver disease. *Clinical Pharmacokinetics*. **37**(1): 17–40. (R, 257 refs)

200 Labroo RB, Paine MF, Thummel KE, Kharasch ED. (1997) Fentanyl metabolism by human hepatic and intestinal cytochrome P450 3A4: implications for interindividual variability in disposition, efficacy, and drug interactions. *Drug Metabolism and Disposition*. **25**(9): 1072–80. (LS)

201 Tallgren M, Olkkola KT, Seppala T, Hockerstedt K, Lindgren L. (1997) Pharmacokinetics and ventilatory effects of oxycodone before and after liver transplantation. *Clinical Pharmacology and Therapeutics*. **61**(6): 655–61. (CS-6)

202 Davis MP, Varga J, Dickerson D, Walsh D, LeGrand SB, Lagman R. (2003) Normal-release and controlled-release oxycodone: pharmacokinetics, pharmacodynamics, and controversy. *Supportive Care in Cancer*. **11**(2): 84–92. (R, 78 refs)

203 Rhee C, Broadbent AM. (2007) Palliation and liver failure: palliative medications dosage guidelines. *Journal of Palliative Medicine*. **10**(3): 677–85. (R, 44 refs)

204 Seager JM, Hawkey CJ. (2001) ABC of the upper gastrointestinal tract: indigestion and non-steroidal anti-inflammatory drugs. *British Medical Journal*. **323**(7323): 1236–9. (R)

205 Pecora PG, Kaplan B. (1996) Corticosteroids and ulcers: is there an association? *Annals of Pharmacotherapy*. **30**(7–8): 870–2. (R)

206 Ellershaw JE, Kelly MJ. (1994) Corticosteroids and peptic ulceration. *Palliative Medicine*. **8**(4): 313–19. (R)

207 Hawkey CJ, Karrasch JA, Szczepanski L, Walker DG, Barkun A, Swanell AJ, Yeomans ND for the Omeprazole vs Misoprostol for NSAID-Induced Ulcer Management (OMNIUM) Study Group. (1998) Omeprazole compared with misoprostol for ulcers associated with non steroidal anti inflammatory drugs. *New England Journal of Medicine*. **338**: 727–34.

208 Nandi R, Fitzgerald M. (2005) Opioid analgesia in the newborn. *European Journal of Pain*. **9**(2): 105–8. (R, 15 refs)

209 Tibboel D, Anand KJ, van den Anker JN. (2005) The pharmacological treatment of neonatal pain. *Seminars in Fetal and Neonatal Medicine*. **10**(2): 195–205. (R, 130 refs)

210 Bellu R, de Waal KA, Zanini R. (2008) Opioids for neonates receiving mechanical ventilation. *Cochrane Database of Systematic Reviews*. **1**: CD004212. (SA, 57 refs)

211 Regnard C, Hunter A. (2005) Increasing prescriber awareness of drug interactions in palliative care. *Journal of Pain and Symptom Management*. **29**(3): 219–21. (Let)

212 Todd J, Rees E, Gwilliam B, Davies A. (2002) An assessment of the efficacy and tolerability of a "double dose" of normal-release morphine sulphate at bedtime. *Palliative Medicine*. **16**(6): 507–12. (RCT-20)

213 Dale O, Piribauer M, Kaasa S, Moksnes K, *et al.* (2009) A double-blind, randomized, crossover comparison between single-dose and double-dose immediate release oral morphine at bedtime in cancer patients. *Journal of Pain and Symptom Management*. **37**: 68–76. (RCT-13)

214 Zernikow B, Lindena G. (2001) Long-acting morphine for pain control in paediatric oncology. *Medical and Pediatric Oncology*. **36**(4): 451–8. (RS-95)

215 World health Organization. (1998) *Cancer Pain Relief and Palliative Care in Children*. Geneva: WHO. (B)

216 Good PD, Ravenscroft PJ, Cavenagh J. (2005) Effects of opioids and sedatives on survival in an Australian inpatient palliative care population. *Internal Medicine Journal*. **35**(9): 512–17. (OS)

217 Wilcock A, Chauhan A. (2007) Benchmarking the use of opioids in the last days of life. *Journal of Pain and Symptom Management*. **34**(1): 1–3. (Let, RS-100)

218 Thorns A, Sykes N. (2000) Opioid use in last week of life and implications for end-of-life decision-making. *Lancet*. **356**: 398–9. (Let, RS-238)

219 Challand S, Frew K. (2008) Benchmarking the use of opioids. *Journal of Pain and Symptom Management*. **35**(5): 456. (Let, RS-451)

220 Palliative Care Formulary online: see www.palliativedrugs.com

221 Portenoy K, Hagen N. (1990) Breakthrough pain: definition, prevalence and characteristics. *Pain*. **41**: 273–81.

222 Mercadante S, Radbruch L, Caraceni A, Cherny N, *et al.* (2002) Steering Committee of the European Association for Palliative Care (EAPC) Research Network. Episodic (breakthrough) pain: consensus

conference of an expert working group of the European Association for Palliative Care. *Cancer*. **94**(3): 832–9. (R, 25 refs)

223 Pereira J, Lawlor P, Vigano A, Dorgan M, Bruera E. (2001) Equianalgesic dose ratios for opioids: a critical review and proposals for long-term dosing. *Journal of Pain and Symptom Management*. **22**: 672–87. (R, 46 refs)

224 Anderson R, Saiers JH, Abram S, Schlicht C. (2001) Accuracy in equianalgesic dosing: conversion dilemmas. *Journal of Pain and Symptom Management*. **21**: 397–406. (R, 55 refs)

225 Cherny N, Ripamonti C, Pereira J, Davis C, *et al.* (2001) Expert Working Group of the European Association of Palliative Care Network. Strategies to manage the adverse effects of oral morphine: an evidence-based report. *Journal of Clinical Oncology*. **19**(9): 2542–54. (R, 72 refs)

226 Mercadante S, Bruera E. (2006) Opioid switching: a systematic and critical review. *Cancer Treatment Reviews*. **32**(4): 304–15. (SA, 50 refs)

227 Shaheen PE, Walsh D, Lasheen W, Davis MP, Lagman RL. (2009) Opioid equianalgesic tables: are they all equally dangerous? *Journal of Pain and Symptom Management*. **38**(3): 409–17. (R, 31 refs)

228 Knotova H, Fine PG, Portenoy RK. (2009) Opioid rotation: the science and the limitations of the equianalgesic dose table. *Journal of Pain and Symptom Management*. **38**(3): 426–39. (R, 95 refs)

229 Vascello L, McQuillan RJ. (2006) Opioid analgesics and routes of administration. In: de Leon-Casasola OA, ed. *Cancer Pain: pharmacological, interventional, and palliative care*. Philadelphia: Elsevier Inc. pp. 171–94. (Ch)

230 Fine G, Portenoy RK, for the *ad hoc* expert panel on evidence review and guidelines for opioid rotation. (2009) Establishing "best practices" for opioid rotation: conclusions of an expert panel. *Journal of Pain and Symptom Management*. **38**(3): 418–25. (R, 12 refs)

231 Hunt A, Goldman A, Devine T, Phillips M. (2001) FEN-GBR-14 Study Group. Transdermal fentanyl for pain relief in a paediatric palliative care population. *Palliative Medicine*. **15**(5): 405–12. (OS-41)

232 Regnard C, Pelham A. (2003) Severe respiratory depression and sedation with transdermal fentanyl: four case studies. *Palliative Medicine*. **17**: 714–6.

233 Regnard C, Badger C. (1987) Opioids, sleep and the time of death. *Palliative Medicine*. **1**(2): 107–10. (RS)

234 Cools HJ, Berkhout AM, De Bock GH. (1996) Subcutaneous morphine infusion by syringe driver for terminally ill patients. *Age and Ageing*. **25**(3): 206–8. (RS)

235 Morita T, Tsunoda J, Inoue S, Chihara S. (2001) Effects of high dose opioids and sedatives on survival in terminally ill cancer patients. *Journal of Pain and Symptom Management*. **21**(4): 282–9. (OS-209)

236 Dart RC, Bailey E. (2007) Does therapeutic use of acetaminophen cause acute liver failure? *Pharmacotherapy*. **27**(9): 1219–30. (R, 192 refs)

237 Carey EJ, Vargas HE, Douglas DD, Balan V, *et al.* (2008) Inpatient admissions for drug-induced liver injury: results from a single center. *Digestive Diseases and Sciences*. **53**(7): 1977–82. (RS)

238 Mercadante S. (2001) The use of anti-inflammatory drugs in cancer pain. *Cancer Treatment Reviews*. **27**(1): 51–61. (R, 100 refs)

239 Lundholm K, Daneryd P, Korner U, Hyltander A, Bosaeus I. (2004) Evidence that long-term COX-treatment improves energy homeostasis and body composition in cancer patients with progressive cachexia. *International Journal of Oncology*. **24**(3): 505–12. (RS)

240 Hawkins C, Hanks GW. (2000) The gastroduodenal toxicity of nonsteroidal anti-inflammatory drugs: a review of the literature. *Journal of Pain and Symptom Management*. **20**(2): 140–51. (R)

241 Litalien C, Jacqz-Aigrain E. (2001) Risks and benefits of nonsteroidal anti-inflammatory drugs in children: a comparison with paracetamol. *Paediatric Drugs*. **3**(11): 817–58. (R, 325 refs)

242 Cuzzolin L, Dal Cere M, Fanos V. (2001) NSAID-induced nephrotoxicity from the fetus to the child. *Drug Safety*. **24**(1): 9–18. (R, 98 refs)

243 Laine L. (2003) Gastrointestinal effects of NSAIDs and coxibs. *Journal of Pain and Symptom Management*. **25**(2S): S32–40. (R, 43 refs)

244 Matsumoto T, Kudo T, Esaki M, Yano T, *et al.* (2008) Prevalence of non-steroidal anti-inflammatory drug-induced enteropathy determined by double-balloon endoscopy: a Japanese multicenter study. *Scandinavian Journal of Gastroenterology*. **43**(4): 490–6. (OS, MC-661)

245 Rahme E, Barkun A, Nedjar H, Gaugris S, Watson D. (2008) Hospitalizations for upper and lower GI events associated with traditional NSAIDs and acetaminophen among the elderly in Quebec, Canada. *American Journal of Gastroenterology*. **103**(4): 872–82. (RS)

246 Laine L. (2002) Gastrointestinal safety of coxibs and outcomes studies: what's the verdict? *Journal of Pain and Symptom Management*. **23**(Suppl.): S11–13. (R, 13 refs)

247 Foral PA, Wilson AF, Nystrom KK. (2002) Gastrointestinal bleeds associated with rofecoxib. *Pharmacotherapy*. **22**(3): 384–6. (R)

248 Bjorkman DJ. (2002) Commentary: gastrointestinal safety of coxibs and outcomes studies: what's the verdict? *Journal of Pain and Symptom Management*. **23**(Suppl.): S5–10. (C)

249 Sturmer T, Erb A, Keller F, Gunther KP, Brenner H. (2001) Determinants of impaired renal function with use of nonsteroidal anti-inflammatory drugs: the importance of half-life and other medications. *American Journal of Medicine*. **111**(7): 521–7. (MC, OS-802)

250 Brater DC. (2002) Renal effects of cyclooxygenase-2 selective inhibitors. Commentary: gastrointestinal safety of coxibs and outcomes studies: what's the verdict? *Journal of Pain and Symptom Management*. **23**(Suppl.): S15–20. (C)

251 Gonzalez E, Gutierrez E, Galeano C, Chevia C, de Sequera P, *et al.* (2008) Early steroid treatment improves the recovery of renal function in patients

with drug-induced acute interstitial nephritis. *Kidney International.* **73**(8): 940–6. (MC, RS-61)

252 Ardoin SP, Sundy JS. (2006) Update on nonsteroidal anti-inflammatory drugs. *Current Opinion in Rheumatology.* **18**(3): 221–6. (R, 58 refs)

253 Haag MD, Bos MJ, Hofman A, Koudstaal PJ, *et al.* (2008) Cyclooxygenase selectivity of nonsteroidal anti-inflammatory drugs and risk of stroke. *Archives of Internal Medicine.* **168**(11): 1219–24. (OS-7636)

254 Mukherjee D. (2008) Nonsteroidal anti-inflammatory drugs and the heart: what is the danger? *Congestive Heart Failure.* **14**(2): 75–82. (R, 48 refs)

255 Abraham NS, Hartman C, Castillo D, Richardson P, Smalley W. (2008) Effectiveness of national provider prescription of PPI gastroprotection among elderly NSAID users. *American Journal of Gastroenterology.* **103**(2): 323–32. (RS-481,980)

256 Koch M, Capurso L, Dezi A, Ferrario F, Scarpignato C. (1995). Prevention of NSAID-induced gastroduodenal mucosal injury: meta-analysis of clinical trials with misoprostol and H_2 antagonists. *Digestive Diseases.* **1**: 62–74.

257 Kart T, Christrup LL, Rasmussen M. (1997) Recommended use of morphine in neonates, infants and children based on a literature review: Part 2 – Clinical use. *Paediatric Anaesthesia.* **7**(2): 93–101. (R, 82 refs)

258 Hu WY, Chiu TY, Cheng SY, Chen CY. (2004) Morphine for dyspnea control in terminal cancer patients: is it appropriate in Taiwan? *Journal of Pain and Symptom Management.* **28**(4): 356–63. (OS-136)

259 Mazzocato C, Buclin T, Rapin CH. (1999) The effects of morphine on dyspnea and ventilatory function in elderly patients with advanced cancer: a randomized double-blind controlled trial. *Annals of Oncology.* **10**(12): 1511–4. (CT-9)

260 Clemens KE, Quednau I, Klaschik E. (2008) Is there a higher risk of respiratory depression in opioid-naive palliative care patients during symptomatic therapy of dyspnea with strong opioids? *Journal of Palliative Medicine.* **11**(2): 204–16. (OS-27)

261 Boyd KJ, Kelly M. (1997) Oral morphine as symptomatic treatment of dyspnoea in patients with advanced cancer. *Palliative Medicine.* **11**(4): 277–81. (OS-15)

262 Bruera E, Macmillan K, Pither J, MacDonald RN. (1990) Effects of morphine on the dyspnea of terminal cancer patients. *Journal of Pain and Symptom Management.* **5**(6): 341–4. (OS-20)

263 Clemens KE, Klaschik E. (2008) Morphine in the management of dyspnoea in ALS: a pilot study. *European Journal of Neurology.* **15**(5): 445–50. (OS-6)

264 Finkelstein Y, Schechter T, Garcia-Bournissen F, Kirby M, *et al.* (2007) Is morphine exposure associated with acute chest syndrome in children with vaso-occlusive crisis of sickle cell disease? A 6-year case-crossover study. *Clinical Therapeutics.* **29**(12): 2738–43. (RS-17)

265 Chan JD, Treece PD, Engelberg RA, Crowley L, *et al.* (2004) Narcotic and benzodiazepine use after withdrawal of life support: association with time to death? *Chest.* **126**(1): 286–93. (RS-75)

266 Twycross RG. (1999) *Morphine and the Relief of Cancer Pain: information for patients, families and friends.* Beaconsfield: Beaconsfield Publishers. (B)

267 Regnard C, Pelham A. (2003) Severe respiratory depression and sedation with transdermal fentanyl: four case studies. *Palliative Medicine.* **17**: 714–16. (CS-4)

268 Medicines and Healthcare Products Regulatory Agency. (2008) Fentanyl patches: serious and fatal overdose from dosing errors, accidental exposure and inappropriate use. *Drug Safety Update.* **2**(2): 2–3. (Rep)

269 Heiskanen T, Matzke S, Haakana S, Gergov M, Vuori E, Kalso E. (2009) Transdermal fentanyl in cachectic cancer patients. *Pain.* **144**(1–2): 218–22. (OS-20)

270 Sykes N. (1998) The relationship between opioid use and laxative use in terminally ill patients. *Palliative Medicine.* **12**: 375–82. (RS)

271 Wirz S, Wittmann M, Schenk M, Schroeck A, *et al.* (2009) Gastrointestinal symptoms under opioid therapy: a prospective comparison of oral sustained-release hydromorphone, transdermal fentanyl, and transdermal buprenorphine. *European Journal of Pain.* **13**(7): 737–43. (CT-174)

272 Glare P, Walsh D, Sheehan D. (2006) The adverse effects of morphine: a prospective survey of common symptoms during repeated dosing for chronic cancer pain. *American Journal of Hospice and Palliative Medicine.* **23**(3): 229–35. (OS-42)

273 Mercadante S, Villari P, Ferrera P, Casuccio A. (2006) Opioid-induced or pain relief-reduced symptoms in advanced cancer patients? *European Journal of Pain.* **10**(2): 153–9. (OS-35)

274 Harris JD, Kotob F. (2006) Management of opioid-related side effects. In: de Leon-Casasola OA, ed. *Cancer Pain: pharmacological, interventional, and palliative care.* Philadelphia: Elsevier Inc. pp. 207–30. (Ch)

275 Taub A. (1982) Opioid analgesics in the treatment of chronic intractable pain of non-neoplastic origin. In: Kitahata LM, Collins JG, eds. *Narcotic Analgesics in Anaesthesiology.* Baltimore: Williams and Wilkins. pp. 199–208. (Ch)

276 Cherny N, Ripamonti C, Pereira J, Davis C, Fallon M, McQuay H, Mercadante S, Pasternak G, Ventafridda V. Expert Working Group of the European Association of Palliative Care Network. (2001) Strategies to manage the adverse effects of oral morphine: an evidence-based report. *Journal of Clinical Oncology.* **19**(9): 2542–54. (R, 172 refs)

277 Hanks GW, Roberts CJC, Davies AN. (2004) Principles of drug use in palliative medicine. In: Doyle D, Hanks GWC, Cherney N, Calman K, eds. *Oxford Textbook of Palliative Medicine, 3rd ed.* Oxford: Oxford Medical Press. pp. 213–25. (Ch)

278 Goodman A. (1990) Addiction: definition and implications. *British Journal of Addiction.* **85**(11): 1403–8. (R)

279 Passik S, Portenoy R. (1998) Substance abuse issues in palliative care. In: Berger A, ed. *Principles*

and Practice of Supportive Oncology. Philadelphia: Lippincott-Raven. (Ch)

280 Joranson DE, Ryan KM, Gilson AM, Dahl JL. (2000) Trends in medical use and abuse of opioid analgesics. *Journal of the American Medical Association*. **283**(13): 1710–14. (RS)

281 Twycross RG, Wald SJ. (1976) Longterm use of diamorphine in advanced cancer. In: Bonica JJ, ed. *Advances in Pain Research and Therapy, Vol 1*. New York: Raven Press. (Ch)

282 Wilwerding MB, Loprinzi CL, Mailliard JA, O'Fallon JR, *et al.* (1995) A randomized, crossover evaluation of methylphenidate in cancer patients receiving strong narcotics. *Supportive Care in Cancer.* **3**(2): 135–8. (RCT)

283 White ID, Hoskin PJ, Hanks GW, Bliss JM. (1989) Morphine and dryness of the mouth. *British Medical Journal*. **298**(6682): 1222–3. (OS)

284 Smith MT. (2000) Neuroexcitatory effects of morphine and hydromorphone: evidence implicating the 3-glucuronide metabolites. *Clinical and Experimental Pharmacology and Physiology*. **27**(7): 524–8. (R, 30 refs)

285 Sarhill N, Davis MP, Walsh D, Nouneh C. (2001) Methadone-induced myoclonus in advanced cancer. *American Journal of Hospice and Palliative Care*. **18**(1): 51–3. (CS-1)

286 Stuerenburg HJ, Claassen J, Eggers C, Hansen HC. (2000) Acute adverse reaction to fentanyl in a 55 year old man. *Journal of Neurology, Neurosurgery and Psychiatry*. **69**(2): 281–2. (Let, CS-1)

287 Adair JC, el-Nachef A, Cutler P. (1996) Fentanyl neurotoxicity. *Annals of Emergency Medicine*. **27**(6): 791–2. (Let, CS-1)

288 Okon TR, George ML. (2008) Fentanyl-induced neurotoxicity and paradoxic pain. *Journal of Pain and Symptom Management*. **35**(3): 327–33. (CS-1)

289 Glare P, Walsh D, Sheehan D. (2006) The adverse effects of morphine: a prospective survey of common symptoms during repeated dosing for chronic cancer pain. *American Journal of Hospice and Palliative Medicine*. **23**(3): 229–35. (OS-56)

290 Mercadante S. (1995) Dantrolene treatment of opioid-induced myoclonus. *Anesthesia and Analgesia*. **81**(6): 1307–8. (R)

291 Holdsworth MT, Adams VR, Chavez CM, Vaughan LJ, Duncan MH. (1995) Continuous midazolam infusion for the management of morphine-induced myoclonus. *Annals of Pharmacotherapy*. **29**(1): 25–9. (CS-1)

292 Fountain A. (2002) Before you blame the morphine: visual hallucinations in palliative care. *CME Cancer Medicine*. **1**(1): 23–6. (R, 78 refs)

293 Krajnik M, Zylicz Z. (2001) Understanding pruritus in systemic disease. *Journal of Pain and Symptom Management*. **21**(2): 151–68. (R, 142 refs)

294 Ganesh A, Maxwell LG. (2007) Pathophysiology and management of opioid-induced pruritus. *Drugs*. **67**(16): 2323–33. (R, 88 refs)

295 Twycross R, Greaves MW, Handwerker H, Jones EA, *et al.* (2003) Itch: scratching more than the surface. *Quarterly Journal of Medicine*. **96**(1): 7–26. (R, 211 refs)

296 Kuraishi Y, Yamaguchi T, Miyamoto T. (2000) Itch-scratch responses induced by opioids through central mu opioid receptors in mice. *Journal of Biomedical Science*. **7**(3): 248–52. (LS)

297 Maxwell LG, Kaufmann SC, Bitzer S, Jackson EV Jr., *et al.* (2005) The effects of a small-dose naloxone infusion on opioid-induced side effects and analgesia in children and adolescents treated with intravenous patient-controlled analgesia: a double-blind, prospective, randomized, controlled study. *Anesthesia and Analgesia*. **100**(4): 953–8. (RCT-46)

298 Challand S, Frew K, Regnard C. (2008) Is there a problem with oxycodone? *Journal of Pain and Symptom Management*. **36**(6): e1–3. (Let, OS-100)

299 Chu LF, Angst MS, Clark D. (2008) Opioid-induced hyperalgesia in humans: molecular mechanisms and clinical considerations. *Clinical Journal of Pain*. **24**(6): 479–96. (R, 192 refs)

300 Cohen SP, Christo PJ, Wang S, Chen L, *et al.* (2008) The effect of opioid dose and treatment duration on the perception of a painful standardized clinical stimulus. *Regional Anesthesia and Pain Medicine*. **33**(3): 199–206. (CT-382)

301 Harris JD. (2008) Management of expected and unexpected opioid-related side effects. *Clinical Journal of Pain*. **24**(Suppl. 10): S8–13. (R)

302 Davis AM, Inturrisi CE. (1999) d-Methadone blocks morphine tolerance and N-methyl-D-aspartate-induced hyperalgesia. *Journal of Pharmacology and Experimental Therapeutics*. **289**(2): 1048–53. (LS)

303 Gan TJ, Ginsberg B, Glass PS, Fortney J, Jhaveri R, Perno R. (1997) Opioid-sparing effects of a low-dose infusion of naloxone in patient-administered morphine sulfate. *Anesthesiology*. **87**(5): 1075–81. (RCT-60)

304 Cepeda MS, Alvarez H, Morales O, Carr DB. (2004) Addition of ultralow dose naloxone to postoperative morphine PCA: unchanged analgesia and opioid requirement but decreased incidence of opioid side effects. *Pain*. **107**(1–2): 41–6. (265-RCT)

305 Mercadante S, Villari P, Ferrera P. (2003) Naloxone in treating central adverse effects during opioid titration for cancer pain. *Journal of Pain and Symptom Management*. **26**: 691–3. (CS, Let)

306 Twycross R. (1994) The risks and benefits of corticosteroids in advanced cancer. *Drug Safety*. **11**(3): 163–78. (R)

307 Margolin L, Cope DK, Bakst-Sisser R, Greenspan J. (2007) The steroid withdrawal syndrome: a review of the implications, etiology and treatments. *Journal of Symptom Management*. **33**(2): 224–8. (CS-3, R, 20 refs)

Other physical symptoms

NOTES

Ascites

CLINICAL DECISION AND ACTION CHECKLIST

1. Could the symptoms and signs have a different cause?
2. Is the prognosis short?
3. Is the ascites causing distress?
4. Will the patient tolerate diuretics?
5. Is the ascites recurring?

KEY POINTS

- Paracentesis offers immediate relief but poor long-term control.
- Combination diuretics offer useful long-term control in some patients.

INTRODUCTION

The development of ascites usually carries a poorer prognosis in both cancer and liver disease.[1,2] Nevertheless, median survival in malignant ascites is nearly 6 months, and can be longer in ovarian carcinoma.[3] The commonest causes of malignant ascites are primary tumors of breast, ovary, colon, stomach, pancreas, and bronchus. Symptoms of ascites include nausea, vomiting, abdominal distension or pain, edema (legs, perineum or lower trunk), and breathlessness due to diaphragmatic splinting.[4]

TYPES OF ASCITES

Four types can be identified.[5]

Raised hydrostatic pressure: causes include cirrhosis; congestive heart failure; inferior vena cava obstruction; hepatic vein occlusion by thrombus; compression from tumors or metastases in the liver or abdomen.

Decreased osmotic pressure: caused by protein depletion (nephrotic syndrome, protein-losing enteropathy), reduced protein intake (malnutrition), or reduced protein production (cirrhosis).

Fluid production exceeding resorptive capacity: caused by infection or intra-abdominal tumors.

Chylous: due to obstruction and leakage of the lymphatics draining the gut.

TREATMENT

Diuretics, paracentesis, and peritoneovenous shunting are still the mainstays of treatment,[6–8] although the evidence for all three is weak.

Diuretics

Diuretics have long been a useful treatment in cirrhotic ascites.[9] Patients with liver metastases (and resulting portal hypertension) are most likely to respond to diuretics.[9,10] A serum–ascites albumin gradient >11 g/L is a simple way of selecting such patients, especially in non-cirrhotic patients.[8,11,12] Patients with a high-gradient ascites have circulating blood volume depletion and consequent activation of the renin/angiotensin system,[13] so spironolactone is the diuretic of choice. Its use with furosemide is well established.[14–16] The aim is a weight loss of 0.5–1 kg/day and if peripheral edema is present high doses can be tolerated.[17–19] However, diuretics can cause electrolyte disturbances and hypotension. They also need to be used with caution in patients with poor renal or hepatic function.

Paracentesis

This is helpful for short-term symptom relief. Insertion methods vary from using a peritoneal dialysis (PD) catheter attached to a standard PD collection bag, to using a large-bore IV cannula or a suprapubic trochar and catheter. The use of 0.5% bupivacaine or lidocaine as local anesthetic for the puncture site allows pain-free drainage for up to 8 hours if necessary.

Puncture sites should be away from scars, tumor masses, distended bowel, bladder, liver or the inferior epigastric arteries that run 5 cm either side of the anterior midline. The best sites are in the left iliac fossa (at least 10 cm from the midline) and in the midline suprapubically (the bladder must be empty). A lateral approach is advisable in patients with distended bowel – marked distension is a contraindication to paracentesis.

As a check, the needle used for the local anesthetic can be used to determine if ascitic fluid is present before inserting the drainage tube. If there is any uncertainty, ultrasound should be arranged. Ultrasound is being used more and more routinely, especially if the ascites is loculated.[20,21]

Volume drained: in malignant ascites it is safe and effective to drain up to 5 liters over a few hours without intravenous fluid replacement, even in children.[6,22,23] Most symptoms can be relieved after only 2 hours' drainage, although it may take 72 hours after drainage has stopped before severe breathlessness improves.[24] Patients with other causes of ascites can have much larger volumes drained but to avoid hypotension they may need an albumin infusion, the administration of midodrine 5–10 mg,[25] or drainage over several days.[26] However, in patients with distended abdominal organs or intra-abdominal tumor masses, draining to dryness can cause considerable pain and it is best to drain only enough to reduce the discomfort caused by the distension.

After removal of the catheter any leakage of ascites from the puncture site can be collected with a colostomy bag. Leakage usually stops after 2–3 days and so the patient is spared a suture.

<table>
<tr><th>Clinical decision</th><th>If YES carry out the action below</th></tr>
<tr><td>1 Could the symptoms and signs have a different cause?</td><td>Signs of ascites: flank dullness, shifting dullness, fluid thrill.
• Exclude: other causes of abdominal distension such as bowel obstruction, abdominal tumor or hepatomegaly.
• If uncertain, consider an abdominal ultrasound examination.</td></tr>
<tr><td>2 Is the prognosis short? (day-to-day deterioration)</td><td>• If free of symptoms: no further action required.
• If symptoms are troublesome:
Nausea and vomiting: see Nausea and vomiting, p. 167.
Abdominal stretch pain:
— consider a brief paracentesis of 2 liters to reduce discomfort
— acetaminophen or diclofenac may help discomfort. Consider TENS.
Peripheral edema: see cd-6 in Edema and lymphedema, p. 143.</td></tr>
<tr><td>3 Is the ascites causing distress?</td><td>• If dehydrated, hypotensive or the ascites is due to cirrhosis: start IV infusion of Dextran 70.
• In the <u>absence</u> of gross bowel distension or abdominal tumor:
Carry out therapeutic paracentesis (see opposite for details):
— drain 2 liters over 1 hour, then drain up to a further 3 liters over 3–4 hours (larger volumes will need drainage over 24 hours or more)
— remove tube and place ostomy bag over puncture site
— if hypotension develops start IV infusion of Dextran
— stop if pain develops (patients with extensive abdominal cancer are more comfortable if some fluid is left to cushion tumor masses).
• If little or no fluid obtained: the ascites may be loculated. Arrange for drainage under ultrasound control.
• If ascites is too viscous to drain (e.g. ovarian carcinoma): consider paracentesis with suction. Alternatively, ask surgeon to form an artificial fistula.</td></tr>
<tr><td>4 Will the patient tolerate diuretics?</td><td>• For patients able to take oral medication and with good renal function:
Measure abdominal girth at a marked site each week.
If the serum–ascites albumin gradient is >11 g/L start spironolactone 100 mg with furosemide 40 mg PO once daily.
Increase doses up to 300 mg spironolactone and 80 mg furosemide to achieve a weight loss of 0.5–1 kg/day. Patients with peripheral edema may tolerate doses up to furosemide 160 mg + spironolactone 400 mg daily for a limited period.
NB. Spironolactone takes up to two weeks to reach a steady plasma level.[27]
• For patients with impaired renal function:
Ask the advice of the renal physicians.
Use paracentesis to drain sufficient for comfort.
• If hypotension develops: start IV infusion Dextran and reduce diuretic dose. Check serum electrolytes weekly. Continue diuretics at lowest dose that will control symptoms.</td></tr>
<tr><td>5 Is the ascites recurrent?</td><td>• Consider
— systemic octreotide or intraperitoneal triamcinolone (10 mg/kg)
— spironolactone plus clonidine 750 microg 12 hourly
— a semi-permanent indwelling peritoneal catheter (see text opposite).
• Discuss options with
— oncologist, e.g. systemic chemotherapy, immunotherapy
— gastroenterologist or surgeon, e.g. peritoneovenous shunt.</td></tr>
</table>

Adapted from Regnard and Mannix[28]
cd = clinical decision

Catheters and shunts

Peritoneal drainage catheters can be inserted in carefully selected patients[8] and left for prolonged periods.[29] There are reports of using such catheters to drain 2 liters/day for as long as 18 months.[30,31] However, one-third of drainage catheters block and peritonitis is a risk.[32] An alternative is a peritoneal port through which the ascites is drained intermittently at home.[33]

Peritoneovenous shunts drain ascites into a vein. Patients with ovarian and breast cancer have the best response rates (≥50%) to peritoneovenous shunts, those with gastrointestinal malignancies the worst (10–15%).[8] Thus insertion of a shunt in those with gastrointestinal malignancies is generally agreed to be contraindicated. The complication rate is reported by some to be equivalent to or better than that for traditional paracentesis.[34] Shunts can be inserted percutaneously,[35,36] but the long-term use of shunts results in troublesome complications in both cirrhosis and cancer-related ascites.[37–40]

A disadvantage of repeated paracentesis is the steady loss of albumin.[41] This will result in a low serum albumin and the risk of increasing peripheral edema.

Other treatments

In malignancy, systemic or intraperitoneal chemotherapy has been used,[42] but although benefit has been shown in one large study[43] the benefit in advanced disease has not been shown.[6] Intraperitoneal triamcinolone may have a role.[44,45] Octreotide has been reported to reduce ascites in cancer,[46] and cirrhosis.[47] In mucinous ascites that is too viscous for tube drainage, consider either paracentesis with suction, or asking a surgeon to fashion an artificial fistula to drain the ascites. Patients with cirrhotic ascites can be helped by restriction of dietary sodium or using a clonidine-spironolactone combination.[48,49]

REFERENCES: ASCITES

B = book; C = comment; Ch = chapter; CS-n = case study-no. of cases; CT-n = controlled trial-no. of cases; E= editorial; GC = group consensus; I = interviews; Let = Letter; LS = laboratory study; MC = multi-center; OS-n = open study-no. of cases; R = review; RCT-n = randomized controlled trial-no. of cases; RS-n = retrospective survey-no. of cases; SA = systematic or meta analysis.

1 Ayantunde AA, Parsons SL. (2007) Pattern and prognostic factors in patients with malignant ascites: a retrospective study. *Annals of Oncology*. **18**(5): 945–9. (RS)

2 Spadaro A, Luigiano C, De Caro G, Morace C, Tortorella V, Bonfiglio C, Pagano N, Consolo P, Alibrandi A, Ajello A, Ferrau O, Freni MA. (2007) Prognostic factors of survival in complicated viral and alcoholic cirrhosis without hepatocellular carcinoma: a retrospective study. *Minerva Gastroenterologica e Dietologica*. **53**(4): 311–19. (RS-255)

3 Carr BI, Buch SC, Kondragunta V, Pancoska P, Branch RA. (2009). Tumor and liver determinants of prognosis in unresectable hepatocellular carcinoma: a case cohort study. *Journal of Gastroenterology and Hepatology*. **23**(8): 1259–66. (OS-967)

4 Keen J, Fallon M. (2002) Malignant ascites. In: Ripamonti C, Bruera E. *Gastrointestinal Symptoms in Advanced Cancer Patients*. Oxford: Oxford University Press. pp. 279–90. (Ch)

5 Parsons SL, Watson SA, Steele RJC. (1996) Malignant ascites. *British Journal of Surgery*. **83**: 6–14. (R, 92 refs)

6 Aslam N, Marino CR. (2001) Malignant ascites: new concepts in pathophysiology, diagnosis, and management. *Archives of Internal Medicine*. **161**(22): 2733–7. (R, 28 refs)

7 Stephenson J, Gilbert J. (2002) The development of clinical guidelines on paracentesis for ascites related to malignancy. *Palliative Medicine*. **16**(3): 213–18. (R)

8 Becker G, Galandi D, Blum HE. (2006) Malignant ascites: systematic review and guideline for treatment. *European Journal of Cancer*. **42**: 589–97. (R)

9 Leiva JG, Salgado JM, Estradas J, Torre A, Uribe M. (2007) Pathophysiology of ascites and dilutional hyponatremia: contemporary use of aquaretic agents. *Annals of Hepatology*. **6**(4): 214–21. (R, 41 refs)

10 Parsons SL, Lang MW, Steele RJ. (1996) Malignant ascites: a 2-year review from a teaching hospital. *European Journal of Surgical Oncology*. **22**: 237–9. (RS-164)

11 Runyon BA. (1994) Current concepts: care of patients with ascites. *The New England Journal of Medicine*. **330**: 337–42. (R)

12 Khandwalla HE, Fasakin Y, El-Serag HB. (2009) The utility of evaluating low serum albumin gradient ascites in patients with cirrhosis. *American Journal of Gastroenterology*. **104**(6): 1401–5.

13 Becker G. (2007) Medical and palliative management of malignant ascites. *Cancer Treatment and Research*. **134**: 459–67. (R, 53 refs)

14 Jelan R, Hayes PC. (1997) Hepatic encephalopathy and ascites. *Lancet*. **350**: 1309–14. (R, 62 refs)

15 Greenway B, Johnson PJ, Williams R. (1982) Control of malignant ascites with spironolactone. *British Journal of Surgery*. **69**: 441–2. (OS-15)

16 Fogel MR, Sawhney VK, Neal EA, Miller RG, Knauer CM, Gregory PB. (1981) Diuresis in the ascitic patient: a randomised controlled trial of three regimens. *Journal of Clinical Gastroenterology*. **3**(Suppl. 1): 73–80. (RCT-90)

17 Alimentary symptoms. In: Twycross R, Wilcock A, Stark Toller C. (2009) *Symptom Management in Advanced Cancer*. Nottingham: palliativedrugs.com. pp. 61–144. (Ch)

18 Pockros PJ, Reynolds TB. (1986) Rapid diuresis in patients with ascites from chronic liver disease: the importance of peripheral oedema. *Gastroenterology*. **90**: 1827–33. (OS-14)

19 Saravanan R, Cramp ME. (2002) Investigation and treatment of ascites. *Clinical Medicine (Journal of the Royal College of Physicians of London)*. **2**: 310–13. (R)

20 Nazeer SR, Hillary D, Miller AH. (2005) Ultrasound-assisted paracentesis performed by emergency physicians vs the traditional technique: a prospective, randomized study. *American Journal of Emergency Medicine*. **23**(3): 363–7. (RCT – 100)

21 Macdonald R, Kirwan J, Roberts S, Gray D, Allsopp L, Green J. (2006) Ovarian cancer and ascites: a questionnaire on current management in the United kingdom. *Journal of Palliative Medicine*. **9**(6): 1264–70. (OS-492)

22 Forouzandeh B, Konicek F, Sheagren JN. (1996) Large-volume paracentesis in the treatment of cirrhotic patients with refractory ascites: the role of postparacentesis plasma volume expansion. *Journal of Clinical Gastroenterology*. **22**(3): 207–10. (R, 51 refs)

23 Kramer RE, Sokol RJ, Yerushalmi B, Liu E, MacKenzie T, Hoffenberg EJ, Narkewicz MR. (2001) Large-volume paracentesis in the management of ascites in children. *Journal of Pediatric Gastroenterology and Nutrition*. **33**(3): 245–9. (RS-21)

24 McNamara P. (2000) Paracentesis: an effective method of symptom control in the palliative care setting? *Palliative Medicine*. **14**(1): 62–4. (OS)

25 Singh V, Dheerendra PC, Singh B, Nain CK, *et al.* (2008) Midodrine versus albumin in the prevention of paracentesis-induced circulatory dysfunction in cirrhotics: a randomised pilot study. *American Journal of Gastroenterology*. **103**(6): 1399–1405. (RCT-40)

26 Smith GS, Barnard GF. (1997) Massive volume paracentesis (up to 41 liters) for the outpatient management of ascites. *Journal of Clinical Gastroenterology*. **25**(1): 402–3. (CS-1)

27 Sungaila I, Bartle WR, Walker SE, *et al.* (1992) Spironolactone pharmacokinetics and pharmacodynamics in patients with cirrhotic ascites. *Gastroenterology*. **102**: 1680–85. (OS-9)

28 Regnard C, Mannix. (1995) Management of ascites. In: *Flow Diagrams in Advanced Cancer and Other Diseases*. London: Edward Arnold. pp. 36–8. (Ch)

29 Lee A, Lau TN, Yeong KY. (2000) Indwelling catheters for the management of malignant ascites. *Supportive Care in Cancer*. **8**(6): 493–9. (RS-38)

30 Brooks RA, Herzog TJ. (2006) Long-term semi-permanent catheter use for the palliation of malignant ascites. *Gynecologic Oncology*. **101**(2): 360–2. (CS-1)

31 Mercadante S, Intravaia G, Ferrera P, Villari P, David F. (2008) Peritoneal catheter for continuous drainage of ascites in advanced cancer patients. *Supportive Care in Cancer*. **16**(8): 975–8. (OS-40)

32 Fleming ND, Alvarez-Secord A, von Guenigen V, Miller MJ, Abernethy AP. (2009) Indwelling catheters for the management of refractory malignant ascites: a systematic literature review and retrospective chart review. *Journal of Pain and Symptom Management*, **38**(3): 341–49. (SA-15; RS-19)

33 Savin MA, Kirsch MJ, Romano WJ, Wang SK, Arpasi PJ, Mazon CD. (2005) Peritoneal ports for treatment of intractable ascites. *Journal of Vascular and Interventional Radiology*. **16**(3): 363–8. (CS-27)

34 Seike M, Maetani I, Sakai Y. (2007) Treatment of malignant ascites in patients with advanced cancer: peritoneovenous shunt versus paracentesis. *Journal of Gastroenterology and Hepatology*. **22**(12): 2161–6. (CT–69)

35 Mercadante S, Intravaia G, Ferrera P, Villari P, David F. (2008) Peritoneal catheter for continuous drainage of ascites in advanced cancer patients. *Supportive Care in Cancer*. **16**(8): 975–8. (OS-40)

36 Barnett TD, Rubins J. (2002) Placement of a permanent tunneled peritoneal drainage catheter for palliation of malignant ascites: a simplified percutaneous approach. *Journal of Vascular and Interventional Radiology*. **13**(4): 379–83. (RS-29)

37 Zervos EE, McCormick J, Goode SE, Rosemurgy AS. (1997) Peritoneovenous shunts in patients with intractable ascites: palliation at what price? *American Surgeon*. **63**(2): 157–62. (OS-48)

38 Schumacher DL, Saclarides TJ, Staren ED. (1994) Peritoneovenous shunts for palliation of the patient with malignant ascites. *Annals of Surgical Oncology*. **1**: 378–81. (OS-89)

39 Adam RA, Adam YG. (2004) Malignant ascites: past, present, and future. *Journal of the American College of Surgeons*. **198**: 999–1011. (R, 102 refs)

40 Albillos A, Banares R, Gonzalez M, Catalina MV, Molinero LM. (2005) A meta-analysis of transjugular intrahepatic portosystemic shunt versus paracentesis for refractory ascites. *Journal of Hepatology*. **43**(6): 990–6. (SA)

41 Schiano TD, Black M, Hills C, Ter H, Bellary S, Miller LS. (2000) Correlation between increased colloid osmotic pressure and the resolution of refractory ascites after transjugular intrahepatic portosystemic shunt. *Southern Medical Journal*. **93**(3): 305–9. (OS-23)

42 Malik I, Abubakar S, Rizwana I, Alam F, Rizvi J, Khan A. (1991) Clinical features and management of malignant ascites. *Journal of the Pakistan Medical Association*. **41**(2): 38–40. (RS-45)
43 Link KH, Roitman M, Holtappels M, Runnebaum I, Urbanzyk H, Leder G, Staib L. (2003) Intraperitoneal chemotherapy with mitoxantrone in malignant ascites. *Surgical Oncology Clinics of North America*. **12**(3): 865–72 (RS-143)
44 Mackey JR, Wood L, Nabholtz J, Jensen J, Venner P. (2000) A phase II trial of triamcinolone hexacetanide for symptomatic recurrent malignant ascites. *Journal of Pain and Symptom Management*. **19**(3): 193–9. (OS-15)
45 Jenkin RP, Bamford R, Patel V, Kelly L, *et al.* (2009) The use of intraperitoneal triamcinolone acetonide for the management of recurrent malignant ascites in a patient with non-Hodgkin's lymphoma. *Journal of Pain and Symptom Management*. **36**(5): e4–5. (CS-1)
46 Cairns W, Malone R. (1999) Octreotide as an agent for the relief of malignant ascites in palliative care patients. *Palliative Medicine*. **13**(5): 429–30. (CS-3)
47 Kalambokis G, Economou M, Kosta P, Papadimitriou K, Tsianos EV. (2006) The effects of treatment with octreotide, diuretics, or both on portal hemodynamics in nonazotemic cirrhotic patients with ascites. *Journal of Clinical Gastroenterology*. **40**(4): 342–6. (RCT-20)
48 Schouten J, Michielsen PP. (2007) Treatment of cirrhotic ascites. *Acta Gastroenterologica Belgica*. **70**(2): 217–22. (R, 68 refs)
49 Lenaerts A, Codden T, Henry JP, Legros F, Ligny G. (2005) Comparative pilot study of repeated large volume paracentesis vs the combination on clonidine-spironolactone in the treatment of cirrhosis-associated refractory ascites. *Gastroenterologie Clinique et Biologique*. **29**(11): 1137–42. (RCT-20)

Bleeding

CLINICAL DECISION AND ACTION CHECKLIST

1 Is there a risk of bleeding?

If bleeding:
2 Is the patient hypotensive?
3 Is the bleeding site visible?
4 Is the source of bleeding internal?

KEY POINTS

- Catastrophic, external bleeding is uncommon.
- Control of external bleeding is usually possible.
- Exclude coagulation disorders.

SEVERE HEMORRHAGE

Since small, repeated bleeds can herald a major bleed, hemorrhage is a common fear. In reality, death from hemorrhage is rare and even in patients with previous bleeds 10% or fewer will die from hemorrhage.[1–6] Admission may be needed for minor bleeds if the patient and family find these frightening and if they want treatment. Successful treatment of a major hemorrhage is usually only possible in acute hospital settings in non-malignant conditions.

In any setting, use dark green or blue towels to soak up the blood loss as the absorbed blood will appear a less frightening black, not red. Perineal pads will help with the management of vaginal and low gastrointestinal bleeding. The patient will feel cold because of the hypotension, and will need warm blankets. Such an event is frightening for the patient who may need rapid sedation intravenously. The touch and closeness of another person is essential. *The partner, family, and staff will need support after such an experience.*

COAGULATION DISORDERS

The advice of a hematologist is invaluable in many of these conditions and the patient may require admission to hospital. In very advanced disease this is not usually appropriate. Fortunately, such events are uncommon, and usually occur in the last hours or days of life when distressing bleeding can be managed as described opposite.

Warfarin excess: the long half-life of warfarin and its many drug interactions mean that over-anticoagulation can occur easily.[7,8] In the presence of major bleeding give vitamin K 5 mg by slow IV injection and consider giving fresh frozen plasma. For high INR values (5–8) in the absence of troublesome bleeding, vitamin K is only needed if there are other risk factors for bleeding.

Platelet deficiency or malfunction: a number of conditions can deplete platelets (chemotherapy, bone marrow infiltration, heparin, enlarged spleen, liver disease, or drugs). Platelet transfusions may help active bleeding but need to be repeated every few days, and in someone deteriorating daily little will be gained by continuing.

Reduced clotting factors: abnormal clotting due to a failure to produce clotting factors is a sensitive sign of liver failure. It can only be treated by giving fresh frozen plasma on a daily basis. Clotting factors can be depleted by the excessive clotting that occurs in disseminated intravascular coagulation (DIC). DIC can respond to a simple regimen of an antifibrinolytic such as tranexamic acid and low-dose heparin.[9,10]

Vitamin K deficiency: this occurs in malabsorption and can occur in obstructive jaundice and distal small bowel resection. It can be corrected by replacing vitamin K orally or IV.

RADIOTHERAPY

This is helpful in patients with hemoptysis[11,12] and vaginal bleeding.[13] Single treatments are possible in frail patients, and internal radioactive sources (brachytherapy) are being used for bronchial bleeding.[12,14,15] Intravaginal and intrauterine sources can also be used to control bleeding from advanced gynecological tumors.[16]

PHARMACOLOGICAL AGENTS

Topical/locally acting drugs: sucralfate is useful in controlling the bleeding from a gastric carcinoma,[17] or it can be applied topically, directly to the bleeding point if this is visible. Sucralfate enemas have been used to control post-irradiation

Clinical decision	If YES carry out the action below
1 Is there a risk of bleeding?	• **If on warfarin:** keep INR to between 1.5 and 3. • **If this is a coagulation disorder** (e.g. low or abnormal platelets; increased warfarin levels due to reduced warfarin metabolism or displacement by another drug; disseminated intravascular coagulation; renal failure; hepatic impairment; vitamin K or C deficiency): — treatment can be difficult. Vitamin K may help if the patient is over-warfarinized, suffers from severe hepatic impairment or has malabsorption (*see* text above). Otherwise, the advice of a hematologist is essential. • **If rapidly growing and erosive tumor:** keep dark green or blue towel and sedation to hand. Consider referral for radiotherapy or embolization.

Adapted from Regnard and Makin[18]
cd = clinical decision

Clinical decision	If YES carry out the action below
2 Is the patient hypotensive?	• **If treatment is appropriate:** *see* cd-3c in *Emergencies*, p. 333. • **If treatment is not appropriate:** *If the patient is distressed:* give midazolam 5–15 mg titrated IV (if IV access not possible give buccally or into the deltoid muscle). *If hemorrhage is visible* (ulcer, hemoptysis, hematemesis): use dark green or blue towels to make the appearance of blood less frightening to patient, partner or family (*see* cd-3 below). • **Place warm blankets over the patient and do not leave the patient unattended.**
3 Is the bleeding source visible?	• **Promote clotting:** apply sucralfate suspension or a calcium alginate dressing. • **Apply pressure** to stop flow. • **Prevent re-bleeding:** *Topical:* apply sucralfate or tranexamic acid under non-adherent dressing (e.g. Mepitel). The dressing can be left in place for several days, although re-bleeding may need daily applications. NB. Do not use sucralfate in areas currently receiving radiotherapy. *Systemic:* tranexamic acid PO 1 g q8h or aminocaproic acid (US only) PO 5 g initially followed by 1 g four times a day. • **Consider:** radiotherapy, diathermy or embolization.
4 Is the source of bleeding internal?	• **Hemoptysis:** *If minor (streaked sputum):* tranexamic acid PO 1 g q8h or aminocaproic acid (US only) PO 5 g initially followed by 1 g four times a day. *If troublesome (clots, anemia, or frequent bleeds):* radiotherapy, radiofrequency laser, or embolization. • **Hematemesis and/or melena:** *Stop gastric irritants*, e.g. non-steroidal anti-inflammatory drugs. *If minor* (altered blood or positive fecal occult blood): 2 g sucralfate PO q12h. *If troublesome* (fresh blood, melena or anemia): 2 g sucralfate PO q4h *plus* omeprazole 20–40 mg PO daily (absorption of lansoprazole is reduced by sucralfate). NB. If source is non-malignant, refer urgently for endoscopy and surgical opinion. • **Mouth or nasopharynx:** *If anterior nose:* pack with gauze soaked in sucralfate suspension. Refer to ear, nose, and throat surgeons if re-bleeding occurs. *If posterior nose:* refer to ear, nose, and throat surgeons for packing under observation + diathermy. *If oral:* use sucralfate suspension (diluted 1:1 with water) as a mouthwash. • **Rectum or vagina:** *If minor (streaking only):* observe and consider pads. *If troublesome (clots, frequent bleeds, or anemia):* tranexamic acid PO 1 g q8h or aminocaproic acid (US only) PO 5 g initially followed by 1 g q6h. *Consider* radiotherapy, topical sucralfate suspension or topical tranexamic acid. • **Other sources:** *Hematuria: see* cd-3 *Urinary problems and sexual difficulties*, p. 225. *Intrapleural or intra-abdominal:* exclude coagulation disorder or trauma. Start tranexamic acid PO 1 g q8h or aminocaproic acid (US only) PO 5 g initially followed by 1 g four times a day.

Adapted from Regnard and Makin[18]
cd = clinical decision

rectal bleeding.[19,20] A 1% alum solution can reduce bladder hemorrhage (*see* cd-3 in *Urinary problems and sexual difficulties*, p. 225).[21–23] Topical tranexamic acid reduces bleeding from a rectal carcinoma and other sites.[24–26] In the US a topical aminocaproic acid preparation (available from a compounding pharmacy) can also be used.[27] Vasoconstrictors such as adrenalin work for 10–15 minutes but re-bleeding is common after the adrenalin is absorbed.

Dressings: some dressings such as calcium alginate are hemostatic, but leave fibers in the wound that are difficult to clear. Dressings with very low adherence (e.g. Mepitel) are useful as a base for applying sucralfate. These and moist environment dressings (alginate, hydrogels) can be left in place for up to seven days, avoiding any disturbance to the fragile bleeding surface.

Systemic drugs: tranexamic acid and aminocaproic acid inhibit the breakdown of fibrin clots and are well absorbed orally,[28] but should be avoided in hematuria since they can produce hard clots that are difficult to remove and can cause obstruction.[29,30] There is no clear evidence that these drugs increase the risk of thromboembolic disease,[31] but there have been case reports of pulmonary embolism with tranexamic acid.[32] There is a report of using systemic octreotide for bleeding from a gastric malignancy.[33]

PHYSICAL TREATMENTS

Heat and cold: lasers can palliate bleeding from tumors accessible externally or through an endoscope.[34,35] Diathermy can be helpful, but it can make bladder bleeding worse.[21] Radiofrequency ablation heats the tissue using microwave energy and can be helpful in treating hemoptysis.[36] The effects of cryotherapy are usually brief.

Embolization: this can be useful in controlling bleeding,[37] and it has been used in hemoptyses,[38] bleeding from the bladder,[39] prostate,[40] stomach,[41] head and neck cancers,[42] and malignant ulcers.[43] Pain and pyrexia may occur for a few days after embolization. There are risks, especially in the presence of abnormal anatomy,[44] and it needs a radiologist experienced in the procedure.

REFERENCES: BLEEDING

B = book; C = comment; Ch = chapter; CS-n = case study-no. of cases; CT-n = controlled trial-no. of cases; E = editorial; GC = group consensus; I = interviews; Let = Letter; LS = laboratory study; MC = multi-center; OS-n = open study-no. of cases; R = review; RCT-n = randomized controlled trial-no. of cases; RS-n = retrospective survey-no. of cases; SA = systematic or meta analysis.

1 Håkanson E, Konstantinov IE, Fransson S-G, Svedjeholm R. (2002). Management of life-threatening haemoptysis. *British Journal of Anaesthesia*. **88**(2): 291–5. (CS-2)

2 Upile T, Triaridis S, Kirkland P, Archer D, Searle A, Irving C, Rhys Evans P. (2005) The management of carotid artery rupture. *European Archives of Otorhinolaryngology*. **262**(7): 555–60. (RS-11)

3 Flume PA, Yankaskas JR, Ebeling M, Hulsey T, Clark LL. (2005) Massive hemoptysis in cystic fibrosis. *Chest*. **128**(2): 729–38. (RS-28,858)

4 Thompson AB, Teschler H, Rennard SI. (1992) Pathogenesis, evaluation, and therapy for massive hemoptysis. *Clinics in Chest Medicine*. **13**(1): 69–82. (R, 85 refs)

5 Klebl F, Bregenzer N, Schofer L, Tamme W, *et al.* (2005) Risk factors for mortality in severe upper gastrointestinal bleeding. *International Journal of Colorectal Disease*. **20**(1): 49–56. (RS-362)

6 Rios A, Montoya MJ, Rodriguez JM, Serrano A, Molina J, Parrilla P. (2005) Acute lower gastrointestinal hemorrhages in geriatric patients. *Digestive Diseases and Sciences*. **50**(5): 898–904. (RS-43)

7 Soto-Cardenas MJ, Pelayo-Garcia G, Rodriguez-Camacho A, Segura-Fernandez E, *et al.* (2008) Venous thromboembolism in patients with advanced cancer under palliative care: additional risk factors, primary/secondary prophylaxis and complications observed under normal clinical practice. *Palliative Medicine*. **22**(8): 965–8. (RS-71)

8 Noble SI, Shelley MD, Coles B, Williams SM, Wilcock A, Johnson MJ. (2008) Association for Palliative Medicine for Great Britain and Ireland. Management of venous thrombo-embolism in patients with advanced cancer: a systematic review and meta-analysis. *Lancet Oncology*. **9**(6): 577–84. (SA-19, 55 refs)

9 Saba HI, Morelli GA. (2006) The pathogenesis

and management of disseminated intravascular coagulation. *Clinical Advances in Hematology and Oncology*. **4**(12): 919–26. (R)

10 Franchini M. (2005) Pathophysiology, diagnosis and treatment of disseminated intravascular coagulation: an update. *Clinical Laboratory*. **51**(11–12): 633–9. (R, 93 refs)

11 Bhatt ML, Mohani BK, Kumar L, Chawla S, Sharma DN, Rath GK. (2000) Palliative treatment of advanced non small cell lung cancer with weekly fraction radiotherapy. *Indian Journal of Cancer*. **37**(4): 148–52. (OS-47)

12 Mallick I, Sharma SC, Behera D. (2007) Endobronchial brachytherapy for symptom palliation in non-small cell lung cancer: analysis of symptom response, endoscopic improvement and quality of life. *Lung Cancer*. **55**(3): 313–8. (CT-80)

13 Onsrud M, Hagen B, Strickert T. (2001) 10-Gy single-fraction pelvic irradiation for palliation and life prolongation in patients with cancer of the cervix and corpus uteri. *Gynecologic Oncology*. **82**(1): 167–71. (RS-64)

14 Scarda A, Confalonieri M, Baghiris C, Binato S, Mazzarotto R, Palamidese A, Zuin R, Fantoni U. (2007) Out-patient high-dose-rate endobronchial brachytherapy for palliation of lung cancer: an observational study. *Monaldi Archives for Chest Disease*. **67**(3): 128–34. (OS-35)

15 Escobar-Sacristan JA, Granda-Orive JI, Gutierrez Jimenez T, Delgado JM, Rodero Banos A, Saez Valls R. (2004) Endobronchial brachytherapy in the treatment of malignant lung tumours. *European Respiratory Journal*. **24**(3): 348–52. (OS-81)

16 Tan HS. (1994) Use of high dose rate gammamed brachytherapy in the palliative treatment of gynaecological cancer. *Annals of the Academy of Medicine, Singapore*. **23**(2): 231–4. (OS-24)

17 Regnard CFB, Mannix K. (1990) Palliation of gastric carcinoma haemorrhage with sucralfate. *Palliative Medicine*. **4**: 329–30. (Let, CS-1)

18 Regnard C, Makin W. (1995) Bleeding. In: *Flow Diagrams in Advanced Cancer and Other Diseases*. London: Edward Arnold. pp. 44–7. (Ch)

19 Leiper K, Morris AI. (2007) Treatment of radiation proctitis. *Clinical Oncology (Royal College of Radiologists)*. **19**(9): 724–9. (R, 37 refs)

20 Chun M, Kang S, Kil HJ, Oh YT, Sohn JH, Ryu HS. (2004) Rectal bleeding and its management after irradiation for uterine cervical cancer. *International Journal of Radiation Oncology, Biology, Physics*. **58**(1): 98–105. (R)

21 Bullock N, Whitaker RH. (1985) Massive bladder haemorrhage. *British Medical Journal*. **291**: 1522–3. (E)

22 Takashi M, Kondo A, Kato K, Murase T, Miyake K. (1988) Evaluation of intravesical alum irrigation for massive bladder hemorrhage. *Urologia Internationalis*. **43**(5): 286–8. (CS-4)

23 Mukamel E, Lupu A, deKernion JB. (1986) Alum irrigation for severe bladder hemorrhage. *Journal of Urology*. **135**(4): 784–5. (CS-5)

24 McElligot E, Quigley C, Hanks GW. (1992) Tranaxamic acid and rectal bleeding. *Lancet*. **337**: 431. (L, CS-1)

25 Molloy DO, Archbold HA, Ogonda L, McConway J, Wilson RK, Beverland DE. (2007) Comparison of topical fibrin spray and tranexamic acid on blood loss after total knee replacement: a prospective, randomised controlled trial. *Journal of Bone and Joint Surgery – British Volume*. **89**(3): 306–9. (RCT-150)

26 Baric D, Biocina B, Unic D, Sutlic Z, Rudez I, Vrca VB, Brkic K, Ivkovic M. (2007) Topical use of antifibrinolytic agents reduces postoperative bleeding: a double-blind, prospective, randomized study. *European Journal of Cardio-Thoracic Surgery*. **31**(3): 366–71. (RCT-300)

27 Thomas DC, Wormald PJ. (2008) A randomized controlled pilot study of epsilon-aminocaproic acid as a topical hemostatic agent for postoperative bleeding in the sheep model of chronic sinusitis. *American Journal of Rhinology*. **22**: 188–91.

28 Dean A, Tuffin P. (1997) Fibrinolytic inhibitors for cancer-associated bleeding problems. *Journal of Pain and Symptom Management*. **13**(1): 20–4. (CT-16)

29 Schultz M, van der Lelie H. (1995) Microscopic haematuria as a relative contraindication for tranexamic acid. *British Journal of Haematology*. **89**(3): 663–4. (CS-3)

30 Manjunath G, Fozailoff A, Mitcheson D, Sarnak MJ. (2002) Epsilon-aminocaproic acid and renal complications: case report and review of the literature. *Clinical Nephrology*. **58**: 63–7. (R)

31 Lindoff C, Rybo G, Astedt B. (1993) Treatment with tranexamic acid during pregnancy, and the risk of thrombo-embolic complications. *Thrombosis and Haemostasis*. **70**(2): 238–40. (RS-2102)

32 Taparia M, Cordingley FT, Leahy MF. (2002) Pulmonary embolism associated with tranexamic acid in severe acquired haemophilia. *European Journal of Haematology*. **68**(5): 307–9. (CS-1)

33 Sanaka M, Yamamoto T, Kawakami T, Kuyama Y. (2005) Octreotide for palliative treatment of bleeding from unresectable gastric cancer. *Hepato-Gastroenterology*. **52**(64): 2 p preceding I. (CS-1)

34 Ventrucci M, Di Simone MP, Giulietti P, De Luca G. (2001) Efficacy and safety of Nd:YAG laser for the treatment of bleeding from radiation proctocolitis. *Digestive and Liver Disease*. **33**(3): 230–3. (OS-9)

35 Han CC, Prasetyo D, Wright GM. (2007) Endobronchial palliation using Nd:YAG laser is associated with improved survival when combined with multimodal adjuvant treatments. *Journal of Thoracic Oncology*. **2**(1): 59–64. (RS-153)

36 Steinke K. (2008) Radiofrequency ablation of pulmonary tumours: current status. *Cancer Imaging*. **8**: 27–35. (R, 78 refs)

37 Broadley KE, Kurowska A, Dick R, Platts A, Tookman A. (1995) The role of embolization in palliative care. *Palliative Medicine*. **9**(4): 331–5. (CS-3)

38 Corr P, Blyth D, Sanyika C, Royston D. (2001) Efficacy and cost-effectiveness of bronchial arterial embolisation in the treatment of major haemoptysis. *South African Medical Journal*. **91**(10): 861–4. (RS-87)

39 Nabi G, Sheikh N, Greene D, Marsh R. (2003) Therapeutic transcatheter arterial embolization in the management of intractable haemorrhage from pelvic urological malignancies: preliminary experience and long-term follow-up. *BJU International.* **92**(3): 245–7. (CS-6)

40 Appleton DS, Sibley GNA, Doyle PT. (1988) Internal iliac artery embolisation of bladder and prostate haemorrhage. *British Journal of Urology.* **61**: 45–7. (OS-8)

41 Blake MA, Owens A, O'Donoghue DP, MacErlean DP. (1995) Embolotherapy for massive upper gastrointestinal haemorrhage secondary to metastatic renal cell carcinoma: report of three cases. *Gut.* **37**(6): 835–7. (CS-3)

42 Chou WC, Lu CH, Lin G, Hong YS, Chen PT, Hsu HC, Chen JS, Yeh KY, Wang HM, Liaw CC. (2007) Transcutaneous arterial embolization to control massive tumor bleeding in head and neck cancer: 63 patients' experiences from a single medical center. *Supportive Care in Cancer.* **15**(10): 1185–90. (RS)

43 Rankin EM, Rubens RD, Redy JF. (1988) Transcatheter embolisation to control severe bleeding in fungating breast cancer. *European Journal of Surgical Oncology.* **14**: 27–32. (OS-9)

44 McQuillan RE, Grzybowska PH, Finlay IG, Hughes J. (1996) Use of embolisation in palliative care. *Palliative Medicine.* **10**: 169–72. (Let)

Bowel obstruction

CLINICAL DECISION AND ACTION CHECKLIST

1 Is there any doubt this is a bowel obstruction?
2 Is constipation the sole cause?
3 Is a physical blockage absent or unlikely?
4 Is thirst present?
5 Is surgery or stenting possible?
6 Is nausea and/or vomiting present?
7 Is pain present?
8 Is the obstruction complete and continuous?
9 Is the obstruction partial or intermittent?
10 Is adrenal insufficiency present?

KEY POINTS

- Inoperable, complete bowel obstruction can be managed at home.
- Nasogastric tubes and IV hydration are of limited use in many patients but have a role in some patients.

INTRODUCTION

Bowel obstruction can be a dramatic and frightening development but it is not always terminal – the median survival is 3 months.[1] However, if it is complete and untreatable, it indicates a short prognosis, often of only weeks. Medical management will keep the majority of patients comfortably free of nausea and pain,[2] and so enable them to remain at home.[3,4]

CAUSES OF OBSTRUCTION

Recurrent abdominal cancer causes multiple blockages,[5,6] especially with small bowel blockage.[7,8]

Metastatic obstruction from tumors arising from outside the abdomen is usually due to spread from primary melanoma, breast, or lung.[9]

Constipation can mimic obstruction and a supine abdominal X-ray will demonstrate severe constipation.[10]

Benign adhesions may occur in up to 20% of patients with recurrent abdominal cancer,[11] and can be caused by previous surgery[12] or radiotherapy.[13] Adhesions are the commonest cause of small bowel obstruction.[14–16]

Motility disorders can cause the same features as a physical blockage.

SURGERY

This should always be considered since it may be a simple procedure. It can improve outcome,[17,18] but it can also have a significant mortality and morbidity and some studies have shown no difference in survival.[19] An understanding surgical opinion is essential.[20]

STENTS AND TUBES

Stents: these are an option in patients with duodenal[21] or colorectal obstructions[22–24] who are unfit for surgery.

Nasogastric tubes: these are ineffective in controlling postoperative vomiting.[25–27] Symptom control in obstruction can be achieved without using NG tubes in most patients,[28] and antisecretory drugs should be tried first (e.g. hyoscine or hyoscyamine, octreotide).[29–31] However, nasogastric suction or drainage has a place in three situations:

a. *Feculant or fecal vomiting:* feculant vomiting is not the vomiting of feces, but of small bowel contents colonized by colonic bacteria in obstructions lasting a week or more. True fecal vomiting is much less common and is due to a gastrocolic fistula.
b. *Proximal small bowel obstruction:* if this cannot be bypassed surgically or stented, nasogastric suction can be useful in decompressing the stomach. Longer tubes can be placed endoscopically into the jejunum if necessary.[32]
c. *Gastric atony: see* p. 170.

Gastrostomy or jejunostomy: these are alternatives to nasogastric tubes for patients with persistent vomiting due to a proximal bowel obstruction.[20,33,34]

PHARMACOLOGICAL

Nausea: *see Nausea and vomiting*, p. 167. This is a distressing symptom for patients but will respond to dimenhydrinate, diphenhydramine or methotrimeprazine (Canada only), i.e. antiemetics that block the vagal afferent pathway. A secondary onset of nausea (possibly due to invasion of the small bowel by colonic bacteria, causing a release of bacterial toxins that stimulate the dopamine receptors in the chemoreceptor trigger zone) will

Clinical decision	If YES carry out the action below
1 Is there any doubt this is a bowel obstruction?	• **Consider** other causes of nausea and vomiting (*see Nausea and vomiting*, p. 167), abdominal distension (e.g. ascites), colic (e.g. contact stimulant laxatives), or altered bowel habit (e.g. constipation).
2 Is constipation the sole cause?	Bowel history, examination and plain abdominal X-ray will help in deciding. • Clear rectum and start laxative (*see Constipation*, p. 107).
3 Is a physical blockage absent or unlikely?	This may be peristaltic failure (absent or reduced bowel sounds): • **Exclude** peritonitis, septicemia or recent cord compression. • **Stop antiperistaltic drugs** (e.g. antimuscarinics). • **Stop osmotic and macrogol laxatives.** • **Consider adding** a stimulant laxative acting on small and large bowel, e.g. bisacodyl. Alternatively, try neostigmine SC 1–2.5 mg q6h (do not use if these are present: asthma, cardiac problems, hypotension, peptic ulcer, hyperthyroidism, renal problems).

Adapted from Regnard[35]
cd = clinical decision

Clinical decision	If YES carry out the action below
4 Is thirst present?	• **Rehydrate** orally, SC or IV (*see Nutrition and hydration problems*, p. 178).
5 Is surgery or stenting possible?	• **Surgery is possible if** the patient agrees and is in good or reasonable nutritional and medical condition. The prognosis is poor if there has been previous abdominal radiotherapy, there are abdominal masses, multiple blockages, rapidly recurring ascites, poor nutrition or a small bowel blockage. • **Referral for stenting** is an alternative.
6 Is nausea and/or vomiting present?	• **If gastric stasis is suspected:** start metoclopramide SC infusion 30–90 mg/24 hours or 10–20 mg SC q8h. In children, domperidone (in the US available from a compounding pharmacy) is safer (*see Drugs in children: starting doses*, p. 303). If metoclopramide or domperidone make the vomiting worse, reduce the dose. • **If a physical obstruction is likely:** start dimenhydrinate or diphenhydramine 25 mg SC q4h OR haloperidol 1–2 mg q8h SC or 5 mg/24 hours CSCI OR methotrimeprazine (Canada only) 5–12.5 mg SC or PO at bedtime. Start at half these doses for patients >70 years age; for children *see Drugs in children: starting doses*, p. 303. • **If nausea and/or vomiting persist:** replace dimenhydrinate or diphenhydramine with haloperidol 1–2 mg q8h SC or 5 mg/24 hours CSCI OR methotrimeprazine (Canada only) 2.5–5 mg PO or SC once at bedtime. *If vomiting persists:* add octreotide SC 100–600 microg/24 hours. Hyoscine butylbromide SC infusion 60–120 mg/24 hours (in the US hyoscyamine 0.25–0.5 mg SC/IV q4h PRN) is an alternative to octreotide but takes up to 3 days to reach maximum effect.
7 Is pain present?	• **Colic:** *see* cd-4b in *Diagnosing and treating pain*, p. 49. • **Abdominal distension:** acetaminophen 650 mg q4h. If this is insufficient follow the WHO analgesic staircase. • **Celiac plexus pain:** start gabapentin 100 mg q8h and titrate daily until pain controlled.[36] If the pain persists refer to a pain specialist for a celiac plexus block.
8 Is the obstruction complete and continuous?	• **Stop all laxatives.** Treat a dry mouth (*see* cd-4 in *Oral problems*, p. 187). • **If colic is present:** start hyoscine butylbromide SC infusion 60–120 mg/24 hr (in the US hyoscyamine 0.25–0.5 mg SC/IV q4h PRN) (takes up to 3 days to reach maximum effect). • **Allow oral hydration and feeding**, using occasional, small snacks. • **Consider high dose dexamethasone** (16 mg daily) if short-term relief of obstruction is appropriate.
9 Is the obstruction partial or intermittent?	• **Stop osmotic, stimulant, and macrogol laxatives.** • **Start docusate** 100 mg PO q8h and titrate for a comfortable stool without colic. • **Avoid high roughage foods** (e.g. peas, beans, whole fruit): continue oral feeding and hydration with small, frequent low-fiber snacks. • **For intermittent colic** use hyoscine hydrobromide 75–300 microg buccally (max. 900 micrograms in any 24-hour period) as this can be self-administered by the patient. (Canada only. In the US use hyoscyamine 0.125–0.25 mg PO/SL tid-qid PRN.)
10 Is adrenal insufficiency present?	Increasing fatigue, progressive hypotension, persistent nausea, and vomiting. • *See* cd-7a in *Emergencies*, p. 341.

Adapted from Regnard[35]
cd = clinical decision

often respond to haloperidol or methotrimeprazine (Canada only).

Colic: this can radiate to a variety of sites in the abdomen and elsewhere, but the pain usually has the typical periodic nature of colic, recurring regularly every few minutes (*see* cd-4b in *Diagnosing and treating pain*, p. 49). In complete, inoperable obstruction all laxatives should be stopped, and as the risk of producing an ileus with antispasmodics is not relevant these can be used to treat the colic. Partial obstruction is different, with a need to preserve bowel motility and yet prevent colic. The use of a laxative with minimal stimulant activity (docusate), dietary advice (avoiding high-fiber foods) and the cautious use of antispasmodics keeps symptoms to a minimum. In patients with irreversible obstruction, persistent colic can be treated by creating an ileus with continuous infusions of hyoscine butylbromide (Canada), hyoscyamine (US) or octreotide.

Octreotide inhibits many gastrointestinal functions and results in less bowel distension and motility. It is more effective than hyoscine hydrobromide (scopolamine) in controlling symptoms, but the two can be used in combination.[37,38]

Steroids: these have two roles.

a. *Relieving obstruction:* in patients with obstruction caused by tumor, high-dose dexamethasone (8–16 mg daily) can relieve obstruction temporarily in some patients by reducing peritumoral edema.[39,40]
b. *Adrenal insufficiency:* this is can occur in up to half of patients with extensive intra-abdominal cancer,[41] and empirical treatment with corticosteroids may offer a worthwhile improvement.

Dysmotility and ileus: absent motility (ileus) or abnormal bowel motility (dysmotility) can cause obstructive symptoms. Dysmotility is common in cancer and can be caused by retroperitoneal disease, antimuscarinic drugs or autonomic failure. Prokinetics such as metoclopramide and erythromycin have been suggested for a hypoactive bowel,[42] but there is no evidence to support their use.[43–45] In contrast, bisacodyl,[46] or neostigmine may have a role.[47]

PROXIMAL OBSTRUCTIONS

These are more likely to cause vomiting, but less likely to cause distension. In pancreatic carcinoma most are due to poor motility rather than a physical obstruction,[48] and can be treated as for gastric stasis (*see* cd-2a in *Nausea and vomiting*, p. 169). Complete, inoperable, high obstructions may need several approaches:

- a nasogastric tube or gastrostomy (*see* p. 100)
- ranitidine to reduce the volume of gastric secretions (this can be given by continuous subcutaneous infusion – *see* p. 322).

FEEDING AND HYDRATION

Hydration: most patients with distal obstructions will absorb sufficient fluid from their upper gut to prevent symptomatic dehydration. Parenteral feeding is often unnecessary, unless it is a preliminary to surgery.[49] Patients with repeated vomiting or high obstructions proximal to the mid-jejunum will need intravenous or subcutaneous hydration to offset the thirst resulting from the rapid dehydration. However, as patients deteriorate their fluid intake reduces, and parenteral hydration is not usually needed at the end of life (*see Nutrition and hydration problems*, p. 175).

Feeding: most patients with obstruction due to malignancy have advanced disease and are too ill to want or benefit from nutrition. However, some patients obstruct at an earlier stage and can benefit from parenteral nutrition.[50]

REFERENCES: BOWEL OBSTRUCTION

B = book; C = comment; Ch = chapter; CS-n = case study-no. of cases; CT-n = controlled trial-no. of cases; E = editorial; GC = group consensus; I-n = interviews –no. of cases; LS = laboratory study; MC = multi-center; OS-n = open study-no. of cases; R, n = review, no. of references; RCT-n = randomized controlled trial-no. of cases; RS-n = retrospective survey-no. of cases; SA-n = systematic or meta analysis –no. of studies.

1 Pameijer CR, Mahvi DM, Stewart JA, Weber SM. (2005) Bowel obstruction in patients with metastatic cancer: does intervention influence outcome? *International Journal of Gastrointestinal Cancer.* **35**(2): 127–33. (RS-114)

2 Frank C. (1997) Medical management of intestinal obstruction in terminal care. *Canadian Family Physician.* **43**: 259–65. (R, 29refs)

3 Platt V. (2001) Malignant bowel obstruction: so much more than symptom control. *International Journal of Palliative Nursing.* **7**(11): 547–54. (R, 47 refs)

4 Lynch B, Sarazine J. (2006) A guide to understanding malignant bowel obstruction. *International Journal of Palliative Nursing.* **12**(4): 164–6, 168–71. (R, 21 refs)

5 Miller G, Boman J, Shrier I, Gordon PH. (2000) Small-bowel obstruction secondary to malignant disease: an 11-year audit. *Canadian Journal of Surgery.* **43**(5): 353–8. (RS-32)

6 Ripamonti C, Mercandante S. (2004). Pathophysiology and management of malignant bowel obstruction. In: Doyle D, Hanks G, Cherney NI, Calman K. *Oxford Textbook of Palliative Medicine, 3rd ed.* Oxford: Oxford University Press. (Ch)

7 Tunca JC, Buchler DA, Mack EA, *et al.* (1981) The management of ovarian-cancer-caused bowel obstruction. *Gynaecological Oncology.* **12**: 186–92.

8 Landercasper J, Cogbill TH, Merry WH, Stolee RT, Strutt PJ. (1993) Long-term outcome after hospitalization for small-bowel obstruction. *Archives of Surgery.* **128**(7): 765–70. (RS-309)

9 Telerman A, Gerard B, Van den Heule B, Bleiberg H. (1985) Gastrointestinal metastases from extra-abdominal tumours. *Endoscopy.* **17**: 99–101. (RS)

10 Lagman RL, Walsh D. (2009) Are abdominal X-rays useful in palliative medicine? *European Journal of Palliative Care.* **16**(1): 6–10. (R, 37 refs)

11 Ketcham AS, Hoye RC, Pilch YH, Morton DL. (1970) Delayed intestinal obstruction following treatment for cancer. *Cancer.* **25**: 406–10.

12 Duron JJ, Silva NJ, du Montcel ST, Berger A, Muscari F, Hennet H, Veyrieres M, Hay JM. (2006) Adhesive postoperative small bowel obstruction: incidence and risk factors of recurrence after surgical treatment: a multicenter prospective study. *Annals of Surgery.* **244**(5): 750–7. (OS-286)

13 Baxter NN, Hartman LK, Tepper JE, Ricciardi R, Durham SB, Virnig BA. (2007) Postoperative irradiation for rectal cancer increases the risk of small bowel obstruction after surgery. *Annals of Surgery.* **245**(4): 553–9. (RS-5606)

14 Miller G, Boman J, Shrier I, Gordon PH. (2000) Etiology of small bowel obstruction. *American Journal of Surgery.* **180**(1): 33–6. (RS, 552)

15 Moran BJ. (2007) Adhesion-related small bowel obstruction. *Colorectal Disease.* **9**(Suppl. 2): 39–44. (R, 23 refs)

16 Attard JA, MacLean AR. (2007) Adhesive small bowel obstruction: epidemiology, biology and prevention. *Canadian Journal of Surgery.* **50**(4): 291–300. (R, 76 refs)

17 Mangili G, Aletti G, Frigerio L, Franchi M, Panacci N, Vigano R, DE Marzi P, Zanetto F, Ferrari A. (2005) Palliative care for intestinal obstruction in recurrent ovarian cancer: a multivariate analysis. *International Journal of Gynecological Cancer.* **15**(5): 830–5. (RS-47)

18 Guenaga KF, Lustosa SA, Saad SS, Saconato H, Matos D. (2007) Ileostomy or colostomy for temporary decompression of colorectal anastomosis. *Cochrane Database of Systematic Reviews.* **1**: CD004647. (SA-5, 39 refs)

19 Feuer DJ, Broadley KE, Shepherd JH, Barton DP. (2000) Surgery for the resolution of symptoms in malignant bowel obstruction in advanced gynaecological and gastrointestinal cancer. *Cochrane Database of Systematic Reviews.* **4**: CD002764. (SA, 89 refs)

20 Ripamonti C, Twycross R, Baines M, Bozzetti F, Capri S, De Conno F, Gemlo B, Hunt TM, Krebs HB, Mercadante S, Schaerer R, Wilkinson P. (2001) Working Group of the European Association for Palliative Care. Clinical-practice recommendations for the management of bowel obstruction in patients with end-stage cancer. *Supportive Care in Cancer.* **9**(4): 223–33. (GC)

21 Park HS, Do YS, Suh SW, Choo SW, Lim HK, Kim SH, Shim YM, Park KC, Choo IW. (1999) Upper gastrointestinal tract malignant obstruction: initial results of palliation with a flexible covered stent. *Radiology.* **210**(3): 865–70. (OS-21)

22 Khot UP, Lang AW, Murali K, Parker MC. (2002) Systematic review of the efficiency and safety of colorectal stents. *British Journal of Surgery.* **89**(9): 1096–102. (R, 48 refs).

23 Bittinger M, Messman H. (2007) Self-expanding metal stents as nonsurgical palliative therapy for malignant colonic obstruction: time to change the standard of care? *Gastrointestinal Endoscopy.* **66**: 928–9. (E)

24 Alcantara M, Serra X, Bombardo J, Falco J, Perandreu J, Ayguavives I, Mora L, Hernando R, Navarro S. (2007) Colorectal stenting as an effective therapy for preoperative and palliative treatment of large bowel obstruction: 9 years' experience. *Techniques in Coloproctology.* **11**(4): 316–22. (OS-95)

25 Koukouras D, Mastronikolis NS, Tzoracoleftherakis E, Angelopoulou E,

Kalfarentzos F, Androulakis J. (2001) The role of nasogastric tube after elective abdominal surgery. *Clinica Terapeutica*. **152**(4): 241–4. (RCT-100)

26 Pearl ML, Valea FA, Fischer M, Chalas E. (1996) A randomized controlled trial of postoperative nasogastric tube decompression in gynecologic oncology patients undergoing intra-abdominal surgery. *Obstetrics and Gynecology*. **88**(3): 399–402. (RCT-110)

27 Cunningham J, Temple WJ, Langevin JM, Kortbeek J. (1992) A prospective randomized trial of routine postoperative nasogastric decompression in patients with bowel anastomosis. *Canadian Journal of Surgery*. **35**(6): 629–32. (RCT-102)

28 Laval G, Arvieux C, Stefani L, Villard ML, Mestrallet JP, Cardin N. (2006) Protocol for the treatment of malignant inoperable bowel obstruction: a prospective study of 80 cases at Grenoble University Hospital Center. *Journal of Pain and Symptom Management*. **31**(6): 502–12. (CT-80)

29 Ripamonti C, Mercadante S, Groff L, Zecca E, De Conno F, Casuccio A. (2001) Role of octreotide, scopolamine butylbromide, and hydration in symptom control of patients with inoperable bowel obstruction and nasogastric tubes: a prospective randomized trial. *Journal of Pain and Symptom Management*. **19**(1): 23–34. (RCT-17)

30 Mangili G, Franchi M, Mariani A, Zanaboni F, Rabaiotti E, Frigerio L, Bolis PF, Ferrari A. (1996) Octreotide in the management of bowel obstruction in terminal ovarian cancer. *Gynecologic Oncology*. **61**(3): 345–8. (OS-21)

31 Mercadante S, Spoldi E, Caraceni A, Maddaloni S, Simonetti MT. (1993) Octreotide in relieving gastrointestinal symptoms due to bowel obstruction. *Palliative Medicine*. **7**(4): 295–9. (OS-14)

32 Gowen GF. (2007) Rapid resolution of small-bowel obstruction with the long tube, endoscopically advanced into the jejunum. *American Journal of Surgery*. **193**(2): 184–9. (OS-23)

33 Meyer L, Pothuri B. (2006) Decompressive percutaneous gastrostomy tube use in gynecologic malignancies. *Current Treatment Options in Oncology*. **7**(2): 111–20. (R, 30 refs)

34 Pothuri B, Montemarano M, Gerardi M, Shike M, Ben-Porat L, Sabbatini P, Barakat RR. (2005) Percutaneous endoscopic gastrostomy tube placement in patients with malignant bowel obstruction due to ovarian carcinoma. *Gynecologic Oncology*. **96**(2): 330–4. (OS-94)

35 Regnard C. (1995) Bowel obstruction. In: *Flow Diagrams in Advanced Cancer and Other Diseases*. London: Edward Arnold. pp. 29–31. (Ch)

36 Pelham A, Lee MA, Regnard CBF. (2002) Gabapentin for coeliac plexus pain. *Palliative Medicine* **16**: 355–6. (CS-3)

37 Mystakidou K, Tsilika E, Kalaidopoulou O, Chondros K, Georgaki S, Papadimitriou L. (2002) Comparison of octreotide administration vs conservative treatment in the management of inoperable bowel obstruction in patients with far advanced cancer: a randomized, double-blind, controlled clinical trial. *Anticancer Research*. **22**(2B): 1187–92. (RCT-68)

38 Mercadante S, Ripamonti C, Casuccio A, Zecca E, Groff L. (2000) Comparison of octreotide and hyoscine butylbromide in controlling gastrointestinal symptoms due to malignant inoperable bowel obstruction. *Supportive Care in Cancer*. **8**(3): 188–91. (RCT-18)

39 Feuer DJ, Broadley KE. (2000) Corticosteroids for the resolution of malignant bowel obstruction in advanced gynaecological and gastrointestinal cancer. *Cochrane Database of Systematic Reviews*. **2**: CD001219. (SA-3, 10 refs)

40 Mercadante S, Casuccio A, Mangione S. (2007) Medical treatment for inoperable malignant bowel obstruction: a qualitative systematic review. *Journal of Pain and Symptom Management*. **33**(2): 217–23. (SA-5)

41 Poon D, Cheung YB, Tay MH, Lim WT, Lim ST, Wong NS, Koo WH. (2005) Adrenal insufficiency in intestinal obstruction from carcinomatosis peritonei: a factor of potential importance in symptom palliation. *Journal of Pain and Symptom Management*. **29**(4): 411–18. (OS-29)

42 Mercadante S, Ferrera P, Villari P, Marrazzo A. (2004) Aggressive pharmacological treatment for reversing malignant bowel obstruction. *Journal of Pain and Symptom Management*. **28**(4): 412–16. (OS-15)

43 Cheape JD, Wexner SD, James K, Jagelman DG. (1991) Does metoclopramide reduce the length of ileus after colorectal surgery? A prospective randomized trial. *Diseases of the Colon and Rectum*. **34**(6): 437–41. (RCT-100)

44 Traut U, Brugger L, Kunz R, Pauli-Magnus C, Haug K, Bucher HC, Koller MT. (2008) Systemic prokinetic pharmacologic treatment for postoperative adynamic ileus following abdominal surgery in adults. *Cochrane Database of Systematic Reviews*. **1**: CD004930. (R, 130 refs)

45 Lightfoot AJ, Eno M, Kreder KJ, O'Donnell MA, Rao SS, Williams RD. (2007) Treatment of postoperative ileus after bowel surgery with low-dose intravenous erythromycin. *Urology*. **69**(4): 611–15. (RCT-22)

46 Wiriyakosol S, Kongdan Y, Euanorasetr C, Wacharachaisurapol N, Lertsithichai P. (2007) Randomized controlled trial of bisacodyl suppository versus placebo for postoperative ileus after elective colectomy for colon cancer. *Asian Journal of Surgery*. **30**(3): 167–72. (RCT-20)

47 Batke M, Cappell MS. (2008) Adynamic ileus and acute colonic pseudo-obstruction. *Medical Clinics of North America*. **92**(3): 649–70. (R, 113 refs)

48 Alimentary symptoms. In: Twycross RG, Wilcock A, Stark Toller C. (2009). *Symptom Management in Advanced Cancer*. Nottingham: palliativedrugs.com. pp. 61–144. (Ch)

49 Mercadante S. (1996) Nutrition in cancer patients. *Supportive Care in Cancer*. **4**(1): 10–20. (R)

50 Fan BG. (2007) Parenteral nutrition prolongs the survival of patients associated with malignant gastrointestinal obstruction. *Journal of Parenteral and Enteral Nutrition.* **31**(6): 508–10. (OS-115)

NOTES

Constipation

CLINICAL DECISION AND ACTION CHECKLIST

1 Is this bowel obstruction?
2 Have the feces been easy and comfortable to pass?
3 Ensure privacy
4 Is there a treatable cause?
5 Is the rectum or stoma full?
6 Is the colon full?
7 Is the constipation persisting?

KEY POINTS

- Constipation can mimic some features of advanced disease.
- Give appropriate laxatives regularly and titrate to maintain a comfortable stool. The aim is quality, not quantity!
- Diarrhea can be a symptom of constipation.

INTRODUCTION

Constipation is a common and distressing problem in cancer, AIDS, cardiac disease respiratory disease, and renal disease.[1,2] It is often due to analgesics, but can be caused by many other drugs, biochemical abnormalities such as hypercalcemia, metabolic problems such as diabetes, and is a higher risk at the extremes of age, in those with severe neurological diseases and people with severe intellectual disability.[3–17] Constipation tends to worsen as an illness progresses, but eases in the last days of life.[18,19] The key to its management is anticipation, and treatment often indicates a failure in prevention.

SYMPTOMS AND CAUSES

Definition: constipation is the passage of small, hard feces infrequently and with difficulty.[1] This is usually accompanied by additional symptoms.

Symptoms: reduced frequency of stool is common in advanced disease and patients often need reassurance that this is normal. However, patients with constipation often notice a sense of incomplete evacuation after defecation. Other symptoms are abdominal pain, flatulence, distension, nausea, vomiting, halitosis, overflow diarrhea, malaise, fecal incontinence, and anorexia. Constipation is a common cause of distress and may increase agitation in confused patients or precipitate seizures in children with neurological impairment.

Assessment: the patient's history is important and several assessment scales are available.[17,20] Clinical assessment of the abdomen and hydration status is essential. In children, fecal masses are easily felt. Some patients may need an abdominal X-ray.[21,22]

Causes: a hard stool is a dry stool. Factors that reduce water in the stool are dehydration (common in children and frail older people), reduced bowel transit (drugs, immobility, depression, hypercalcemia, hypothyroidism, and neurological gut dysmotility), reduced secretions into the gut (drugs, dehydration) and the inability of the stool to retain water (reduced fiber intake due to anorexia or feeding difficulties). Other causes include painful defecation (local tumor, anal fissure) or a fear of defecation.

Constipating drugs include those that reduce forward peristalsis and increase muscle tone (opioids); those that reduce secretions into the gut (opioids and drugs with antimuscarinic action, including tricyclic antidepressants, hyoscine hydrobromide or butylbromide, methotrimeprazine); and drugs that reduce all bowel contractions (antimuscarinic drugs and some anticonvulsants).

TREATMENT

Examination: rectal examination provides useful information but should always be done gently and correctly:

- Ask the patient to lie on their side with their knees drawn up towards their chest.
- Place a lubricated, gloved finger pad flat over the anus (i.e. finger is horizontal to the anus, not vertical).
- Gently pull back on the posterior anal margin (i.e. towards the coccyx).
- As the anus relaxes, gently move the finger to the vertical position allowing the finger to slowly enter the anus.
- Gradually insert the finger into the rectum.
- If it is necessary to rotate the examining finger, do this slowly.

Rectal examination technique in adults

However, in children rectal examination can be traumatic and should only be done when absolutely necessary, by experienced staff and using the little finger for younger children. Abdominal examination often provides more information in children than in adults.

Opioid-induced constipation does not usually respond to changes in diet/fluids, and laxatives are nearly always needed.[23] This is usually successful. In a few patients, switching to alternative opioids may help and both fentanyl and methadone have been claimed to have a lower incidence of causing constipation.[24–29] Opioid antagonists are an alternative (*see* p. 111).

Rectal measures: these can be useful if stool is present in the rectum or sigmoid colon. Phosphate enemas can sometimes

Clinical decision	If YES carry out the action below
1 Is this bowel obstruction?	• *See Bowel obstruction*, p. 99. Consider abdominal X-ray.
2 Have the feces been easy and comfortable to pass?	• **If constipation is a risk, and if feasible and possible:** — correct dehydration and ensure good hydration — change to drugs with less constipating action — encourage mobility and exercise — review food content and presentation to increase fiber content (*see* cd-6 in *Nutrition and hydration problems*, p. 179). — if the risk persists (e.g. starting opioids): start a laxative. • **If the stool frequency is less than usual:** this is common and normal in advanced disease because of reduced intake, but is often misinterpreted as constipation. Reassurance and explanation is needed. • **If this is diarrhea:** exclude overflow diarrhea caused by constipation (an X-ray may be needed). *See Diarrhea*, p. 115.
3 Ensure privacy: in a double or four-bed room help to get to a toilet is preferable to a bedside commode behind curtains that are transparent to sounds and smells.	
4 Is there a treatable cause?	• **Examples:** constipating drug (change to less constipating drug); hypercalcemia (*see* cd-7b in *Emergencies*, p. 341); spinal cord compression (*see* cd-9a in *Emergencies*, p. 345); depression (*see Withdrawal and depression*, p. 253).
5 Is the rectum or stoma full?	• **If the feces are hard:** — avoid phosphate enemas — encourage fluids and start a combination of a stimulant laxative (sennosides or bisacodyl) *plus* a softening laxative (docusate or lactulose) — a bisacodyl suppository will increase rectal tone within 45 min, and encourage rectal emptying, but it must be in contact with the rectal wall to be effective. A docusate enema (100 mg docusate liquid rectally) may also help in evacuating the rectum and colon — for colostomies, a suppository can be held in place with a gloved finger for 10 min, or an enema can be retained for 10 min by using an inflated Foley catheter. • **If the feces are soft:** stimulate the colon with sennosides or bisacodyl PO (6–12 hour delay). • **If there is no success in emptying the rectum or stoma:** carry out a manual evacuation using topical anesthetic gel and sedative cover (e.g. IV or buccal midazolam).
6 Is the colon full?	• **If colic is present:** start docusate 100–300 mg PO q8h. Consider a high mineral oil enema. • **If colic is absent:** start a combination of a regular stimulant plus softening laxative.

Adapted from Regnard[30]
cd = clinical decision

cause water and electrolyte disturbances, more so in the very young or the over 65 age group and when co-morbidities are present. They should therefore be used with caution.[31] Most suppositories stimulate rectal emptying simply through the physical stimulation of insertion, but bisacodyl can produce direct stimulation of rectal contraction.[32,33]

Laxatives: some laxatives should not be used in the context of advanced disease:

Bulking agents (e.g. bran, psyllium): can precipitate obstruction if dehydrated
Mineral oil: risk of lipid pneumonia

Laxatives to be avoided

Most common laxatives are well tolerated.[23,34] Lactulose is a safe laxative,[35] but when used as the sole laxative higher doses have to be used which can cause symptomatic dehydration and abdominal bloating.[23,36] Evidence is scarce on which laxatives to use in palliative care.[37,38] In opioid-induced constipation lactulose is as effective as sennosides,[39] or a macrogol.[40]

However, there are problems with using single laxatives. Sennosides cause more adverse effects than lactulose;[41] lactulose can be too sweet for some patients; and the evidence of the efficacy of oral docusate alone is lacking.[42] Using a macrogol alone requires large volumes of 250–500 mL daily or more. These volumes are poorly tolerated,[43] especially in patients with advanced disease.

Consequently, it is common practice to use a combination of laxatives, usually a contact stimulant (e.g. sennosides) plus either a softener (e.g. docusate) or an osmotic agent (e.g. lactulose).[44,45] Commercially available combinations are convenient but less flexible and more expensive than two single laxatives given separately. Bisacodyl is a useful stimulant laxative in that it is hydrolyzed to BHPM (bis(4-hydroxyphenyl)phenylmethane), a stimulant that acts on both the small and large bowels.[46] Sodium picosulfate is no better than bisacodyl.[47]

Dose titration: proportionately less laxative is required at higher opioid doses.[1,44] Each patient requires individual titration since the dose range is wide with some patients needing 10 tablets (86 mg) of sennosides daily in addition to a softener such as lactulose or docusate.

All laxatives and rectal measures have a delay before they act and their effect can be assessed:[1]

Rectal measures:	
docusate enema	5–20 min
bisacodyl suppository	15–60 min
glycerine suppository	15–60 min
arachis oil enema	1 hour
Injectable opioid reversal agent:	
methylnaltrexone SC	20 min–4 hours
Contact stimulants (oral):	
sennosides	8–12 hours
bisacodyl	6–12 hours
Softening laxatives (oral)	
lactulose	1–2 days
docusate	1–3 days
macrogols	1–3 days

Time to wait for constipation treatments

Diet and exercise: One study showed that to achieve a 50% increase in bowel frequency, a patient would have to take over four times as much fiber.[48] The correlation between activity and exercise is weak.[49] In the context of cachexia, reduced intake, and fatigue these are not a realistic prospect for most patients.

Patients with colostomies: gently inserting a finger will show if feces are present. If feces are present, treat as for feces in rectum (*see* cd-5 on the previous page). If feces are absent, exclude obstruction and follow the clinical decisions 6 and 7 in the tables.

Clinical decision	If YES carry out the action below
7 Is the constipation persisting?	• **If defecation is painful:** exclude anal fissure, painful hemorrhoids or local tumor. • **If opioid-induced:** — consider switching to fentanyl or methadone — consider naloxone at 10% of daily morphine dose, with maximum single dose of 5 mg PO q8h, or methylnaltrexone 8–12 mg (0.15 mg/kg) SC once every 2–3 days (latter can precipitate severe colic). • **If neurological gut dysmotility is present** (paraplegia, autonomic insufficiency, children with neurological impairment): consider a once or twice daily dose of bisacodyl 5 mg. • **If impaction is present despite rectal measures:** — start a macrogol, e.g. polyethylene glycol (Golytely) 250 mL — q6h for 1–3 days if the patient can tolerate the high fluid volume — if this is ineffective carry out a manual evacuation under mild midazolam sedation.

Adapted from Regnard[30]
cd = clinical decision

Patients with neurological impairment: there are few adequate trials in patients with paraplegia or cerebral palsy,[9] but rectal stimulation with a bisacodyl suppository will encourage evacuation.[50,51] Evacuation is easier if the feces are made firmer by using a contact laxative alone (e.g. sennosides). A firmer stool also reduces the risk of accidents due to diarrhea or unexpected defecation.

Impaction: this can develop if constipation is left untreated and defecation is difficult because of frailty, disability, or reduced rectal sensation. It is therefore common in elderly adults or disabled children. It can cause discomfort, pain, fecal incontinence, urinary retention, and bowel obstruction. Rectal measures may help, but manual evacuation may be needed which should be done under mild sedation for comfort. An alternative is the use of macrogols, which has been shown in children to be a more effective and cheaper alternative to manual evacuations and with fewer adverse effects.[52] There is only modest evidence that this might be useful in adults.[53] In addition, high doses have to be used which can be poorly tolerated in ill patients.

Systemic drugs

Opioid antagonists: these may have a role in opioid-induced constipation, but evidence for their efficacy is poor.[54] Oral naloxone has been used to reverse opioid-induced constipation,[55,56] but the incidence of analgesic reversal is uncertain.[57,58] Naloxone is widely available but needs to be given in doses of 2–5 mg if given orally.[59,60] Methylnaltrexone is a new preparation but has only been tested in a small number of patients,[61–66] has to be given subcutaneously, is expensive, and long-term effects are unknown. It should be used only in opioid-induced constipation that is resistant to conventional laxative combinations, or in patients unable to take enteral laxatives.[1,62] For example, it may have a role in patients taking opioids with no oral or enteral route for laxatives. It can cause severe colic in some patients.

Prokinetics such as metoclopramide and erythromycin have been suggested as a means of treating constipation,[67] but further work has failed to show any useful effect on gut motility.[68–70]

REFERENCES: CONSTIPATION

B = book; C = comment; Ch = chapter; CS-n = case study-no. of cases; CT-n = controlled trial-no. of cases; E = editorial; GC = group consensus; I-n = interviews-no. of cases; LS = laboratory study; MC = multi-center; OS-n = open study-no. of cases; R, refs = review, no. of references; RCT-n = randomized controlled trial-no. of cases; RS-n = retrospective survey-no. of cases; SA-n = systematic or meta analysis-no. of studies.

1 Larkin PJ, Sykes NP, Centeno C, Ellershaw JE, *et al.* on behalf of the European Consensus Group on Constipation in Palliative Care (2008). The management of constipation in palliative care. *Palliative Medicine*. **22**: 796–807. (SA, GC, 43 refs)

2 Solano JP, Gomes B, Higginson IJ. (2006) A comparison of symptom prevalence in far advanced cancer, AIDS, heart disease, chronic obstructive pulmonary disease and renal disease. *Journal of Pain and Symptom Management.* **31**(1): 58–69. (SA-64)

3 Meuser T, Pietruck C, Radbruch L, Stute P, Lehmann KA, Grond S. (2001) Symptoms during cancer pain treatment following WHO-guidelines: a longitudinal follow-up study of symptom prevalence, severity and etiology. *Pain.* **93**(3): 247–57. (OS-593)

4 Edmonds P, Karlsen S, Khan S, Addington-Hall J. (2001) A comparison of the palliative care needs of patients dying from chronic respiratory diseases and lung cancer. *Palliative Medicine.* **15**(4): 287–95. (I-636)

5 Walsh D, Donnelly S, Rybicki L. (2000) The symptoms of advanced cancer: relationship to age, gender, and performance status in 1,000 patients. *Supportive Care in Cancer.* **8**(3): 175–9. (OS-1000)

6 Fallon MT, Hanks GW. (1999) Morphine, constipation and performance status in advanced cancer patients. *Palliative Medicine.* **13**(2): 159–60. (OS)

7 Sykes NP. (1998) The relationship between opioid use and laxative use in terminally ill cancer patients. *Palliative Medicine.* **12**(5): 375–82. (OS-498)

8 Mitchell SL, Kiely DK, Hamel MB. (2004) Dying with advanced dementia in the nursing home. *Archives of Internal Medicine.* **164**: 321–6. (RS-2492)

9 Wiesel PH, Norton C, Brazzelli M. (2001 and 2006) Management of faecal incontinence and constipation in adults with central neurological diseases. *Cochrane Database of Systematic Reviews*. 2001 **4**: CD002115. Update in *Cochrane Database of Systematic Reviews*. 2006; **2**: CD002115. (R, 53 refs)

10 Krogh K, Christensen P, Laurberg S. (2001) Colorectal symptoms in patients with neurological diseases. *Acta Neurologica Scandinavica.* **103**(6): 335–43. (R, 80 refs)

11 Wiesel PH, Norton C, Glickman S, Kamm MA. (2001) Pathophysiology and management of bowel dysfunction in multiple sclerosis. *European Journal of Gastroenterology and Hepatology.* **13**(4): 441–8. (R, 86 refs)

12 Bennett M, Cresswell H. (2003) Factors influencing constipation in advanced cancer patients: a prospective study of opioid dose, dantron dose and physical functioning. *Palliative Medicine.* **17**(5): 418–22. (OS-50)

13 Bohmer CJ, Taminiau JA, Klinkenberg-Knol EC, Meuwissen SG. (2001) The prevalence of constipation in institutionalized people with intellectual disability. *Journal of Intellectual Disability Research.* **45**(3): 212–8. (OS-215)

14 Krogh K, Christensen P, Laurberg S. (2001) Colorectal symptoms in patients with neurological diseases. *Acta Neurologica Scandinavica.* **103**(6): 335–43. (R, 80 refs)

15 Sellin JH, Chang EB. (2008) Therapy insight: gastrointestinal complications of diabetes – pathophysiology and management. *Nature Clinical Practice. Gastroenterology and Hepatology.* **5**(3): 162–71. (R, 74 refs)

16 Tobias N, Mason D, Lutkenhoff M, Stoops M, Ferguson D. (2008) Management principles of organic causes of childhood constipation. *Journal of Pediatric Health Care.* **22**(1): 12–23. (R, 32 refs)

17 Goodman M, Low J, Wilkinson S. (2005) Constipation management in palliative care: a survey of practices in the United Kingdom. *Journal of Pain and Symptom Management.* **29**: 238–44. (OS-475)

18 Mercadante S, Fulfaro F, Casuccio A. (2000) The impact of home palliative care on symptoms in advanced cancer patients. *Supportive Care in Cancer.* **8**(4): 307–10. (OS-211)

19 Mercadante S, Casuccio A, Fulfaro F. (2000) The course of symptom frequency and intensity in advanced cancer patients followed at home. *Journal of Pain and Symptom Management.* **20**(2): 104–12. (CT-370)

20 Longstreth GF, Thompson WG, Chey WD, Houghton LA, Mearin F, Spiller RC. (2006) Functional bowel disorders. *Gastroenterology.* **130**(5): 1480–91. (R, 95 refs)

21 Bruera E, Suarez-Almanzor M, Velasco A, Bertolino M, MacDonald SM, Hanson J. (1994) The assessment of constipation in terminal cancer patients admitted to a palliative care unit: a retrospective review. *Journal of Pain and Symptom Management.* **9**(8): 515–9. (RS-122)

22 Lagman RL, Walsh D. (2009) Are abdominal X-rays useful in palliative medicine? *European Journal of Palliative Care.* **16**(1): 6–10. (R, 37 refs)

23 Thorpe DM. (2001) Management of opioid-induced constipation. *Current Pain and Headache Reports.* **5**(3): 237–40. (R, 7 refs)

24 Mercadante S, Casuccio A, Fulfaro F, Groff L, Boffi R, Villari P, Gebbia V, Ripamonti C. (2001) Switching from morphine to methadone to improve analgesia and tolerability in cancer patients: a prospective study. *Journal of Clinical Oncology.* **19**(11): 2898–904. (CT-52)

25 Gourlay GK. (2001) Treatment of cancer pain with transdermal fentanyl. *Lancet Oncology.* **2**(3): 165–72. (R, 51 refs)

26 Nugent M, Davis C, Brooks D, Ahmedzai SH. (2001) Long-term observations of patients receiving transdermal fentanyl after a randomized trial. *Journal of Pain and Symptom Management.* **21**(5): 385–91. (RCT-73)

27 Radbruch L, Sabatowski R, Loick G, Kulbe C, Kasper M, Grond S, Lehmann KA. (2000) Constipation and the use of laxatives: a comparison between transdermal fentanyl and oral morphine. *Palliative Medicine*. **14**(2): 111–19. (MC, CT-46)

28 Ahmedzai S, Brooks D. (1997) Transdermal fentanyl versus sustained-release oral morphine in cancer pain: preference, efficacy, and quality of life. The TTS-Fentanyl Comparative Trial Group. *Journal of Pain and Symptom Management*. **13**(5): 254–61. (MC, RCT)

29 Daeninck PJ, Bruera E. (1999) Reduction in constipation and laxative requirements following opioid rotation to methadone: a report of four cases. *Journal of Pain and Symptom Management*. **18**(4): 303–9. (CS-4)

30 Regnard C. (1995) Constipation. In: *Flow Diagrams in Advanced Cancer and Other Diseases*. London: Edward Arnold. pp. 11–13. (Ch)

31 Mendoza J, Legido J, Rubio S, Gisbert JP. (2007) Systematic review: the adverse effects of sodium phosphate enema. *Alimentary Pharmacology and Therapeutics*. **26**(1): 9–20. (R, 75 refs)

32 Gosselink MJ, Hop WC, Schouten WR. (2000) Rectal tone in response to bisacodyl in women with obstructed defecation. *International Journal of Colorectal Disease*. **15**(5–6): 297–302. (CT-60)

33 Flig E, Hermann TW, Zabel M. (2000) Is bisacodyl absorbed at all from suppositories in man? *International Journal of Pharmaceutics*. **196**(1): 11–20. (OS-15)

34 Xing JH, Soffer EE. (2001) Adverse effects of laxatives. *Diseases of the Colon and Rectum*. **44**(8): 1201–9. (R, 107 refs)

35 Hallmann F. (2000) Toxicity of commonly used laxatives. *Medical Science Monitor*. **6**(3): 618–28. (R, 110 refs)

36 Kyle G. (2006) Assessment and treatment of older patients with constipation. *Nursing Standard*. **21**(8): 41–6.

37 Miles CL, Fellowes D, Goodman ML, Wilkinson S. (2006) Laxatives for the management of constipation in palliative care patients. *Cochrane Database of Systematic Reviews*. **4**: CD003448. (R, 60 refs)

38 Coggrave M, Wiesel PH, Norton C. (2006) Management of faecal incontinence and constipation in adults with central neurological diseases. *Cochrane Database of Systematic Reviews*. **(2)**: CD002115. (R, 87refs)

39 Agra Y, Sacristan A, Gonzalez M, Ferrari M, Portugues A, Calvo MJ. (1998) Efficacy of senna versus lactulose in terminal cancer patients treated with opioids. *Journal of Pain and Symptom Management*. **15**(1): 1–7. (RCT-91)

40 Freedman MD, Schwartz HJ, Roby R, Fleisher S. (1997) Tolerance and efficacy of polyethylene glycol 3350/electrolyte solution versus lactulose in relieving opiate induced constipation: a double-blinded placebo-controlled trial. *Journal of Clinical Pharmacology*. **37**(10): 904–7. (RCT-57)

41 Sykes NP. (1996) A volunteer model for the comparison of laxatives in opioid-related constipation. *Journal of Pain and Symptom Management*. **11**(6): 363–9. (CT-10)

42 Hurdon V, Viola R, Schroder C. (2000) How useful is docusate in patients at risk for constipation? A systematic review of the evidence in the chronically ill. *Journal of Pain and Symptom Management*. **19**(2): 130–6. (SA)

43 Lichtenstein GR, Grandhi N, Schmalz M, Lottes SR, Forbes WP, Walker K, Zhang B. (2007) Clinical trial: sodium phosphate tablets are preferred and better tolerated by patients compared to polyethylene glycol solution plus bisacodyl tablets for bowel preparation. *Alimentary Pharmacology and Therapeutics*. **26**(10): 1361–70. (RCT-411)

44 Maddi VI. (1979) Regulation of bowel function by a laxative/stool softener preparation in aged nursing home patients. *Journal of the American Geriatrics Society*. **27**(10): 464–8. (OS-42)

45 Sykes NP. (1991) A clinical comparison of laxatives in a hospice. *Palliative Medicine*. **5**: 307–14. (OS)

46 Roth W, Beschke K. (1988) Pharmacokinetics and laxative effect of bisacodyl following administration of various dosage forms. [German] *Arzneimittel-forschung*. **38**(4): 570–4. (RCT-12)

47 Kienzle-Horn S, Vix JM, Schuijt C, Peil H, Jordan CC, Kamm MA. (2007) Comparison of bisacodyl and sodium picosulphate in the treatment of chronic constipation. *Current Medical Research and Opinion*. **23**(4): 691–9. (RCT-144)

48 Mumford SP. (1986) Can high fibre diets improve the bowel function in patients on radiotherapy ward? In: Twycross RG, Lack SA, eds. *Control of Alimentary Symptoms in Far Advanced Cancer*. Edinburgh: Churchill Livingstone. p. 183.

49 Tuteja AK, Talley NJ, Joos SK, Woehl JV, Hickam DH. (2005) Is constipation associated with decreased physical activity in normally active subjects? *American Journal of Gastroenterology*. **100**(1): 124–9. (Q-1069)

50 Stiens SA, Luttrel W, Binard JE. (1998) Polyethylene glycol versus vegetable oil based bisacodyl suppositories to initiate side-lying bowel care: a clinical trial in persons with spinal cord injury. *Spinal Cord*. **36**(11): 777–81. (CT-14)

51 House JG, Stiens SA. (1997) Pharmacologically initiated defecation for persons with spinal cord injury: effectiveness of three agents. *Archives of Physical Medicine and Rehabilitation*. **78**(10): 1062–5. (RCT)

52 Guest JF, Candy DC, Clegg JP, Edwards D, *et al.* (2007) Clinical and economic impact of using macrogol 3350 plus electrolytes in an outpatient setting compared to enemas and suppositories and manual evacuation to treat paediatric faecal impaction based on actual clinical practice in England and Wales. *Current Medical Research and Opinion*. **23**(9): 2213–25. (RS-112)

53 Culbert P, Gillett H, Ferguson A. (1998) Highly effective new oral therapy for faecal impaction. *British Journal of General Practice*. **48**(434): 1599–600. (OS-13)

54 McNicol ED, Boyce D, Schumann R, Carr DB. (2008) Mu-opioid antagonists for opioid-induced

bowel dysfunction. *Cochrane Database of Systematic Reviews*. **2**: CD006332. (SA-33, 74 refs)

55 Meissner W, Schmidt U, Hartmann M, Kath R, Reinhart K. (2000) Oral naloxone reverses opioid-associated constipation. *Pain*. **84**(1): 105–9. (OS-22)

56 Sykes NP. (1996) An investigation of the ability of oral naloxone to correct opioid-related constipation in patients with advanced cancer. *Palliative Medicine*. **10**(2): 135–44. (RCT-17)

57 Meissner W, Ullrich K. (2002) Naloxone, constipation and analgesia. *Journal of Pain and Symptom Management*. **24**(3): 276–7. (Let)

58 Liu M. (2002) Naloxone, constipation and analgesia: author's response. *Journal of Pain and Symptom Management*. **24**(3): 277–9. (Let)

59 Liu M, Wittbrodt E. (2002) Low-dose oral naloxone reverses opioid-induced constipation and analgesia. *Journal of Pain and Symptom Management*. **23**(1): 48–53. (OS)

60 Sykes NP. (1996) An investigation of the ability of oral naloxone to correct opioid-related constipation in patients with advanced cancer. *Palliative Medicine*. **10**(2): 135–44. (OS-17)

61 Thomas J, Karver S, Cooney GA, Chamberlain BH, *et al*. (2008) Methylnaltrexone for opioid-induced constipation in advanced illness. *New England Journal of Medicine*. **358**(22): 2332–43. (RCT-133)

62 Portenoy RK, Thomas J, Moehl Boatwright ML, Tran D, *et al*. (2008) Subcutaneous methylnaltrexone for the treatment of opioid-induced constipation in patients with advanced illness: a double-blind, randomized, parallel group, dose-ranging study. *Journal of Pain and Symptom Management*. **35**(5): 458–68. (RCT-33)

63 Stephenson J. (2002) Methylnaltrexone reverses opioid-induced constipation. *Lancet Oncology*. **3**(4): 202. (CT)

64 Becker G, Galandi D, Blum HE. (2007) Peripherally acting opioid antagonists in the treatment of opiate-related constipation: a systematic review. *Journal of Pain and Symptom Management*. **34**(5): 547–65. (SA-20)

65 Shaiova L, Rim F, Friedman D, Jahdi M. (2007) A review of methylnaltrexone, a peripheral opioid receptor antagonist, and its role in opioid-induced constipation. *Palliative and Supportive Care*. **5**(2): 161–6. (R, 30 refs)

66 Yuan CS. (2007) Methylnaltrexone mechanisms of action and effects on opioid bowel dysfunction and other opioid adverse effects. *Annals of Pharmacotherapy*. **41**(6): 984–93. (R, 88 refs)

67 Sharma SS, Bhargava N, Mathur SC. (1995) Effect of oral erythromycin on colonic transit in patients with idiopathic constipation: a pilot study. *Digestive Diseases and Sciences*. **40**(11): 2446–9. (OS-11)

68 Cheape JD, Wexner SD, James K, Jagelman DG. (1991) Does metoclopramide reduce the length of ileus after colorectal surgery? A prospective randomized trial. *Diseases of the Colon and Rectum*. **34**(6): 437–41. (RCT-100)

69 Traut U, Brugger L, Kunz R, Pauli-Magnus C, Haug K, Bucher HC, Koller MT. (2008) Systemic prokinetic pharmacologic treatment for postoperative adynamic ileus following abdominal surgery in adults. *Cochrane Database of Systematic Reviews*. 1: CD004930. (R, 130 refs)

70 Lightfoot AJ, Eno M, Kreder KJ, O'Donnell MA, Rao SS, Williams RD. (2007) Treatment of postoperative ileus after bowel surgery with low-dose intravenous erythromycin. *Urology*. **69**(4): 611–5. (RCT-22)

Diarrhea

CLINICAL DECISION AND ACTION CHECKLIST

1. Is the patient dehydrated?
2. Is constipation present?
3. Are drugs or diet the cause?
4. Is previous bowel surgery the cause?
5. Is this a secretory diarrhea?
6. Is the stool mixed with blood or discharge?
7. Are the stools very dark or very pale?
8. Is a fistula the cause?
9. Is there clear fluid in the stool?
10. Is the diarrhea persisting?

KEY POINTS

- Rehydration is an essential part of management.
- Infection should be excluded.
- Constipation with overflow can be a cause.

INTRODUCTION

Diarrhea occurs in up to 10% of cancer patients,[1] but up to 38% of people with AIDS.[2] It is exhausting and distressing. Any fecal incontinence can create a loss of dignity for the patient and high stress on the carer. At home, washing clothes and sheets becomes a major problem. In any setting odor adds to everyone's distress. It is not surprising, therefore, that persisting diarrhea can have severe effects on image, mood, and relationships that will need support and help.

There are numerous causes and a systematic approach to diagnosis and treatment is essential.[3] Managing the patient at home is possible,[4] but severe or persistent diarrhea often requires inpatient care. Risk factors for fecal incontinence include advancing age, immobility, neurological disease, spinal injury, previous obstetric trauma, pelvic prolapse, previous colonic or rectal surgery, hospitalized patients, diabetes, fecal impaction, stroke, and severe cognitive impairment.[5,6]

ASSESSMENT

Dehydration must be excluded:

Mild dehydration

Thirst, reduced urine output, reduced skin turgor.

Severe dehydration (clinical shock)

Decreased or altered level of consciousness, delirium, pale or mottled skin, cold peripheries, weak pulse, tachycardia, hypotension.

Warning signs in children suggesting a risk of shock:[7] altered responsiveness, lethargy, sunken eyes, tachycardia, tachypnea.

Signs and symptoms of dehydration

Abdominal and rectal examination may indicate constipation or obstruction. Blood biochemistry will indicate the severity of dehydration and renal impairment, but clinical signs can be helpful (*see* table). A plain abdominal X-ray will help differentiate hard stool from tumor masses. Stool culture is necessary if infection is suspected and should include testing for *C. difficile* toxin if the patient has been on antibiotics. Some patients will need a colonoscopy to find the cause.

TREATMENT

Rehydration: for adults, rehydration powders offer no advantages for those able to maintain oral intake.[8] For children, reduced-osmolarity oral solutions (ORS) are safer and more effective than the traditional WHO formula.[9,10] Oral rehydration is as effective as parenteral hydration.[11,12] The latter is necessary if the fluid loss is severe and should be 0.9% sodium chloride with 5% glucose to encourage intracellular rehydration.

Drugs: a wide range of drugs can cause diarrhea[13] (*see* cd-3 opposite) and the drugs usually need to be stopped. Infective colitis is more common in older patients on antibiotics such as broad-spectrum cephalosporins, and those using proton pump inhibitors.[14]

Diet: if there is no excess of roughage in the diet (e.g. large amounts of fruit), malabsorption and dietary intolerance (e.g. lactose or gluten sensitivity) should be considered since the diet will have to be modified. For patients who are being fed enterally, using a fiber-supplemented feed can reduce diarrhea.[15]

Previous surgery can cause diarrhea through a number of mechanisms. Gastrectomy patients can suffer from food being "dumped" into the bowel causing nausea, bloating, and diarrhea – this can respond to octreotide.[16] If the terminal ileum has been resected, bile salts escape into the colon and cause local irritation.[17]

Steatorrhea is due to excessive fat in the stool. In pancreatic insufficiency enteric coated replacement enzymes must be used to ensure the enzyme is delivered unaltered to the small intestine.[18] Reducing gastric acid with a proton pump inhibitor (PPI) such as lansoprazole or omeprazole produces a less acid environment in the bowel, which improves fat absorption. This resolves steatorrhea in up to 40% of patients with pancreatic insufficiency.[19,20] This is particularly important where alkaline pancreatic secretions are reduced (e.g. pancreatitis, cystic fibrosis), and following small bowel resection (where gastric acid output increases due to raised gastrin).

Blood loss into the upper gastrointestinal tract irritates the bowel producing a loose, dark or black stool. *See* cd-4 in *Bleeding*, p. 95.

Loperamide increases water absorption by slowing forward peristalsis, resulting in increased absorption of fluid and

Clinical decision	If YES carry out the action below
1 Is the patient dehydrated?	• **Rehydration treatment:** reduced osmolality solution PO or NG; or 0.9% saline plus 5% glucose solution IV. Severely dehydrated adults may need as much as 6–8 L/24 hours as long as the loss continues.
2 Is constipation present?	• **Consider overflow diarrhea:** abdominal and rectal examination may uncover the presence of hard stool. On occasions a plain abdominal X-ray is needed to differentiate hard stool from tumor masses.
3 Are drugs or diet the cause?	• **Consider these drugs as a cause:** β-blockers, H_2 blockers (e.g. ranitidine), chemotherapy, diuretics, oral iron, laxatives, magnesium-containing antacids, NSAIDs, octreotide, ondansetron, PPIs. • **Antibiotic-induced colitis:** should be excluded by identifying *C. difficile* toxin in the stool. • **Consider these dietary causes:** malabsorption of carbohydrates, lactose intolerance, disaccharide deficiency, gluten sensitivity, zinc deficiency. • **Related to nasogastric feeding:** dilute feeds or increase length of feeding time. Using a fiber-supplemented feed can reduce diarrhea. If the symptoms persist discuss a change of feed type with the dietician.
4 Is previous bowel surgery the cause?	• **Post gastrectomy** (dumping syndrome): small, frequent snacks. Consider octreotide. • **Intestinal resection** (bile salts irritate colon): cholestyramine 12–16 g daily + ranitidine. • **Blind loop** (causing bacterial overgrowth): tetracycline (or metronidazole) for 2–4 weeks.
5 Is this a secretory diarrhea?	• **Consider infection:** Send stool for *C. difficile* toxin test and culture. Once antibiotics have started loperamide can be given. • **Diabetic autonomic failure:** clonidine (50–150 microg/24 hours) may help in diabetes. • **For Zollinger-Ellison syndrome:** high-dose lansoprazole or omeprazole. • **Tumor secreting vasoactive intestinal peptide (VIPoma):** octreotide 150–1500 microg/24 hours. • **Carcinoid:** start lansoprazole or omeprazole. Consider octreotide SC q8h or CSCI 150–1500 microg/24 hours.
6 Is the stool mixed with blood or discharge?	• **Fungating rectal or colonic tumor:** topical corticosteroids (hydrocortisone or betamethasone enema) plus metronidazole 500 mg q12h. Use topical sucralfate or tranexamic acid to control bleeding close to anal margin. Consider radiotherapy. • **Infection** (e.g. clostridium, shigella, salmonella): identify and treat. • **Inflammatory bowel disease:** assess cause (e.g. Crohn's disease) and treat.

Adapted from Regnard and Mannix[21]
cd = clinical decision

nutrients. It can be used in infective diarrhea as long as treatment of the infection has started. In children over 3 years it can be a useful adjunct to oral rehydration but should be avoided in children with severe dehydration or bloody diarrhea.[22] It is also important to exclude overflow diarrhea due to constipation before starting loperamide.

Cancer treatment diarrhea. Radiotherapy-induced diarrhea can respond to *L. acidophilus* cultures taken orally,[23] or $5HT_3$ antagonists.[24,25] Opioids such as codeine are more effective than bulking agents.[26] If pelvic radiotherapy causes a proctitis, adjust laxatives to keep the stool soft.

Octreotide has been used successfully in AIDS-related diarrhea,[27] cancer,[28] in postgastrectomy dumping,[29] carcinoid,[30,31] and may also have a role to play in other causes of severe refractory diarrhea,[32,33] although more evidence of efficacy is needed.[34] Octreotide does not reduce diarrhea due to radiotherapy or chemotherapy.[35,36] Side-effects of octreotide include diarrhea and steatorrhea.

Infection has become an increasingly common cause with the rising frequency of *Clostridium difficile* infection.[37,38] The presence of the *C. difficile* toxin in the stool confirms the diagnosis. Mild infection often resolves without treatment.[39] For more persistent or severe infection, oral metronidazole remains the first line treatment, although other antibiotics may have to be used.[39,40]

Dietary supplements: probiotics (live bacteria such as "live yoghurt") can reduce diarrhea due to radiotherapy, acute gastroenteritis, rotavirus, antibiotics, enteral feeds and inflammatory bowel disease such as Crohn's disease, although not all probiotics are equally effective.[23,41–44] Zinc supplements may also have a role.[45–47]

Skin protection: ointments and silicone creams are useful to protect the skin. However, in the presence of pads they will reduce or prevent the pads from absorbing fluid, and if stoma or adhesive stool-collecting bags are used they will prevent adhesion. In these situations water-based creams can be used (e.g. Conotrane, Cavilon).

Physical devices

Very fluid stool and discharge can be managed by different systems:

Stool collecting bags: some are empty stoma-like bags with a folded adhesive patch that adheres to the perianal area. They require an intact perianal skin, but can be kept in place for up to a week since the bag can be drained and flushed with water for cleaning.[48,49] Others are bags containing an absorbent gel that solidifies on contact with fluid and which can be used inside commodes or bed pans, or simply held against the perineum to collect the diarrhea.[50] Both types are only suitable for bed-bound patients. Although expensive, they can be used for a week or more.

Rectal tubes: these are appliances consisting of soft tubes with an inflatable balloon that sits in the rectum, allowing stool to drain into an attached bag. The diarrhea must be very fluid with no solid matter, and patients must be bed bound with little or no mobility. The tubes can stay in place for up to 30 days. Although expensive, they are cheaper than the cost of the care, laundry, and skin damage of fecal incontinence.

Clinical decision	If YES carry out the action below
7 Are the stools very dark or very pale?	• **If the stools are very pale:** consider if this is steatorrhea (pale, malodorous stools that are difficult to flush away). Start loperamide (2 mg with each loose stool, up to 16 mg daily). *For pancreatic insufficiency:* enteric coated pancreatin plus a PPI (lansoprazole or omeprazole). *For obstructive jaundice:* enteric coated pancreatin plus a PPI (lansoprazole or omeprazole). Consider high-dose dexamethasone, bypass surgery, or endoscopic stent. • **If the stools are very dark:** test the stool for the presence of blood: *If fecal occult blood test negative:* consider oral dye (e.g. beetroot) or iron supplements as possible cause. Reassure the patient. *If fecal occult test positive:* consider upper gastrointestinal blood loss (*see Bleeding*, cd-4, p. 95). Heme-based tests are unaffected by oral iron.
8 Is a fistula the cause?	• **Urine** (vesicocolic or vesicorectal fistula): catheter (urethral or suprapubic). Consider desmopressin at night (*see* cd-7 in *Urinary problems and sexual difficulties*, p. 229). • **Gastrocolic or enterorectal fistula:** consider arranging for a colostomy.
9 Is there clear fluid in the stool?	• **Secretory diarrhea:** *see* causes in cd-5 on p. 117. • **Mucus** (total bowel obstruction/blind rectum/rectal or colonic tumor secreting mucus): exclude overflow due to constipation, otherwise hyoscine butylbromide may help (SC infusion 60–300 mg/24 hours) (US hyoscyamine 0.25–0.5 mg IV/SC q4h PRN).
10 Is the diarrhea persisting?	• **Exclude:** *Chemotherapy or radiotherapy* causing irritation and damage to bowel mucosa. Start with loperamide. If this is ineffective *add* ondansetron 4–8 mg PO or SC. *Constipation* causing spurious diarrhea. *Pelvic floor abnormalities*, e.g. prolapse, poor anal tone. *Infection:* send 3 stool specimens (in AIDS up to 6 stool specimens may be needed, and for CMV or adenovirus a rectal biopsy or upper GI endoscopy may be required).[51] Ask laboratory to check stool for candida. *Irritable colon:* increase dietary fiber. *Anxiety, fear: see Anxiety*, p. 239. *Fecal incontinence due to neurological or sphincter dysfunction:* consider a colostomy. If time is available, start a bowel management program. *Autonomic failure:* clonidine (50–150 microg/24 hours) may help in diabetes. • **Treat symptomatically:** *Loperamide* 2–4 mg with each loose stool (up to 32 mg daily may be needed in AIDS-related diarrhea). Stop laxatives and magnesium-containing antacids. *Consider:* — hyoscine butylbromide SC infusion 60–300 mg/24 hr or in US hyoscyamine 0.25–0.5 mg SC/IV q4h PRN — octreotide SC q8h or infusion 150–1500 microg/24 hr — probiotics and zinc as a dietary adjuncts. *If pads or adhesive collecting bags are used:* avoid ointments or silicone-based creams. *If diarrhea or discharge is very fluid:* consider stool collecting devices (*see* text). • **Ask for advice** from a continence nurse specialist.

Adapted from Regnard and Mannix[21]
cd = clinical decision

Rectal plugs are made of a porous absorbent foam which expands when inserted into the rectum. It can be left in place for up to 12 hours and therefore has a role in more mobile patients who can insert and hold the device in place.

Bowel management program: this is an individualized plan aimed at preventing incontinence and encouraging effective bowel transit.[52] The input of a continence specialist is essential.

Laundry: cleaning soiled clothes and bed sheets can be unpleasant and exhausting for relatives and access to an effective laundry service is essential.

REFERENCES: DIARRHEA

B = book; C = comment; Ch = chapter; CS-n = case study-no. of cases; CT-n = controlled trial-no. of cases; E = editorial; GC = group consensus; I = interviews; LS = laboratory study; MC = multi-center; OS-n = open study-no. of cases; R = review; RCT-n = randomized controlled trial-no. of cases; RS-n = retrospective survey-no. of cases; SA = systematic or meta analysis.

1 Solomon R, Cherny NI. (2006) Constipation and diarrhea in patients with cancer. *Cancer Journal.* **12**(5): 355–64. (R, 71 refs)

2 Willoughby VR, Sahr F, Russell JB, Gbakima AA. (2001) The usefulness of defined clinical features in the diagnosis of HIV/AIDS infection in Sierra Leone. *Cellular and Molecular Biology.* **47**(7): 1163–7. (OS-124)

3 Schiller LR. (2007) Management of diarrhea in clinical practice: strategies for primary care physicians. *Reviews in Gastroenterological Disorders.* **7**(Suppl. 3): S27–38. (R, 27 refs)

4 Nazarko L. (2007) Managing diarrhoea in the home to prevent admission. *British Journal of Community Nursing.* **12**(11): 508–12. (R, 16 refs)

5 Roach M, Christie JA. (2008) Fecal incontinence in the elderly. *Geriatrics.* **63**(2): 13–22. (R, 56 refs)

6 National Institute for Clinical Excellence (NICE). (2007) *Faecal Incontinence: the management of faecal incontinence in adults.* London: NICE.

7 Khanna R, Lakhanpaul M, Burman-Roy S, Murphy MS. (2009) Diarrhoea and vomiting caused by gastroenteritis in children: summary of NICE guidance. *British Medical Journal.* **338**: 1009–12. (R, 4 refs)

8 Wingate D, Phillips SF, Lewis SJ, Malagelada JR, *et al.* (2001) Guidelines for adults on self-medication for the treatment of acute diarrhoea. *Alimentary Pharmacology and Therapeutics.* **15**(6): 773–82. (R, 79 refs)

9 Hahn S, Kim S, Garner P. (2002) Reduced osmolarity oral rehydration solution for treating dehydration caused by acute diarrhoea in children. *Cochrane Database of Systematic Reviews.* **1**: CD002847. (R, 61 refs)

10 Sentongo TA. (2004) The use of oral rehydration solutions in children and adults. *Current Gastroenterology Reports.* **6**(4): 307–13. (R, 45 refs)

11 Spandorfer PR, Alessandrini EA, Joffe MD, Localio R, Shaw KN. (2005) Oral versus intravenous rehydration of moderately dehydrated children: a randomized, controlled trial. *Pediatrics.* **115**(2): 295–301. (RCT-73)

12 Bellemare S, Hartling L, Wiebe N, Russell K, *et al.* (2004) Rehydration versus intravenous therapy for treating dehydration due to gastroenteritis in children: a meta-analysis of randomised controlled trials. *BMC Medicine.* **2**: 11. (SA-14)

13 Trinh C, Prabhakar K. (2007) Diarrheal diseases in the elderly. *Clinics in Geriatric Medicine.* **23**(4): 833–56. (R, 153 refs)

14 Baxter R, Ray GT, Fireman BH. (2008) Case-control study of antibiotic use and subsequent Clostridium difficile-associated diarrhea in hospitalized patients. *Infection Control and Hospital Epidemiology.* **29**(1): 44–50. (OS-4493)

15 Elia M, Engfer MB, Green CJ, Silk DB. (2008) Systematic review and meta-analysis: the clinical and physiological effects of fibre-containing enteral formulae. *Alimentary Pharmacology and Therapeutics.* **27**(2): 120–45. (R, 92 refs)

16 Vecht J, Masclee AA, Lamers CB. (1997) The dumping syndrome: current insights into pathophysiology, diagnosis and treatment. *Scandinavian Journal of Gastroenterology.* **223**(Suppl.): 21–7. (R, 95 refs)

17 Robb BW, Matthews JB. (2005) Bile salt diarrhea. *Current Gastroenterology Reports.* **7**(5): 379–83. (R, 33 refs)

18 Safdi M, Bekal PK, Martin S, Saeed ZA, Burton F, Toskes PP. (2006) The effects of oral pancreatic enzymes (Creon 10 capsule) on steatorrhea: a multicenter, placebo-controlled, parallel group trial in subjects with chronic pancreatitis. *Pancreas.* **33**(2): 156–62. (RCT)

19 DiMagno EP. (2001) Gastric acid suppression and treatment of severe exocrine pancreatic insufficiency. *Best Practice and Research in Clinical Gastroenterology.* **15**(3): 477–86. (R, 20 refs)

20 Tran TM, Van den Neucker A, Hendriks JJ, Forget P, Forget PP. (1998) Effects of a proton-pump inhibitor in cystic fibrosis. *Acta Paediatrica.* **87**(5): 553–8. (OS-15)

21 Regnard C, Mannix K. (1995) The control of diarrhoea. In: *Flow Diagrams in Advanced Cancer and Other Diseases.* London: Edward Arnold. pp. 32–5. (Ch)

22 Li ST, Grossman DC, Cummings P. (2007) Loperamide therapy for acute diarrhea in children: systematic review and meta-analysis. *PLoS Medicine/Public Library of Science.* **4**(3): e98. (SA)

23 Urbancsek H, Kazar T, Mezes I, Neumann K. (2001) Results of a double-blind, randomized study to evaluate the efficacy and safety of Antibiophilus in patients with radiation-induced diarrhoea.

European Journal of Gastroenterology and Hepatology. **13**(4): 391–6. (RCT-206)

24 Sorbe B, Berglind AM, De Bruijn K. (1992) Tropisetron, a new 5-HT3 receptor antagonist, in the prevention of irradiation-induced nausea, vomiting and diarrhoea. *European Journal of Gynaecological Oncology*. **13**(5): 382–9. (OS-20)

25 Henriksson R, Lomberg H, Israelsson G, Zackrisson B, Franzen L. (1992) The effect of ondansetron on radiation-induced emesis and diarrhoea. *Acta Oncologica*. **31**(7): 767–9. (OS-33)

26 Lodge N, Evans ML, Wilkins M, Blake PR, Fryatt I. (1995) A randomized cross-over study of the efficacy of codeine phosphate versus Ispaghulahusk in patients with gynaecological cancer experiencing diarrhoea during pelvic radiotherapy. *European Journal of Cancer Care*. **4**(1): 8–10. (RCT-10)

27 Cello JP, Grendall JH, Basuk P, Simon D, Weiss L, Wittner M, Rood RP, Wilcox CM, Forsmark CE, Read AE. (1991) Effect of octreotide on refractory AIDS-associated diarrhea. *Annals of Internal Medicine*. **115**: 705–10. (MC, CT-51)

28 Dean A, Bridge D, Lickiss JN. (1994) The palliative effects of octreotide in malignant disease. *Annals of the Academy of Medicine, Singapore*. **23**(2): 212–15. (R, 38 refs)

29 Mackie CR, Jenkins SA, Hartley MN. (1991) Treatment of severe postvagotomy/postgastrectomy symptoms with the somatostatin analogue octreotide. *British Journal of Surgery*. **78**: 1338–43. (OS-14)

30 Harris AG, Redfern JS. (1995) Octreotide treatment of carcinoid syndrome: analysis of published dose-titration data. *Alimentary Pharmacology and Therapeutics*. **9**(4): 387–94. (SA, 83 refs)

31 Rohaizak M, Farndon JR. (2002) Use of octreotide and lanreotide in the treatment of symptomatic non-resectable carcinoid tumours. *ANZ Journal of Surgery*. **72**(9): 635–8. (CS-10)

32 Mercadante S. (1995) Diarrhea in terminally ill patients: pathophysiology and treatment. *Journal of Pain and Symptom Management*. **10**(4): 298–309. (R, 37 refs)

33 Fried M. (1999) Octreotide in the treatment of refractory diarrhea. *Digestion*. **60**(Suppl. 2): S42–6. (R, 38 refs)

34 Szilagyi A, Shrier I. (2001) Systematic review: the use of somatostatin or octreotide in refractory diarrhoea. *Alimentary Pharmacology and Therapeutics*. **15**(12): 1889–97. (R, 58 refs)

35 Rosenoff SH, Gabrail NY, Conklin R, Hohneker JA, Berg WJ, Warsi G, Maloney J, Benedetto JJ, Miles EA, Zhu W, Anthony L. (2006) A multicenter, randomized trial of long-acting octreotide for the optimum prevention of chemotherapy-induced diarrhea: results of the STOP trial. *The Journal of Supportive Oncology*. **4**(6): 289–94. (RCT-147)

36 Martenson JA, Halyard MY, Sloan JA, Proulx GM, *et al.* (2008) Phase III, double-blind study of depot octreotide versus placebo in the prevention of acute diarrhea in patients receiving pelvic radiation therapy: results of North Central Cancer Treatment Group N00CA. *Journal of Clinical Oncology*. **26**(32): 5248–53. (RCT-125)

37 Bartlett JG, Gerding DN. (2008) Clinical recognition and diagnosis of Clostridium difficile infection. *Clinical Infectious Diseases*. **46**(Suppl. 1): S12–18. (R, 48 refs)

38 Crogan NL, Evans BC. (2007) Clostridium difficile: an emerging epidemic in nursing homes. *Geriatric Nursing*. **28**(3): 161–4. (R, 14 refs)

39 Nelson R. (2007) Antibiotic treatment for Clostridium difficile-associated diarrhea in adults. *Cochrane Database of Systematic Reviews*. **3**: CD004610. (R, 44 refs)

40 Balagopal A, Sears CL. (2007) Clostridium difficile: new therapeutic options. *Current Opinion in Pharmacology*. **7**(5): 455–8. (R, 30 refs)

41 Gill H, Prasad J. (2008) Probiotics, immunomodulation, and health benefits. *Advances in Experimental Medicine and Biology*. **606**: 423–54. (R, 155 refs)

42 Sazawal S, Hiremath G, Dhingra U, Malik P, Deb S, Black RE. (2006) Efficacy of probiotics in prevention of acute diarrhoea: a meta-analysis of masked, randomised, placebo-controlled trials. *The Lancet Infectious Diseases*. **6**(6): 374–82. (SA, 58 refs)

43 Whelan K. (2007) Enteral-tube-feeding diarrhoea: manipulating the colonic microbiota with probiotics and prebiotics. *Proceedings of the Nutrition Society*. **66**(3): 299–306. (R, 92 refs)

44 Canani RB, Cirillo P, Terrin G, Cesarano L, *et al.* (2007) Probiotics for treatment of acute diarrhoea in children: randomised clinical trial of five different preparations. *British Medical Journal*. **335**: 340. (RCT-571)

45 Hoque KM, Binder HJ. (2006) Zinc in the treatment of acute diarrhea: current status and assessment. *Gastroenterology*. **130**(7): 2201–5. (R, 37 refs)

46 Lukacik M, Thomas RL, Aranda JV. (2008) A meta-analysis of the effects of oral zinc in the treatment of acute and persistent diarrhea. *Pediatrics*. **121**(2): 326–36. (SA-22)

47 Awasthi S, INCLEN Childnet Zinc Effectiveness for Diarrhea (IC-ZED) Group. (2006) Zinc supplementation in acute diarrhea is acceptable, does not interfere with oral rehydration, and reduces the use of other medications: a randomized trial in five countries. *Journal of Pediatric Gastroenterology and Nutrition*. **42**(3): 300–5. (RCT-2002)

48 Le Lievre S. (2002) An overview of skin care and faecal incontinence. *Nursing Times Plus*. **98**(4): 58–9. (R, 15 refs)

49 Addison R. (1987) Faecal collection. *Journal of District Nursing*. **7**: 20–2. (CS-6)

50 Evans D. (2006) Faecal incontinence products and quality of life. *Nursing Times*. **102**(2): 44–5, 47. (R, 4 refs)

51 Gane EJ, Thomas MG, Nicholson GI, Lane MR. (1992) Upper gastrointestinal endoscopy in patients with human immunodeficiency virus infection: is it worthwhile? *New Zealand Medical Journal*. **105**(946): 475–6. (OS-21)

52 Pierce E, Cowan P, Stokes M. (2001) Managing faecal retention and incontinence in neurodisability. *British Journal of Nursing*. **10**(9): 592–601. (R, 18 refs)

Dyspepsia

CLINICAL DECISION AND ACTION CHECKLIST

1 Are any alarm symptoms present?
2 Could this be structural (acid-related) dyspepsia?
3 Could this be a functional (dysmotility or non-ulcer) dyspepsia?
4 Could this be gastroesophageal reflux disease (GERD)?
5 Is the dyspepsia persisting?

KEY POINTS

- Dyspepsia can be caused by acid-induced damage, abnormal motility, or esophageal reflux.
- Adults and children with severe neurological impairment are particularly prone to dyspepsia.
- "Alarm" symptoms should usually prompt urgent investigation.
- Prokinetic agents and proton pump inhibitors are important treatments in dyspepsia.

INTRODUCTION

There has long been disagreement on the definition of dyspepsia.[1] The difficulty is that dyspepsia is a syndrome with several very different causes. The current view is that dyspepsia is a syndrome whose symptoms arise in the upper gastrointestinal tract (i.e. duodenum to esophagus),[2] with upper abdominal pain as the commonest feature.[3,4] Three types are now recognized: structural dyspepsia, functional dyspepsia, and gastroesophageal reflux disease (GERD).

Whatever the cause, dyspepsia is a common problem, especially in children with complex disabilities. Although pain is common, in adults and children with communication difficulties, the only symptoms may be food refusal, weight loss, or failure to thrive.

TYPES OF DYSPEPSIA

Structural (acid-related) dyspepsia is due to acid-related damage of the stomach or duodenum, e.g. peptic ulcer. NSAIDs and *H. pylori* infection are common causes.[5–7] A common symptom is epigastric pain that is worse at night and relieved by antacids.[4]

Functional (dysmotility or non-ulcer) dyspepsia is due to abnormal motility of the stomach and duodenum, or of the esophagus. It has a wide range of causes,[8] and is now defined by two symptom entities: epigastric pain (epigastric pain syndrome) and meal-related symptoms (post-prandial distress syndrome).[9] Thus, pain is relieved by vomiting in gastroduodenal dysmotility, but in esophageal dysmotility the pain develops after meals.[4] Gastric stasis and cancer-associated dyspepsia syndrome (CADS) are part of this type of dyspepsia.[10–12] It is more common in neurologically impaired children and often associated with GERD (*see* next type).[13]

Gastroesophageal reflux disease (GERD) is caused by reflux of gastric contents into the esophagus sufficient to cause local damage and symptoms.[14] It occurs in up to 75% of neurologically impaired children.[13,15] Other causes include hiatus hernia, adoption of a prolonged supine position, and increased intra-abdominal pressure secondary to tumor, ascites, hepatomegaly, spasticity, scoliosis, or seizures.[16] GERD symptoms can be worsened by overfeeding, especially through a gastrostomy in neurologically impaired adults and children, whose energy needs are less than active patients. Symptoms are intermittent and often non-specific. They may include heartburn (especially on bending and lying flat), dysphagia, epigastric pain, with atypical symptoms of vomiting, dental enamel erosion, respiratory symptoms (e.g. nocturnal post-prandial asthma, aspiration, chest infections), eating-related problems (e.g. irritability, hyperextensive posture, choking, dysphagia), and ear, nose and throat problems (e.g. cough, hoarseness).[16–20] Sandifer's syndrome (neck extension and head rotation during or after meals) can occur in infants or young children and is associated with iron deficiency anemia and severe esophagitis.

TREATMENT

Alarm symptoms: these are symptoms that would normally require prompt investigation and treatment (*see* cd-1 opposite). Some patients will be too ill for transfer or will have made clear their wish to remain at home or hospice. These patients need adequate analgesia, antiemetics, comfort, and company for their last days and hours.

Structural dyspepsia: first-line treatment is a proton pump inhibitor (PPI),[21] even if an ulcer is bleeding.[22] If the patient is vomiting or has swallowing problems pantoprazole can be given intravenously, or omeprazole through a feeding tube (*see Drug information*, p. 318).

If gastric bleeding is occurring, sucralfate is an effective hemostatic agent.[23–25] Infection with *H. pylori* is common and should be treated if present.[26,27] NSAIDs are another common cause of mucosal damage and should be stopped or changed to an NSAID less likely to cause damage (*see Managing the adverse effects of analgesics*, p. 70).

Functional dyspepsia: this often needs a prokinetic agent that will have to be given by a non-oral route if vomiting is present.[28–31] In standard doses metoclopramide is as effective as domperidone (available in US from

Clinical decision	If YES carry out the action below
1 Are any alarm symptoms present?	• **Prompts for urgent investigation:** chronic gastrointestinal bleeding, unintentional weight loss, dysphagia, persistent vomiting, iron deficiency anemia, epigastric mass, suspicious findings after a barium meal, patients over 55 years with recent, persistent, or unexplained dyspepsia. • **Prompts for immediate investigation and management:** *Rapid clinical deterioration: see* cd-1 in *Emergencies*, p. 331. *Persistent vomiting causing dehydration or electrolyte disturbance: see Nausea and vomiting*, p. 167. *Hematemesis* (from bleeding ulcer or severe gastritis): *see* cd-4 in *Bleeding*, p. 95. *Melena* (upper gastrointestinal hemorrhage): *see* cd-4 in *Bleeding*, p. 95. *Persistent and worsening pain* (perforation or other intra-abdominal crisis): *see* cd-5d in *Emergencies*, p. 335. *Severe dysphagia* (esophageal obstruction): *see Dysphagia*, p. 131.
2 Could this be structural (acid-related)? e.g. peptic ulcer: epigastric pain or heartburn worse at night and eased by antacids	• **Start a PPI**, e.g. lansoprazole 30 mg PO daily or pantoprazole 40 mg daily PO (or 40 mg IV infusion over 15 minutes). Stop any drugs causing upper GI mucosal irritation, such as iron or an NSAID. Review other irritant drugs such as SSRIs. Arrange for *H. pylori* test (breath test or stool antigen). If positive, treat as in cd-5 on p. 127. • **If bleeding** *(hematemesis or melena):* add sucralfate suspension 10 mL q6h. Do not give within two hours of lansoprazole, warfarin, ketoconazole, or phenytoin.
3 Could this be functional (dysmotility)? e.g. pain eased by vomiting or occurring after meals	• **Reduce the size of meals or feeds** and give more frequently. • **Stop or reduce the dose of antimuscarinic drugs.** • **Start a prokinetic**, e.g. metoclopramide or domperidone (available in US from a compounding pharmacy – 10 mg, 20 mg) 10 mg q6h. Use domperidone for children (*see Drug doses in children: starting doses*, p. 307). If vomiting is present, start metoclopramide SC infusion 30 mg/24 hours or 10 mg SC q6-8h (or domperidone PR 30 mg q6h). Titrate the dose and change to oral domperidone once vomiting is controlled. • **Consider adding simethicone** liquid 20–40 mg before meals or feeds to help trapped gastric air to be brought up.
4 Could this be GERD? e.g. heartburn or epigastric pain worse on bending or lying flat.	• **Start the following** — alginate 250–500 mg, e.g. Gaviscon after each meal or feed (*see Drug doses in children: starting doses*, p. 306). — a prokinetic, e.g. metoclopramide or domperidone (available in US from a compounding pharmacy – 10 mg, 20 mg) 10 mg q6h. Use domperidone for children (*see Drug doses in children: starting doses*, p. 307). • **If dysphagia and/or aspiration are present:** *see Dysphagia*, p. 131. • **If the patient is immobile:** elevate upper body to 30 degrees. • **If NG/gastrostomy fed:** alter feeding regime from large bolus, to frequent small-volume feeds. Continuous feeding can be tried but this sometimes aggravates symptoms.

cd = clinical decision

compounding pharmacy – 10 mg, 20 mg), but in children domperidone is safer.[32,33] In persistent cases erythromycin can help, but can cause nausea, and tolerance may develop.[34–36] Mirtazapine may help resistant gastric stasis.[37] Taking meals as frequent snacks rather than large meals may also help, in addition to correcting the positioning of the patient. In a tube-fed patient smaller, more frequent boluses may help. Activated simethicone is a defoaming agent, which reduces gastric distension.[38,39]

GERD: if dysphagia is a predominant symptom this should be investigated, especially as aspiration occurs silently in up to 40% of patients (*see Dysphagia*, p. 131). In patients unable to position themselves, elevating the upper body to at least 30 degrees of hip-flexion can help. Alginates float on the stomach contents and reduce reflux symptoms.[40] As with dysmotility dyspepsia, prokinetics are an important treatment and altering the size and frequency of meals and feeds can also help. However, a role for PPI drugs may also exist in GERD, and these may need to be continued long term.[41]

PERSISTENT DYSPEPSIA

***H. pylori* infection:** this can coexist with functional dyspepsia and GERD and respond to PPIs,[42–44] or to infection eradication. For palliative care patients with a prognosis of months a PPI will be sufficient, but eradication should be attempted for patients with *H. pylori* who have a longer prognosis.[45,46]

Bile reflux: this can be eased by substances that bind bile acids such as cholestyramine.

Infection: in addition to *H. pylori*, infections such as candida, CMV and herpes (zoster or simplex) can cause the same symptoms as dyspepsia. Treatment will resolve the symptoms.

Referral for investigation and treatment: the opinion of a gastroenterologist can be invaluable. In children with persistent GERD, fundoplication +/- pyloroplasty is effective in over 80%, but surgery has a high morbidity with 26–59% having postoperative complications, 60–75% getting recurrence of GERD (the higher figure in neurological impairment), and 5–15% needing repeat surgery.[15,47] An effective alternative is to consider a jejunal feeding tube.[48,49]

Clinical decision	If YES carry out the action below
5 Is the dyspepsia persisting?	• **Consider infection:** Test for *H. pylori* (stool antigen test or a urea breath test). If positive, start a PPI and use either a) metronidazole 400 mg + clarithromycin 250 mg (both twice daily), or b) amoxicillin 1 g + clarithromycin 500 mg (both twice daily) in addition to a PPI. Consider other infections such as gastric candida, CMV, or herpes: treat the infection. • **If not on PPI:** start pantoprazole 40 mg daily PO or NG (or 40 mg IV infusion over 15 minutes) or lansoprazole 30 mg PO daily. This can help in all types of dyspepsia. Ranitidine is an alternative, but is less effective and can cause problematic rebound nocturnal acid secretion. It can, however, be given as a SC infusion 150–200 mg/24 hr. • **If mucosal ulceration is causing pain:** start a mucosal protecting agent (e.g. sucralfate suspension 10 mL q6h to q8h). • **If bile reflux is the problem:** use cholestyramine 1–2 g after meals. • **If dysphagia or an NG tube is present:** consider gastrostomy. *See Dysphagia*, p. 131 and *Nutrition and hydration problems*, p. 175. • **If dysmotility persists:** consider erythromycin 100–250 mg (10 mg/kg in children) q12h, but if this fails consider mirtazapine 15–30 mg daily. • **If GERD is present:** consider referral for gastroenterological opinion for consideration of a jejunal feeding tube or surgery. • **If symptoms persist:** consider referral for investigation.

cd = clinical decision

REFERENCES: DYSPEPSIA

B = book; C = comment; Ch = chapter; CS-n = case study-no. of cases; CT-n = controlled trial-no. of cases; E = editorial; GC = group consensus; I = interviews; LS = laboratory study; MC = multi-center; OS-n = open study-no. of cases; R = review; RCT-n = randomized controlled trial-no. of cases; RS-n = retrospective survey-no. of cases; SA = systematic or meta analysis.

1 Chiba N. (1998). Definitions of dyspepsia: time for a reappraisal. *European Journal of Surgery Supplement*. **583**: 14–23.

2 Logan R, Delaney B. (2001) Implications of dyspepsia for the NHS. *British Medical Journal*. **323**: 675–7. (R)

3 Meinechie-Schmidt V, Christensen E. (1998) Classification of dyspepsia. *Scandinavian Journal of Gastroenterology*. **33**: 1262–72. (CT-7270)

4 Grainger SL, Klass HJ, Rake MO, Williams JG. (1994) Prevalence of dyspepsia: the epidemiology of overlapping symptoms. *Postgraduate Medical Journal*. **70**: 154–61. (R, 25 refs)

5 Childs S, Roberts A, Meineche-Schmidt V, de Wit N, Rubin G. (2000) The management of Helicobacter pylori infection in primary care: a systematic review of the literature. *Family Practice*. **17**(Suppl. 2): S6–11. (SA, 59 refs)

6 Hawkey CJ. (2000) Non-steroidal anti-inflammatory drug gastropathy. *Gastroenterology*. **119**: 521–35. (R, 143 refs)

7 Weil J, Langamn MJS, Wainwright P, Lawson DH, Rawlins M, *et al.* (2000) Peptic ulcer bleeding: accessory risk factors and interactions with non-steroidal anti-inflammatory drugs. *Gut*. **46**: 27–31. (MC, CT)

8 Mimidis K, Tack J. (2008) Pathogenesis of dyspepsia. *Digestive Diseases*. **26**(3): 194–202. (R, 32 refs)

9 Talley NJ, Ruff K, Jiang X, Jung HK. (2008) The Rome III Classification of dyspepsia: will it help research? *Digestive Diseases*. **26**(3): 203–9. (R, 45 refs)

10 Nelson K, Walsh T, O'Donovan P, Sheehan F, Falk G. (1993) Assessment of upper gastrointestinal motility in the cancer-associated dyspepsia syndrome (CADS). *Journal of Palliative Care*. **9**: 27–31.

11 Armes PJ, Plant HJ, Allbright A, Silverstone T, Slevin ML. (1992) A study to investigate the incidence of early satiety in patients with advanced cancer. *British Journal of Cancer*. **65**: 481–4.

12 Bruera E, Catz Z, Hooper R, Lentle B, MacDonald RN. (1987) Chronic nausea and anorexia in advanced cancer patients: a possible role for autonomic dysfunction. *Journal of Pain and Symptom Management*. **2**: 19–21.

13 Perez ME, Youssef NN. (2007) Dyspepsia in childhood and adolescence: insights and treatment considerations. *Current Gastroenterology Reports*. **9**(6): 447–55. (R, 78 refs)

14 Vandenplas Y, Ashkenazi A, Belli D, Boige N, *et al.* (1993) A proposition for the diagnosis and treatment of gastro-oesophageal reflux disease in children: a report from a working group on gastro-oesophageal reflux disease. Working Group of the European Society of Paediatric Gastro-enterology and Nutrition (ESPGAN). *European Journal of Pediatrics*. **152**(9): 704–11. (R, 44 refs)

15 Martinez DA, Ginn-Pease ME, Caniano DA. (1992) Recognition of recurrent gastroesophageal reflux following antireflux surgery in the neurologically disabled child: high index of suspicion and definitive evaluation. *Journal of Pediatric Surgery*. **27**(8): 983–8. (OS-240)

16 Bagwell CE. (1995) Gastro-oesophageal reflux in children. *Surgery Annual*. **27**: 133–63. (R)

17 de Caestecker J. (2001) ABC of the upper gastrointestinal tract. Oesophagus: heartburn. *British Medical Journal*. **323**: 736–9.

18 Wasowska-Krolikowska K, Toporowska-Kowalska E, Krogulska A. (2002) Asthma and gastroesophageal reflux in children. *Medical Science Monitor*. **8**(3): RA64–71. (R, 45 refs)

19 Mendell DA, Logemann JA. (2002) A retrospective analysis of the pharyngeal swallow in patients with a clinical diagnosis of GERD compared with normal controls: a pilot study. *Dysphagia*. **17**(3): 220–6. (CT-18)

20 Irwin RS, Madison JM. (2002) Diagnosis and treatment of chronic cough due to gastro-esophageal reflux disease and postnasal drip syndrome. *Pulmonary Pharmacology and Therapeutics*. **15**(3): 261–6. (R, 42refs)

21 Moayyedi P, Soo S, Deeks J, Delaney B, Innes M, Forman D. (2006) Pharmacological interventions for non-ulcer dyspepsia. *Cochrane Database of Systematic Reviews*. **4**: CD001960. (SA-73, 190 refs)

22 Leontiadis GI, Sreedharan A, Dorward S, Barton P, *et al.* (2007) Systematic reviews of the clinical effectiveness and cost-effectiveness of proton pump inhibitors in acute upper gastrointestinal bleeding. *Health Technology Assessment*. **11**(51): iii–iv, 1–164. (SA, 266 refs)

23 Lam SK. (1990) Why do ulcers heal with sucralfate? *Scandinavian Journal of Gastroenterology*. **25**(Suppl. 173): 6–16. (R, 106 refs)

24 Caldwell JR, Roth SH, Wu WG, Semble EL, *et al.* (1987) Sucralfate treatment of nonsteroidal anti-inflammatory drug-induced gastrointestinal symptoms and mucosal damage. *American Journal of Medicine*. **83**(Suppl. 3B): 74–82. (RCT-143)

25 Regnard CFB, Mannix K. (1990) Palliation of gastric carcinoma haemorrhage with sucralfate. *Palliative Medicine*. **4**: 329–30. (Let, CS-1)

26 Ford AC, Delaney BC, Forman D, Moayyedi P. (2006) Eradication therapy for peptic ulcer disease in Helicobacter pylori positive patients. *Cochrane Database of Systematic Reviews*. **2**: CD003840. (SA-63, 108 refs)

27 Moayyedi P, Soo S, Deeks J, Delaney B, *et al.* (2006) Eradication of Helicobacter pylori for non-ulcer dyspepsia. *Cochrane Database of Systematic Reviews*. **2**: CD002096. (SA-18, 100 refs)

28 Twycross RG. (1995) The use of prokinetic drugs in palliative care. *European Journal of Palliative Care*. **4**: 141–5. (R)

29 Shivshanker K, Bennett RW, Haynie TP. (1983) Tumor-associated gastroparesis: correction with metoclopramide. *American Journal of Surgery*. **145**: 221–5. (OS-10)
30 Kris MG, Yeh SDJ, Gralla RJ, Young CW. (1985) Symptomatic gastroparesis in cancer patients. A possible cause of cancer-associated anorexia that can be improved with oral metoclopramide. *Proceedings of the American Society of Clinical Oncology*. **4**: 267.
31 Hiyama T, Yoshihara M, Matsuo K, Kusunoki H, *et al.* (2007) Meta-analysis of the effects of prokinetic agents in patients with functional dyspepsia. *Journal of Gastroenterology and Hepatology*. **22**(3): 304–10. (SA-27)
32 Sanger GJ, King FD. (1988) From metoclopramide to selective gut motility stimulants and 5HT3 receptor antagonists. *Drug Design and Delivery*. **3**: 273–95. (R, 143 refs)
33 Loose FD. (1979) Domperidone in chronic dyspepsia: a pilot open study and a multicentre general practice crossover comparison with metoclopramide and placebo. *Pharmatheripeutica*. **2**(3): 140–6.
34 Berne JD, Norwood SH, McAuley CE, Vallina VL, *et al.* (2002) Erythromycin reduces delayed gastric emptying in critically ill trauma patients: a randomized, controlled trial. *Journal of Trauma Injury, Infection and Critical Care*. **53**(3): 422–5. (RCT-68)
35 Booth CM, Heyland DK, Paterson WG. (2002) Gastrointestinal promotility drugs in the critical care setting: a systematic review of the evidence. *Critical Care Medicine*. **30**(7): 1429–35. (SA, 70 refs)
36 Costalos C, Gounaris A, Varhalama E, Kokori F, Alexiou N, Kolovou E. (2002) Erythromycin as a prokinetic agent in preterm infants. *Journal of Pediatric Gastroenterology and Nutrition*. **34**(1): 23–5. (RCT-20)
37 Kim SW, Shin IS, Kim JM, Kang HC, *et al.* (2006) Mirtazapine for severe gastroparesis unresponsive to conventional prokinetic treatment. *Psychosomatics*. **47**(5): 440–2. (CS-1)
38 Bernstein J, Kasich M. (1974) A double-blind trial of simethicone in functional disease of the upper gastrointestinal tract. *Journal of Clinical Pharmacology*. **14**: 614–23. (CT)
39 Ogilvie AL, Atkinson M. (1986) Does dimethicone increase the efficacy of antacids in the treatment of reflux oesophagitis? *Journal of the Royal Society of Medicine*. **79**(10): 584–7. (RCT-45)
40 Mandel KG, Daggy BP, Brodie DA, Jacoby HI. (2000) Review article: alginate-raft formulations in the treatment of heartburn and acid reflux. *Alimentary Pharmacology and Therapeutics*. **14**(6): 669–90. (R, 106 refs)
41 Mayer EA, Tillisch K, Bradesi S. (2006) Review article: modulation of the brain-gut axis as a therapeutic approach in gastrointestinal disease. *Alimentary Pharmacology and Therapeutics*. **24**(6): 919–33. (R, 158 refs)
42 Wang WH, Huang JQ, Zheng GF, Xia HH, *et al.* (2007) Effects of proton-pump inhibitors on functional dyspepsia: a meta-analysis of randomized placebo-controlled trials. *Clinical Gastroenterology and Hepatology*. **5**(2): 178–85. (SA-7)
43 Moayyedi P, Soo S, Deeks J, Delaney B, Innes M, Forman D. (2006) Pharmacological interventions for non-ulcer dyspepsia. *Cochrane Database of Systematic Reviews*. **4**: CD001960. (SA-73, 190 refs)
44 Kusano M, Shimoyama Y, Kawamura O, Maeda M, *et al.* (2007) Proton pump inhibitors improve acid-related dyspepsia in gastroesophageal reflux disease patients. *Digestive Diseases and Sciences*. **52**(7): 1673–7. (CT-66)
45 Ang TL, Fock KM, Teo EK, Chan YH, *et al.* (2006) Helicobacter pylori eradication versus prokinetics in the treatment of functional dyspepsia: a randomized, double-blind study. *Journal of Gastroenterology*. **41**(7): 647–53. (RCT-130)
46 Jarbol DE, Kragstrup J, Stovring H, Havelund T, Schaffalitzky de Muckadell OB. (2006) Proton pump inhibitor or testing for Helicobacter pylori as the first step for patients presenting with dyspepsia? A cluster-randomized trial. *American Journal of Gastroenterology*. **101**(6): 1200–8. (RCT-722)
47 Norrashidah AW, Henry RL. (2002) Fundoplication in children with gastro-oesophageal reflux disease. *Journal of Paediatrics and Child Health*. **38**(2): 156–9. (RS-79)
48 Doede T, Faiss S, Schier F. (2002) Jejunal feeding tubes via gastrostomy in children. *Endoscopy*. **34**(7): 539–42. (OS-52)
49 Wales PW, Diamond IR, Dutta S, Muraca S, *et al.* (2002) Fundoplication and gastrostomy versus image-guided gastrojejunal tube for enteral feeding in neurologically impaired children with gastroesophageal reflux. *Journal of Pediatric Surgery*. **37**(3): 407–12. (RS-111)

NOTES

Dysphagia

CLINICAL DECISION AND ACTION CHECKLIST

1. Is there doubt about the need for hydration and/or feeding?
2. Is a complete obstruction present?
3. Is aspiration causing troublesome symptoms?
4. Is mucosal infection or a dry mouth the cause?
5. Are drugs the cause?
6. Is pain affecting swallowing?
7. Is the dysphagia persisting?

KEY POINTS

- Careful assessment may uncover problems with simple solutions.
- The advice of a specialist speech therapist is invaluable.

INTRODUCTION

For food and fluid to enter the stomach they must be

a) Transferred from table or plate to mouth. Problems with this transfer are often missed and can be caused by any physical impairment (e.g. paralysis, abnormal coordination, weakness, exhaustion) or psychological impairment (e.g. delirium, depression).

b) Transferred from mouth to stomach. This occurs in four phases:

Oral preparatory phase in which food is mixed with saliva and chewed to break down larger particles.

Oral swallowing phase in which the lips are closed to prevent leakage and the anterior tongue retracts and elevates in a wave that pushes the bolus into the oropharynx.

Pharyngeal phase which is triggered by the bolus reaching the posterior tongue. This triggers breathing to stop temporarily and elevates the larynx against the epiglottis to protect the airway and prevent aspiration. A peristaltic wave moves the bolus into the esophagus in under one second. These complex actions are necessary to protect the airway because the pharynx is a shared passage for air and food.

Esophageal phase in which reflex peristalsis carries the bolus down the esophagus, the lower esophageal sphincter relaxes, and the bolus enters the stomach.

Any abnormality in one or more of these four phases is covered by the term dysphagia.

Dysphagia is often seen in cancer, especially in the head and neck or lung,[1] but is much more common in patients with neurological disease such as amyotrophic lateral sclerosis (ALS), stroke, multiple sclerosis, dementia, Parkinson's disease and severe cerebral palsy.[2–7] It is also more common in old age,[8,9] in children with complex problems,[10] and in people with mental health problems.[11] Around 60% of patients with ALS have dysphagia,[2] but aspiration is not a common cause of death in this condition.[3] The prevalence of dysphagia also depends on the site affected, so that it is only 4% in patients with anterior oral cancer, rising to 100% with postcricoid cancer lesions.[12,13] Anything which alters the anatomy or the control of swallowing can affect the oral, pharyngeal, and esophageal phases.[14]

CAUSES

Disease: including local cancer and neurological diseases.

Treatment: surgery and radiotherapy can have short- and long-term effects. Drugs can cause extrapyramidal disorders (antimuscarinic drugs, metoclopramide, haloperidol), increased lower esophageal tone (metoclopramide, domperidone), altered upper esophageal tone (dantrolene), or mucosal damage (cytotoxics, non-steroidal anti-inflammatory drugs).

Advanced disease: dry mouth, weakness and mucosal infection can all cause problems. Candidiasis can involve any part of the gastrointestinal tract.[15] Infection below the pharynx may produce local pain, vomiting or diarrhea but signs of oral candidiasis are present in only 50% of patients with esophageal candidiasis.[16] For treatment *see* cd-3 in *Oral problems*, p. 185.

Concurrent conditions: examples are dyspepsia and stroke. Other factors can compromise swallowing such as local pain, age, missing teeth, unappetizing food, dry mouth, lack of help, drowsiness, depression, and anxiety.

HISTORY AND EXAMINATION

Localization by the patient is accurate in over 90% of cases;[17] however, patients find it difficult to estimate the severity of their dysphagia.[18] Food consistencies are unreliable indicators,[19] and the gag reflex is of little value.[20,21] A basic evaluation can be done at the bedside, but if abnormalities are found or suspected, they should be assessed by a professional qualified in dysphagia assessment and management, usually a speech and language therapist trained in swallowing disorders.[22,23]

It is important to note the oral-to-pharyngeal transit time (OPT) when checking for oropharyngeal causes of dysphagia. It is the time from the first movement of the tongue to the last movement of the larynx measured by placing one finger below the jaw and one over the larynx.[17] In the *dry test swallow*, the patient is asked to swallow without fluid, and in the *wet test swallow* the test is repeated with 5 mL water. The OPT is usually less than one second. Speaking immediately after swallowing will uncover laryngeal penetration by the "gargle" quality to the voice, or by coughing. Some laryngeal penetration by liquids is common and causes no problems,[24] and in 40% of patients aspiration beyond the vocal cords is minor with no symptoms.[17] This challenges the usual view that aspiration is always a serious, life-threatening event and suggests the airways cope with low levels of aspiration.

Clinical decision	If YES carry out the action below
1 Is there doubt about the need for hydration and/or feeding?	*See also Nutrition and hydration problems*, p. 175. • **If the prognosis is short (day-by-day deterioration):** hydrate and feed for comfort or pleasure (moistening the mouth may be all that is needed). • **If dysphagia is due to exhaustion caused by cancer:** consider non-oral feeding only if active cancer treatment is planned. However, non-oral hydration is useful to prevent thirst in some patients with symptomatic dehydration.
2 Is a complete obstruction present?	• **If the prognosis is short (day-by-day deterioration):** consider high-dose dexamethasone 8–16 mg daily (IV or SC in divided doses) if short-term improvement would be helpful. • **If the prognosis is longer (week-by-week deterioration or slower):** start IV or SC hydration and refer for urgent endoscopy. If stenting is not possible, consider referral for a feeding gastrostomy.
3 Is aspiration causing troublesome symptoms?	NB. 40% of patients with aspiration due to oropharyngeal dysphagia can only be identified on videofluoroscopy or fiber-optic endoscopy in the presence of a swallowing therapist. • **If gastroesophageal reflux is suspected:** *see Dyspepsia*, p. 125. • **If a tracheoesophageal fistula is suspected:** refer to the gastroenterologists or interventional radiologists for a covered wall stent. • **If symptoms are distressing** (e.g. choking, coughing, copious secretions, or frequent chest infections): consider stenting for esophageal lesions or a feeding gastrostomy.
4 Is mucosal infection or a dry mouth the cause?	• **If this is infection:** for candidiasis *see* cd-3 in *Oral problems*, p. 185. Viral (e.g. herpes zoster, herpes simplex, CMV): treat according to local antiviral policy. • **If this is dry mouth:** *see* cd-4 in *Oral problems*, p. 187.
5 Are drugs the cause?	*See* the text opposite for examples of drugs that may cause dysphagia. • Reduce dose, change, or stop drug.

Adapted from Regnard[25]
cd = clinical decision

However, such symptomless aspiration does indicate a potential risk of more serious aspiration. The advice of a speech and language therapist trained in swallowing disorders is essential.[26]

INVESTIGATIONS

Oropharyngeal dysphagia is best assessed by videofluoroscopy or fiber-optic nasal endoscopy under the advice of a specialist speech and language therapist.[27–30] A barium swallow is of minimal value and may cause barium aspiration. For esophageal causes endoscopy is essential and manometry can diagnose motility problems.[30]

TREATMENT

Supportive measures: small portions of attractively presented food are essential.[31] Some patients will need the advice of physiotherapist and occupational therapist for posture and physical aids.[32]

Dexamethasone reduces peritumor edema, improves neurological function when perineural tumor invasion has occurred,[33] and may reduce bulbar palsy caused by direct tumor invasion of the skull base.

Radiotherapy can be given as a single intracavity dose. In esophageal carcinoma it can relieve dysphagia in up to 54%

of patients for a median of 4 months.[34] External beam treatment over several sessions can also relieve dysphagia but can itself cause temporary dysphagia via a radiation-induced esophagitis.

Dilatation is effective in malignant obstruction but only lasts a few weeks.[35]

Laser can be used as first line and has advantages over intubation.[36–38]

Stenting: small, expandable metal stents are increasingly being used.[39,40] Covered stents are necessary if a fistula is present.[41] Laser and stenting can be combined with good effect.[42]

Non-oral feeding and hydration will be necessary in patients with long oropharyngeal transit times (diagnosed clinically), those with more than 10% of swallowed material aspirated (diagnosed radiologically), and those who require more nutrition than they can manage orally. Nasogastric feeding, even with fine-bore tubes, is poorly tolerated by patients,[43] does not increase survival,[44,45] but does not appear to worsen aspiration.[46]

Percutaneous gastrostomy has advantages over nasogastric feeding,[47–49] with less aspiration.[50,51] Major complications of a percutaneous endoscopic gastrostomy (PEG) tube are low (<3%) but minor problems (blockage, leakage, local infection) occur in up to one-third.[52] It can have a lower complication rate in some patients,[53,54] but not in advanced cancer.[55] In head and neck cancer patients, complications are five times higher if the gastrostomy is radiologically placed, rather than endoscopically.[56] Despite this, the median survival times in selected advanced cancer patients after PEG placement is 61 days,[55] and PEGs are superior to NG tubes in stroke.[57] Even in elderly patients with dementia the median survival with a PEG can be nearly 6 months,[58] and prognosis is not worsened.[59] It can be inserted through an endoscope or under X-ray control if access is not possible with an endoscope.[60–63] Neither NG tube nor PEG feeding greatly reduce the sensation of hunger,[64,65] although hunger is not common in advanced disease.

Advantages of gastrostomy

Reduced risk of aspiration compared with nasogastric feeding
Preferred by patients to nasogastric tubes
Less pressure to eat orally for survival
Increasingly able to eat for pleasure
Shorter and less distressing mealtimes
Easier administration of medication
Reduced need for hospitalization

Disadvantages of gastrostomy

Serious adverse effect in 3%
Minor complications in one-third
Refeeding syndrome a risk
Gastric stasis needs to be treated
Feeding requires training or help

Advantages and disadvantages of gastrostomy

Pain: this is usually due to mucosal inflammation or damage (e.g. infection, dyspepsia, tumor) or muscle spasm. Mucosal pain can be difficult to treat, but topical treatments can help.[66]

Persisting dysphagia: other causes need to be considered such as neurological problems,[67–69] dental problems,[70–72] dyspepsia due to esophageal dysmotility or gastroesophageal reflux disease, and causes of chronic dysphagia.[27] It is also important to ensure attractive food presentation, privacy, and adequate staffing.[73]

At the end of life: hunger is not usually a problem,[74,75] and unwanted feeding by any route may increase distress.[76] Dehydration causes few symptoms at the end of life,[77] but may contribute to an agitated (hyperalert) delirium which will need non-oral hydration.[78,79] If the

Clinical decision	If YES carry out the action below
6 Is pain affecting swallowing?	• **For oral pain:** *see* cd-5 in *Oral problems*, p. 187. • **For head or neck cancer pain with a rapid onset** (i.e. developing over a few hours): consider occult infection and start metronidazole and cephalexin. • **Soft tissue pain:** use WHO analgesic ladder (*see Choosing an analgesic*, p. 57). • **Esophageal mucosal pain:** — treat any infection present (e.g. candidiasis, herpes, CMV) — for protection try sucralfate suspension 10 mL as required — if still troublesome use mixture of viscous lidocaine 2% 10 mL mixed with 20 mL of antacid ("pink lady"). An alternative is to use the topical action of opioids by swallowing a low dose of an opioid solution (e.g. 2.5–5 mg, or 10% of the 24-hour opioid dose).
7 Is the dysphagia persisting?	• **Does the patient feel the problem is at the level of the chest or abdomen?** In cancer, consider dexamethasone 8–16 mg once daily PO or SC to temporarily open the lumen. Otherwise arrange a barium swallow (but if aspiration is suspected ask for a small-volume gastrograffin swallow). If an abnormality is found on X-ray, refer to the gastroenterologists for endoscopy and manometry. • **Does the patient feel the problem is at the level of the mouth or throat?** Exclude oral problems: *see Oral problems*, p. 183. Check the oral to pharyngeal transit time (OPT) (= time from the first movement of the tongue to the last movement of the larynx). If the OPT is greater than 1 sec refer to a specialist speech and language therapist who can carry out a fuller assessment, and advise on management. OPT of >10 seconds means non-oral feeding is needed. • **Consider the following causes:** **Functional dyspepsia:** *see* cd-3 in *Dyspepsia*, p. 125. **Lambert–Eaton myasthenic syndrome (LEMS)** – seen in 3% of lung cancers. *See* p. 142 and cd-6 in *Fatigue, drowsiness, lethargy and weakness*, p. 155. **Pseudobulbar palsy** (e.g. ALS): refer to ENT team for consideration of a cricopharyngeal myotomy. **Stroke:** refer to the stroke team if available. **Dental problems** (e.g. missing teeth or dentures): refer to dentist. **Environmental:** good food presentation, privacy and adequate staffing are necessary if dysphagic patients are to keep up their fluid and nutritional intake.

Adapted from Regnard[25]
cd = clinical decision

dysphagia is due to exhaustion or fatigue caused by cancer, non-oral hydration and feeding are only appropriate if active cancer treatment is planned with the anticipation of full or partial recovery, or if the patient is thirsty (not just a dry mouth). In cases of doubt it is often possible to delay for several days. It is easier not to start a treatment than to stop it a short time later.

REFERENCES: DYSPHAGIA

B = book; C = comment; Ch = chapter; CS-n = case study-no. of cases; CT-n = controlled trial-no. of cases; E = editorial; GC = group consensus; I = interviews; LS = laboratory study; MC = multi-center; OS-n = open study-no. of cases; R, n refs = review, no. of references; RCT-n = randomized controlled trial-no. of cases; RS-n = retrospective survey-no. of cases; SA = systematic or meta analysis.

1 Roe JW, Leslie P, Drinnan MJ. (2007) Oropharyngeal dysphagia: the experience of patients with non-head and neck cancers receiving specialist palliative care. *Palliative Medicine*. **21**(7): 567–74. (OS-11)

2 Saunders C, Walsh TD, Smith M. (1981) *A Review of 100 Cases of Motor Neurone Disease in a Hospice*. London: Edward Arnold. (RS)

3 O'Brian T, Kelly M, Saunders C. (1992) Motor neurone disease: a hospice perspective. *British Medical Journal*. **304**: 471–3. (R)

4 Fuh JL, Lee RC, Lin CH, Wang SJ, Chiang JH, Liu HC. (1997) Swallowing difficulty in Parkinson's disease. *Clinical Neurology and Neurosurgery*. **99**: 106–12. (CT-109)

5 Thomas FJ, Wiles CM. (1999) Dysphagia and nutritional status in multiple sclerosis. *Journal of Neurology*. **246**: 677–82. (OS-78)

6 Wasson K, Tate H, Hayes C. (2001) Food refusal and dysphagia in older people with dementia: ethical and practical issues. *International Journal of Palliative Nursing*. **7**(10): 465–71. (R)

7 Foley N, Teasell R, Salter K, Kruger E, Martino R. (2008) Dysphagia treatment post stroke: a systematic review of randomised controlled trials. *Age and Ageing*. **37**(3): 258–64. (SA-15)

8 Rademaker AW, Pauloski BR, Colangelo LA, Logemann JA. (1998) Age and volume effects on liquid swallowing function in normal women. *Journal of Speech, Language and Hearing Research*. **41**: 275–84. (OS-167)

9 Kayser-Jones J, Pengilly K. (1999) Dysphagia among nursing home residents. *Geriatric Nursing*. **20**: 77–82. (OS-82)

10 Lefton-Greif MA, Arvedson JC. (2008) Schoolchildren with dysphagia associated with medically complex conditions. *Language, Speech and Hearing Services in the Schools*. **39**(2): 237–48. (CS)

11 Regan J, Sowman R, Walsh I. (2006) Prevalence of dysphagia in acute and community mental health settings. *Dysphagia*. **21**(2): 95–101. (OS-60)

12 Robertson MS, Hornibrook J. (1982) The presenting symptoms of head and neck cancer. *New Zealand Medical Journal*. **95**: 337–41.

13 Aird DW, Bihari J, Smith C. (1983). Clinical problems in the continuing care of head and neck cancer patients. *Ear Nose and Throat Journal*. **62**: 10–30.

14 Regnard CFB. (2003) Dysphagia, dyspepsia and hiccups. In: Calman K, Doyle D, Hanks GWC, eds. *Oxford Textbook of Palliative Medcine, 3rd ed.* Oxford: Oxford University Press. (Ch)

15 Trier JS, Bjorkman DJ. (1984) Esophageal, gastric and intestinal candidiasis. *American Journal of Medicine*. **77**: 39–43. (R)

16 Sheft DJ, Shrago G. (1970) Esophageal moniliasis, the spectrum of the disease. *Journal of the American Medical Association*. **213**: 1859–62. (R)

17 Logemann JA. (1983) *Evaluation and Treatment of Swallowing Disorders*. San Diego: College Hill Press. (B)

18 Ding R, Logemann JA. (2008) Patient self-perceptions of swallowing difficulties as compared to expert ratings of videofluorographic studies. *Folia Phoniatrica et Logopedica*. **60**(3): 142–50. (OS-103)

19 Logemann JA. (1985) Aspiration in head and neck surgical patients. *Annals of Otology, Rhinology and Laryngology*. **94**: 373–6.

20 Farell Z, O'Neill D. (1999) Towards better screening and assessment of oropharyngeal swallow disorders in the general hospital. *Lancet*. **354**: 355–6.

21 Hughes TA, Wiles CM. (1996) Palatal and pharyngeal reflexes in health and in motor neurone disease. *Journal of Neurology, Neurosurgery and Psychiatry*. **61**: 96–8. (CT-214)

22 Eckman S, Roe J. (2005). Speech and language therapists in palliative care: what do we have to offer? *International Journal of Palliative Nursing*. **11**(4): 179–81.

23 Pollens R. (2004). Role of the speech-language pathologist in palliative hospice care. *Journal of Palliative Medicine*. **7**(5): 694–702.

24 Ramsey D, Smithard D, Kalra L. (2005). Silent aspiration: what do we know? *Dysphagia*. **20**(3): 218–25.

25 Regnard C. (1995) Dysphagia. In: *Flow Diagrams in Advanced Cancer and Other Diseases*. London: Edward Arnold. pp. 19–21. (Ch)

26 Poertner LC, Coleman RF. (1998) Swallowing therapy in adults. *Otolaryngologic Clinics of North America*. **31**: 561–79. (R, 31 refs)

27 Leslie P, Carding PN, Wilson JA. (2003) Investigation and management of chronic dysphagia. *British Medical Journal*. **326**: 433–6. (R, 40 refs)

28 Tohara H, Saitoh E, Mays K, Kuhlemeier, Palmer JB. (2003). Three tests for predicting aspiration without videofluoroscopy. *Dysphagia*. **18**: 126–34.

29 Logemann JA, Gensler G, Robbins J, Lindblad AS, *et al.* (2008) A randomized study of three interventions for aspiration of thin liquids in patients with dementia or Parkinson's disease. *Journal of Speech Language and Hearing Research*. **51**(1): 173–83. (RCT-711)

30 Perie S, Laccourreye L, Flahault A, Hazebroucq V, Chaussade S, St. Guily J. (1998) Role of videoendoscopy in assessment of pharyngeal function in oropharyngeal dysphagia: comparison with videofluoroscopy and manometry. *Laryngoscope*. **108**: 1712–6. (OS-34)

31 Unsworth J. (1994) *Coping with the Disability of Established Disease*. London: Chapman and Hall Medical. (B)

32 Hargrove R. (1980) Feeding the severely dysphagic patient. *Journal of Neurosurgical Nursing*. **12**: 102–7. (R)

33 Carter RL, Pittam MR, Tanner NSB. (1982) Pain and dysphagia in patients with squamous carcinomas of the head and neck: the role of perineural spread. *Journal of the Royal Society of Medicine*. **75**: 598–606. (OS)

34 Brewster AE, Davidson SE, Makin WP, Stout R, Burt PA. (1995) Intraluminal brachytherapy using the high dose rate microselectron in the palliation of carcinoma of the oesophagus. *Clinical Oncology*. **7**: 102–5. (OS-197)

35 Aste H, Munizzi F, Martines H, Pugliese V. (1985) Esophageal dilation in malignant dysphagia. *Cancer.* **11**: 2713–5. (OS-38)

36 Carter R, Smith JS, Anderson JR. (1992) Laser recanalization *versus* endoscopic intubation in the palliation of malignant dysphagia: a randomized prospective study. *British Journal of Surgery*. **79**: 1167–70. (RCT-40)

37 Lewis-Jones CM, Sturgess R, Ellershaw JE. (1995) Laser therapy in the palliation of dysphagia in oesophageal malignancy. *Palliative Medicine*. **9**: 327–30. (R, 15 refs)

38 Tietjen TG, Pankaj JP, Kalloo AN. (1994) Management of malignant oesophageal stricture with oesophageal dilatation and oesophageal stents. *The Esophagus*. **4**: 851–62. (R, 45 refs)

39 Conio M, Repici A, Battaglia G, De Pretis G, *et al.* (2007) A randomized prospective comparison of self-expandable plastic stents and partially covered self-expandable metal stents in the palliation of malignant esophageal dysphagia. *American Journal of Gastroenterology*. **102**(12): 2667–77. (RCT-101)

40 Sundelof M, Ringby D, Stockeld D, Granstrom L, Jonas E, Freedman J. (2007) Palliative treatment of malignant dysphagia with self-expanding metal stents: a 12-year experience. *Scandinavian Journal of Gastroenterology*. **42**(1): 11–16. (RS-149)

41 Mason R. (1996) Palliation of malignant dysphagia: an alternative to surgery. *Annals of the Royal College of Surgeons of England*. **78**: 457–62. (RCT-474)

42 Singhvi R, Abbasakoor F, Manson JM. (2000) Insertion of self-expanding metal stents for malignant dysphagia: assessment of a simple endoscopic method. *Annals of the Royal College of Surgeons of England*. **82**: 243–8. (OS-50)

43 Scott AG, Austin HE. (1994) Nasogastric feeding in the management of severe dysphagia in motor neurone disease. *Palliative Medicine*. **8**: 45–9. (CT-31)

44 Mitchell SL, Kiely DK, Lipsitz LA. (1997) The risk factors and impact on survival of feeding tube placement in nursing home residents with severe cognitive impairment. *Archives of Internal Medicine*. **157**: 327–32. (OS-1386)

45 Finucane TE, Bynum JPW. (1996) Use of tube feeding to prevent aspiration pneumonia. *The Lancet*. **348**: 1421–4. (R, 28 refs)

46 Leder SB, Suiter DM. (2008) Effect of nasogastric tubes on incidence of aspiration. *Archives of Physical Medicine and Rehabilitation*. **89**(4): 648–51. (CT-1260)

47 Norton B, Homer-Ward M, Donelly MT, Long RG, Holmes GKT. (1996). A randomised prospective comparison of percutaneous endoscopic gastrostomy and nasogastric tube feeding after dysphagic stroke. *British Medical Journal*. **312**: 13–16.

48 Park RHR, Allison MC, Lang J, *et al.* (1992) Randomised comparison of percutaneous gastrostomy and nasogastric tube feeding in patients with persisting neurological dysphagia. *British Medical Journal*. **304**: 1406–9. (RCT-40)

49 Dwolatzky T, Berezovski S, Friedmann R, Paz J, Clarfield AM, Stessman J, Hamburger R, Jaul E, Friedlander Y, Rosin A, Sonnenblick M. (2001). A prospective comparison of the use of nasogastric and percutaneous endoscopic gastrostomy tubes for long-term enteral feeding in older people. *Clinical Nutrition*. **20**(6): 535–40.

50 Dwolatzky T, Berezovski S, Friedmann R, Paz J, *et al.* (2001) A prospective comparison of the use of nasogastric and percutaneous endoscopic gastrostomy tubes for long-term enteral feeding in older people. *Clinical Nutrition*. **20**(6): 535–40. (CT-122)

51 Gray DS, Kimmel D. (2006) Enteral tube feeding and pneumonia. *American Journal of Mental Retardation*. **111**(2): 113–20. (RS-93)

52 Keeley P. (2002) Feeding tubes in palliative care. *European Journal of Palliative Care*. **9**(6): 229–31. (R, 19 refs)

53 Hull MA, Rawlings J, Murray J, Murray FE, *et al.* (1993) Audit of outcome of long-term enteral nutrition by percutaneous endoscopic gastrostomy. *Lancet*. **341**: 869–72. (OS-49)

54 Dutta D, Bannerjee M, Chambers T. (2004) Is tube feeding associated with altered arterial oxygen saturation in stroke patients? *Age and Ageing*. **33**(5): 493–6. (CT-38)

55 Goncalves F, Mozes M, Saraiva I, Ramos C. (2006) Gastrostomies in palliative care. *Supportive Care in Cancer*. **14**(11): 1147–51. (RS-154)

56 Grant DG, Bradley PT, Pothier DD, Bailey D, *et al.* (2009) Complications following gastrostomy tube insertion in patients with head and neck cancer: a prospective multi-institution study, systematic review and meta-analysis. *Clinical Otolaryngology*. **34**(2): 103–12. (R, 44 refs)

57 Hamidon BB, Abdullah SA, Zawawi MF, Sukumar N, Aminuddin A, Raymond AA. (2006) A prospective comparison of percutaneous endoscopic gastrostomy and nasogastric tube feeding in patients with acute dysphagic stroke. *Medical Journal of Malaysia*. **61**(1): 59–66. (RCT-23)

58 Rimon E, Kagansky N, Levy S. (2005) Percutaneous endoscopic gastrostomy: evidence of different prognosis in various patient subgroups. *Age and Ageing*. **34**(4): 353–7. (OS-674)

59 Higaki F, Yokota O, Ohishi M. (2008) Factors predictive of survival after percutaneous endoscopic gastrostomy in the elderly: is dementia really a risk factor? *American Journal of Gastroenterology*. **103**(4): 1011–6. (CT-311)

60 Ashby M, Game P, Devitt P, Britten-Jones R, *et al.* (1991) Percutaneous gastrostomy as a venting procedure in palliative care. *Palliative Medicine*. **5**: 147–50.

61 Boyd KJ, Beeken L. (1994) Tube feeding in palliative care: benefits and problems. *Palliative Medicine*. **8**: 156–8. (CS-1)
62 Laing B, Smithers M, Harper J. (1994) Percutaneous fluoroscopic gastrostomy: a safe option? *Medical Journal of Australia*. **161**: 308–10. (RS-70)
63 Myssiorek D, Siegel D, Vambutas A. (1998) Fluoroscopically placed gastrostomies in the head and neck patient. *Laryngoscope*. **108**: 1557–60. (OS-35)
64 Stratton RJ, Stubbs RJ, Elia M. (1998) Interrelationship between circulating leptin concentrations, hunger, and energy intake in healthy subjects receiving tube feeding. *Journal of Parenteral and Enteral Nutrition*. **22**(6): 335–9. (CT-6)
65 Stratton RJ, Elia M. (1999) The effects of enteral tube feeding and parenteral nutrition on appetite sensations and food intake in health and disease. *Clinical Nutrition*. **18**(2): 63–70. (R, 79 refs)
66 Gairard-Dory AC, Schaller C, Mennecier B, *et al.* (2005) Chemoradiotherapy-induced esophagitis pain relieved by topical morphine: three cases. *Journal of Pain and Symptom Management*. **30**(2): 107–9. (CS-3)
67 Elrington G. (1992) The Lambert–Eaton myaesthenic syndromes. *Palliative Medicine*. **6**: 9–17. (R)
68 Leighton SEJ, Burton MJ, Lund WS, Cochrane GM. (1994) Swallowing in motor neurone disease. *Journal of the Royal Society of Medicine*. **87**: 801–5. (OS-92)
69 Daniels SK, Foundas AL. (1999) Lesion localization in acute stroke patients with risk of aspiration. *Journal of Neuroimaging*. **9**(2): 91–8. (OS-54)
70 Hildebrandt GH, Dominguez L, Schork MA, Loesche WJ. (1997) Functional units, chewing, swallowing and food avoidance among the elderly. *Journal of Prosthetic Dentistry*. **77**: 588–95. (OS-602)
71 Caruso AJ, Max L. (1997) Effects of aging on neuromotor processes of swallowing. *Seminars in Speech and Language*. **18**: 181–92. (R, 68 refs)
72 Aviv JE. (1997) Effects of aging on sensitivity of the pharyngeal and supraglottic areas. *American Journal of Medicine*. **103**(5A): S74–6. (CT-80)
73 Kayser-Jones J, Schell ES, Porter C, Barbaccia JC, Shaw H. (1999) Factors contributing to dehydration in nursing homes: inadequate staffing and lack of professional supervision. *Journal of the American Geriatrics Society*. **47**: 1187–94. (OS-40)
74 McCann RM, Hall WJ, Groth-Juncker A. (1994). Comfort care for terminally ill patients: the appropriate use of nutrition and hydration. *Journal of the American Medical Association*. **272**(16): 1263–6.
75 Parkash R, Burge F. (1997). The family's perspective on issues of hydration in terminal care. *Journal of Palliative Care*. **13**(4): 23–7.
76 Winter SM. (2000). Terminal nutrition: framing the debate for the withdrawal of nutritional support in terminally ill patients. *American Journal of Medicine*. **109**(9): 723–6.
77 Dunphy K, Finlay I, Rathbone G, Gilbert J, Hicks F. (1995). Rehydration in palliative and terminal care: if not – why not? *Palliative Medicine*. **9**(3): 221–8.
78 Fainsinger RL, Bruera E. (1997). When to treat dehydration in a terminally patient? *Supportive Care in Cancer*. **5**: 205–11.
79 Lawlor PG, Gagnon B, Mancini IL, Pereira JL, Hanson J, Suarez-Almazor ME, Bruera ED. (2000). Occurrence, causes, and outcome of delirium in patients with advanced cancer: a prospective study. *Archives of Internal Medicine*. **160**(6): 786–94.

Edema and lymphedema

CLINICAL DECISION AND ACTION CHECKLIST

1 Is there a cause of swelling other than edema?
2 Initiate skin care, gentle positioning and elevation.
3 Was the onset of the edema sudden?
4 Are there other reversible causes?
5 Encourage normal use and limb function.
6 Is massage indicated?
7 Is containment indicated?

KEY POINTS

- Edema is common in advanced disease, and assessing the cause is a prerequisite of treatment.
- Many signs and symptoms of edema suggest the cause, and some suggest the need for urgent investigation and treatment.
- Treatment is centered on skin care and limb positioning, together with support, exercise, massage, and containment bandaging or hosiery.

INTRODUCTION

Edema is the accumulation of excess fluid in the interstitial space of the tissues and occurs whenever the capillary filtration rate exceeds lymphatic drainage. Lymphedema is a specific term given to edema caused by impairment of lymph drainage.

Edema is a common problem of advanced disease, particularly malignancy. It can affect any part of the body, most commonly occurs in the limbs, but can also affect the trunk, genitalia and neck. It can also be a distressing symptom leading to immobility, pain, and discomfort, loss of function, altered body image, sexual difficulties, anxiety and depression.[1,2] In rare cases it can be associated with malignancy, a lymphangiosarcoma.[3–5]

CAUSES OF EDEMA

Under normal physiological conditions, there is a net filtration of fluid out of the capillaries into tissues. Some fluid returns to the capillaries while the excess is removed by the lymphatic system. In advanced disease there are often multiple factors at work that affect capillary filtration and lymphatic drainage.[6,7]

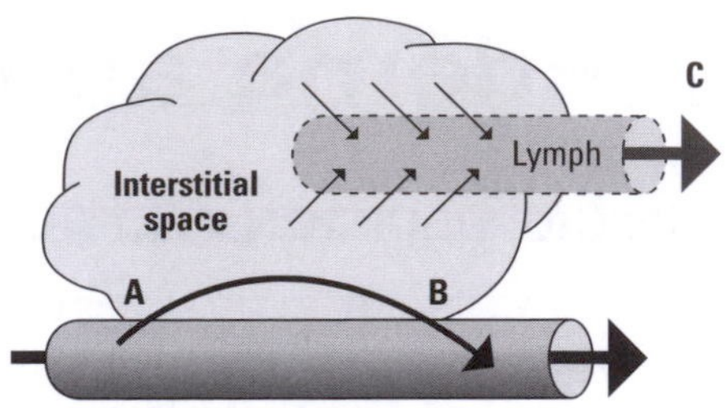

Capillary filtration and re-uptake of fluid

Causes of edema (adapted from CLiP)[11] (*see* text for explanation)

A. Increased filtration

Inflammation in the tissues (e.g. injury, infection) causes capillaries to leak, resulting in increased tissue fluid. Raised venous pressure leads to back pressure on the capillaries and a net increase in fluid filtration from the capillaries. Causes include heart failure, salt/water retention (which may be related to medication), venous thrombosis, venous stasis, and immobility leading to gravitational edema.

B. Reduced capillary re-uptake

If the serum protein level falls the blood cannot retain water as effectively and less water is removed from the interstitial space, resulting in fluid accumulating in the tissues. Causes of reduced protein include cachexia, malnutrition, malabsorption, nephrotic syndrome, and liver failure.

C. Reduced lymphatic drainage

In the northern hemisphere this is most commonly caused by damage or blockage of the lymphatics due to cancer and/or its treatment.[8,9] This reduces their ability to remove tissue fluid, which then accumulates. Lymphatic function can also be compromised by absent, insufficient, or poorly functioning lymphatics (e.g. congenital "primary lymphedema")[10] or by immobility leading to reduced muscle action on the lymphatics. If any cause of edema is present for long enough it will lead to secondary lymphedema, especially with repeated episodes of cellulitis.

FEATURES OF EDEMA

Assessment of the edema should include:

- its speed of onset and distribution
- appearance of the skin (color, temperature, integrity, consistency)
- associated symptoms (pain, sensory changes, breathlessness).

Features suggesting urgent investigation

These include the sudden onset of edema, pain (edema is not usually painful), new distended veins, skin color changes, and breathlessness.

Acute vena cava obstruction: features include sudden onset (hours to days), bilateral limb edema (with or without midline edema of head or genitals), soft pitting edema, and a dusky purplish hue. Headache is a feature of superior vena cava obstruction (SVCO).

Venous thrombosis: This often presents with a sudden onset of unilateral or asymmetrical tense edema which may be painful or tender.[12] There may be a dusky purplish hue and distended veins which persist on elevation.

Heart failure: acute or uncontrolled chronic heart failure may present with

Clinical decision	If YES carry out the action below
1 Is there a cause of swelling other than edema?	• **Consider other causes of swelling:** e.g. tumor, lipedema, steroid-induced truncal obesity, hematoma, surgical emphysema, organomegaly, ascites, and hypertrophy.
2 Establish treatment priority in the context of what is happening to the patient, and consider the likely causes. Initiate skin care, gentle positioning, and elevation.	
3 Was the onset of edema sudden?	• **Venous thrombosis** (sudden, localized, tense edema which may be painful or tender, dusky purplish hue, distended veins despite limb elevation): — arrange urgent ultrasound. If a thrombosis is confirmed consider immediate treatment with low molecular weight heparin (e.g. tinzaparin) unless anticoagulation is contraindicated (e.g. bleeding tendency). • **Cellulitis** (skin red or flushed, usually warmer than surrounding skin): — start oral amoxicillin 500 mg q8h for a minimum of 2 weeks. Use clindamycin 300 mg q6h for patients who are allergic to penicillin or where there is a poor response to oral amoxicillin after 48 hours. Consider intravenous antibiotics if there are signs of septicemia. — avoid exercise in the acute phase — edema treatment (as described in text) can be used under specialist advice and monitoring. • **Acute vena cava obstruction** (bilateral edema, midline edema, dusky color to skin, headache in SVCO): *see* cd-9d in *Emergencies*, p. 345. • **Arterial insufficiency** (white or mottled skin, poor capillary filling, poor or absent pulses): — transfer urgently to vascular surgeons, but if too ill for surgery ensure adequate analgesia (*see* cd-8 in *Diagnosing and treating pain*, p. 53) — avoid containment bandaging or compression hosiery.
4 Are there other reversible causes?	• **Lymphatic obstruction by tumor:** consider dexamethasone, initially 6 mg PO once daily. Consider chemotherapy in sensitive tumors. • **Ventricular (heart) failure:** treat conventionally. • **Drugs** (e.g. NSAIDs, prednisolone, calcium antagonists, gabapentin): change drug if possible. • **Anemia:** treat cause and/or transfuse. • **Ascites:** *see Ascites*, p. 87.
5 Encourage normal use and limb function (*see* text p. 143).	

cd = clinical decision

very soft pitting edema, episodes of breathlessness exacerbated by lying flat, and waking breathless at night.

Cellulitis: this should be considered in all patients with erythema of the skin. It is usually warmer than the surrounding area or other limb, but in patients with edema it can appear as a diffuse rash that is a similar temperature to other areas. It may be associated with pain, a recent increase in swelling and the person may feel systemically unwell or have a pyrexia.

Local malignancy: this may present as demarcated lesions in the skin, which may have raised edges or satellite lesions. These may advance quite rapidly over days or weeks and may ulcerate.

Other causes of edema

Chronic vena cava obstruction: the onset of edema may be more gradual, but because of the development of collateral circulation, distended prominent veins over the trunk may be visible.

Venous incompetence: in chronic edema of venous origin, the distal limb often has a dusky purplish hue and distended varicose veins which collapse when elevated. Thread veins may occur particularly around the ankle, possibly with skin ulceration.

Dependency/gravitational edema: this tends to start as soft pitting edema of the lower legs and is often associated with reduced mobility.

Lipedema: this is an abnormal distribution of adipose tissue. There are large skin folds, tissues are doughy to palpation, non-pitting, but tender and easily bruised. There is a dimpled appearance and the fat deposition is frequently bilateral, with a "pantaloon" effect at ankles or wrists and a relatively normal shape to the feet and hands.

Features of lymphedema

The limb size increases gradually. In early stages the edema may be soft and pit easily on digital pressure, but does not pit easily in the later stages. Mounds of swelling develop in the dorsum of the feet or hands. Although skin color can be normal or paler, the consistency is very different to normal with thickened skin and deepened skin folds. These changes result in a positive Stemmer's sign – the inability to pick up a fold of tissue at the base of the second toe.

In advanced stages, secondary skin changes progress. Fibrosis results in hardening and thickening of skin and subcutaneous tissues. Papillomatosis occurs with cobblestone-like projections representing dilated skin lymphatics surrounded by fibrosed tissue. Lymphangiectasia (also known as lymphangiomas) are soft fluid-filled projections caused by dilatation of lymphatic vessels. These can lead to lymphorrhea, leakage of lymph through the skin. Hyperkeratosis (build-up of horny scales of keratin on the surface of the skin) is common and in the legs this often starts anterior to the ankles.

TREATMENT

The focus is on skin care, limb positioning and support, exercise, massage, and containment.[13,14] Skin care and limb positioning can be undertaken in all cases, while the introduction of the other components of care needs to be considered in the context of the patient's condition and the underlying cause of the edema.

Clinical decision	If YES carry out the action below
6 Is massage indicated?	Lymphatic drainage (massage) is indicated in truncal and midline edema, lymphedema, and to promote comfort and pain relief. • Refer to lymphedema team or clinic, either to teach simple lymphatic drainage to the carer, or to undergo manual lymph drainage.
7 Is containment indicated?	*NB. Do not use containment without specialist advice if the following are present:* severe ventricular failure, AB (ankle/brachial) blood pressure ratio less than 0.8, sensation is absent, any microcirculatory problems (vasculitis, diabetes), or within 8 weeks of a venous thrombosis. • **If this is uncomplicated edema** (regular shape to limb, intact and healthy skin), and if patient and/or carer can tolerate and manage hosiery: — refer to hosiery specialist who can fit appropriate hosiery. • **If this is complicated edema** (fragile or broken skin, distorted or large limb shape, lymphorrhea): — refer to specialist lymphedema team or clinic.

cd = clinical decision

Skin care

Effective skin care optimizes the skin condition and minimizes the risk of skin problems which can lead to fungal infection and/or cellulitis. This includes, on a daily basis:

Washing using pH neutral soap, carefully drying the skin including any skin folds and areas between the fingers or toes.

Moisturizing: applying an appropriate non-perfumed emollient to hydrate the skin, e.g. Glaxal base.

Minimizing the risk of trauma to the skin, e.g. avoiding venepuncture in the affected limb.[15]

Observing skin condition for signs of potential problems (e.g. fungal infection, cellulitis, skin breaks, folliculitis) and treating them accordingly.

Limb positioning and support

The affected limb should be elevated at least to just above the level of the heart, although any elevation can be helpful. This reduces edema by promoting lymphatic and venous return and prevents further aggravation of swelling by reducing capillary pressure It can also promote comfort in the very ill (e.g. by placing soft pillows beneath the edematous legs of a bed-bound patient).

Exercise

This stimulates lymphatic and venous drainage, and promotes mobility and function in the affected limb.[16] The main principles are:

Encourage normal use and limb function wherever possible. For patients who are severely ill or bed bound, passive movements of a swollen limb can reduce stiffness and discomfort.

Avoid excessive exercise, as this aggravates swelling. The patient should wear any compression stockings or garments prescribed for them, both during exercise and for at least an hour afterwards. Avoid exercise if the patient has cellulitis.

Consider physiotherapy referral for patients with mobility difficulties and joint function/movement problems.

Lymphedema management

Where complicated lymphedema is identified, refer to a specialist service, if available, for further assessment of the patient's lymphedema and review of appropriate management options. These are determined by the site, stage, severity and complexity of the swelling, and require the input of a trained practitioner.

Lymphatic drainage

Massage assists in managing edema and providing comfort by promoting lymph flow from congested areas and protein removal from the tissues.[17,18] It can be particularly beneficial in truncal and midline edema (e.g. head/neck, breast, chest, genital, back, abdomen); as a key part of lymphedema management and to promote comfort and pain relief.

Contraindications are cellulitis, venous thrombosis, vena cava obstruction, and heart failure. In some of these cases massage may be recommended with caution, for example, if the disease is advanced and the potential benefits of massage outweigh any burdens. Active cancer (where the patient is currently undergoing treatment) is often believed to be a contraindication, but there is no evidence that massage stimulates metastatic spread.[19] A trained practitioner will advise.

There are two main recognized forms of massage in edema management:

Manual lymphatic drainage (MLD) is a gentle but highly specialized technique, undertaken by specially trained and accredited practitioners.[20] This has the advantage of producing rapid reductions in edema in the first few days of treatment,[21] and continues to improve quality of life in the subsequent months of treatment.[22,23]

Simple lymphatic drainage (SLD) is a simplified version of MLD that patients, relatives/carers, and health care professionals can be taught by a trained therapist, or by another health care professional with knowledge and experience of SLD.[24]

Containment

Containment, through the use of bandaging or compression hosiery, plays an important role in reducing and controlling swelling.[25] External support, particularly when combined with muscular activity, stimulates lymphatic and venous drainage. Bandaging and containment garments should only be prescribed and applied following a holistic clinical evaluation of the underlying causes of the patient's edema and their physical and psychosocial needs. Doppler ultrasound can be used as part of the vascular assessment but should only be carried out by an appropriately trained practitioner. It is used to measure the arterial systolic pressures at the dorsalis pedis and brachial arteries – the ankle/brachial (AB) blood pressure ratio should be above 0.8 to allow bandaging or hosiery to be applied safely.

Bandages are either inelastic with a low extensibility (applying a lower resting pressure and a higher working pressure) or elastic (applying a higher resting pressure, but a lower working pressure). Bandaging is a specialized technique, and should only be applied by a practitioner/carer who has received an appropriate level of training. The choice of bandaging is dependent on the cause of the edema and the patient's individual condition and needs.[26] Indications for bandaging include fragile, damaged or ulcerated skin, distorted limb shape, pronounced skin folds, a limb that is too large for compression garments, lymphatic leakage (lymphorrhea), and secondary changes in the skin and subcutaneous tissues associated with chronic edema. Bandaging is recognized as relatively contraindicated in cases of severe arterial insufficiency, acute cardiac failure, cellulitis, DVT and severe peripheral neuropathy. However, in some of these situations it is possible for bandaging to be applied with caution, depending on the patient's specific medical condition and with ongoing monitoring and evaluation at frequent intervals.

Compression hosiery may be an appropriate alternative to bandaging where the limb shape is regular with minimal distortion, the skin is intact and resilient, and the patient can tolerate and manage hosiery (if necessary, with carer support). Where edema is labile or fluctuates, suitable garments may be difficult to apply. The general contraindications and cautions are similar to those for bandaging, although additionally compression hosiery is not recommended where the skin is in a fragile condition or there is extensive ulceration, extreme limb shape distortion, very deep skin folds or lymphorrhea. Compression garments are available in a range of different compression classes, sizes and styles, and should therefore only be prescribed by a health care professional with detailed knowledge and appropriate training in their role in edema management. The health care professional should also provide the patient/carer with advice on the correct application and positioning of the garment, the maximum length of time the garment should be worn, when to perform skin care and how to care for the garment to ensure its continued efficacy.

Cellulitis

Acute phase: This needs urgent treatment with antibiotics since it can cause systemic illness and damage lymphatics. Obtaining cultures is difficult, but some evidence and current opinion suggests the usual infective organism is a *Streptococcus* rather than *Staphylococcus* and responds to antistreptococcal antibiotics.[27–30] The standard treatment is therefore amoxicillin. Cloxacillin may be effective, especially in the presence of folliculitis in which *Staphylococcus* is the likely organism. Erythromycin is used for those allergic to penicillins, and clindamycin is reserved for those who fail to respond.

Preventative management: abnormal lymphatic drainage can predispose to infection so improving lymphatic function through exercise, massage, and containment are important adjuncts in preventing infection.[31] Patients who have two or more episodes of cellulitis in a year should be offered antibiotic prophylaxis. Penicillin V 500 mg daily (1 g if weight >70 kg) should be the first choice,[32] with erythromycin 250 mg daily for those allergic to penicillin.

Other treatments

Pneumatic compression is limited to simple edema.[33]

Drugs: diuretics can help simple edema, but not lymphedema.[34] Corticosteroids have a role in lymphatic obstruction due to tumor. Although benzopyrones may be beneficial, the evidence base is poor.[34–36] Sodium selenite has been reported in small trials to reduce lymphedema volume, especially after radiotherapy.[37]

TENS has been shown to reduce primary lymphedema.[38]

Surgery has little place in lymphedema management, except in extreme cases where opinion should be sought from a specialist team.

Kinesio taping: specialized skin tape may also be used in conjunction with other containment treatments and massage to increase the effective superficial lymphatic drainage from a site. It is particularly useful in complicated edema conditions distal to scarring, e.g. following extensive head and neck surgery or in midline edema. This should only be applied by professionals with the appropriate level of training.

Subcutaneous drainage (reverse hypodermoclysis): This has been suggested for patients in the last days of life with distressing lower limb edema.[39,40] However, this has been tried in only a few cases, has not been compared with low compression support, and the risks of infection have not been assessed in patients who survive longer than expected.[41]

Edema in children

Edema can occur in children from all the above-mentioned causes – the commonest being primary or congenital lymphedema – or associated with other connective tissue conditions such as juvenile chronic arthritis, psoriasis, and Turner's syndrome. Edema secondary to cancer and/or treatment is rarer but does occur. The same long-term management principles apply for children (skin care, exercise, elevation, and compression) but referral to specialist lymphedema clinics is strongly recommended. Cellulitis is treated in the same way, using amoxicillin, or clindamycin, but with a low threshold for IV antibiotics if systemically unwell.

REFERENCES: EDEMA AND LYMPHEDEMA

B = book; C = comment; Ch = chapter; CS-n = case study-no. of cases; CT-n = controlled trial-no. of cases; E = editorial; GC = group consensus; I = interviews; LS = laboratory study; MC = multi-center; OS-n = open study-no. of cases; R = review; RCT-n = randomized controlled trial-no. of cases; RS-n = retrospective survey-no. of cases; SA = systematic or meta analysis.

1 Twycross R. (2000) Pain in lymphoedema. In: Twycross R, Jenns K, Todd J, eds. *Lymphoedema*. Oxford: Radcliffe Medical Press. pp. 69–88. (Ch)
2 Woods M. (2000) Psychosocial aspects of lymphoedema. In: Twycross R, Jenns K, Todd J, eds. *Lymphoedema*. Oxford: Radcliffe Medical Press. pp. 89–96. (Ch)
3 Mulvenna P, Gillham L, Regnard CFB. (1995) Lymphangiosarcoma: experience in a lymphoedema clinic. *Palliative Medicine*. **9**: 55–9. (CS-3)
4 Hildebrandt G, Mittag M, Gutz U, Kunze ML, Haustein UF. (2001) Cutaneous breast angiosarcoma after conserving treatment of breast cancer. *European Journal of Dermatology*. **11**(6): 580–3.
5 Majeski J, Austin RM, Fitzgerald RH. (2000) Cutaneous angiosarcoma in an irradiated breast after breast conservation surgery: association with chronic breast lymphoedema. *Journal of Surgical Oncology*. **74**(3): 208–12.
6 Stanton A. (2000) How does tissue swelling occur? The physiology and pathophysiology of interstitial fluid formation. In: Twycross R, Jenns K, Todd J, eds. *Lymphoedema*. Oxford: Radcliffe Medical Press. pp. 11–21. (Ch)
7 Topham EJ, Mortimer PS. (2002) Chronic lower limb oedema. *Clinical Medicine*. **2**(1): 28–31. (R, 4 refs)
8 Keeley V. (2000) Classification of lymphoedema. In: Twycross R, Jenns K, Todd J, eds. *Lymphoedema*. Oxford: Radcliffe Medical Press. pp. 22–43. (Ch)
9 Lee TS, Kilbreath SL, Refshauge KM, Herbert RD, Beith JM. (2008) Prognosis of the upper limb following surgery and radiation for breast cancer. *Breast Cancer Research and Treatment*. **110**(1): 19–37. (R, 57 refs)
10 Connell FC, Ostergaard P, Carver C, Brice G, Williams N, Mansour S, Mortimer PS, Jeffery S. (2009) Lymphoedema Consortium. Analysis of the coding regions of VEGFR3 and VEGFC in Milroy disease and other primary lymphoedemas. *Human Genetics*. **124**(6): 625–31. (OS-52)
11 Regnard C, Hughes A. (2004) Oedema. In: CLiP (Current Learning in Palliative Care). See www.helpthehospices.org.uk/clip (accessed 24 September 2009).
12 Kirkova J, Oneschuk D, Hanson J. (2005) Deep vein thrombosis (DVT) in advanced cancer patients with lower extremity edema referred for assessment. *The American Journal of Hospice and Palliative Care*. **22**(2): 145–9. (RS)
13 Lymphoedema Support Network. Available on www.lymphoedema.org/lsn (accessed January 2009).
14 Karadibak D, Yavuzsen T, Saydam S. (2008) Prospective trial of intensive decongestive physiotherapy for upper extremity lymphedema. *Journal of Surgical Oncology*. **97**(7): 572–7. (OS-62)
15 Smith J. (1998) The practice of venepuncture in lymphoedema. *European Journal of Cancer Care*. **7**(2): 97–8. (OS)
16 Hughes K. (2000) Exercise and lymphoedema. In: Twycross R, Jenns K, Todd J, eds. *Lymphoedema*. Oxford: Radcliffe Medical Press. pp. 140–64. (Ch)
17 Mortimer PS, Simmonds R, Rezvani M, Robbins M, Hopewell JW, Ryan TJ. (1990) The measurement of skin lymph flow by isotope clearance: reliability, reproductibility, injections dynamics and the effect of massage. *Journal of Investigative Dermatology*. **95**: 677–82. (OS)
18 Keeley V. (2009) Lymphoedema. In: Hanks G, Cherney NI, Christakis NA, Fallon M, Kaasa S, Portenoy RK, eds. *Oxford Textbook of Palliative Medicine, 4th ed*. Oxford: Oxford University Press. pp. 972–82. (Ch)
19 Godette K, Mondry TE, Johnstone PA. (2006) Can manual treatment of lymphedema promote metastasis? *Journal of the Society for Integrative Oncology*. **4**(1): 8–12. (R, 34 refs)
20 Leduc A, Leduc O. (2000) Manual lymph drainage.

In: Twycross R, Jenns K, Todd J, eds. *Lymphoedema*. Oxford: Radcliffe Medical Press. pp. 203–16. (Ch)

21 Yamamoto T, Todo Y, Kaneuchi M, Handa Y, Watanabe K, Yamamoto R. (2008) Study of edema reduction patterns during the treatment phase of complex decongestive physiotherapy for extremity lymphedema. *Lymphology*. **41**(2): 80–6. (OS-83)

22 Kim SJ, Yi CH, Kwon OY. (2007) Effect of complex decongestive therapy on edema and the quality of life in breast cancer patients with unilateral lymphedema. *Lymphology*. **40**(3): 143–51. (OS-53)

23 Hamner JB, Fleming MD. (2007) Lymphedema therapy reduces the volume of edema and pain in patients with breast cancer. *Annals of Surgical Oncology*. **14**(6): 1904–8. (OS-135)

24 Bellhouse S. (2000) Simple lymphatic drainage. In: Twycross R, Jenns K, Todd J, eds. *Lymphoedema*. Oxford: Radcliffe Medical Press. pp. 216–35. (Ch)

25 Todd J. (2000) Containment in the management of lymphoedema. In: Twycross R, Jenns K, Todd J, eds. *Lymphoedema*. Oxford: Radcliffe Medical Press. pp. 165–202. (Ch)

26 Badger CM, Peacock JL, Mortimer PS. (2000) A randomized, controlled, parallel-group clinical trial comparing multilayer bandaging followed by hosiery versus hosiery alone in the treatment of patients with lymphedema of the limb. *Cancer*. **88**(12): 2832–7. (RCT-90)

27 Cox NH, Colver GB, Paterson WD. (1998) Management and morbidity of cellulitis of the leg. *Journal of the Royal Society of Medicine*. **91**(12): 634–7. (RS-92)

28 Cox NH. (2006) Oedema as a risk factor for multiple episodes of cellulitis/erysipelas of the lower leg: a series with community follow-up. *British Journal of Dermatology*. **155**(5): 947–50. (RS-171)

29 Lazzarini L, Conti E, Tositti G, de Lalla F. (2005) Erysipelas and cellulitis: clinical and microbiological spectrum in an Italian tertiary care hospital. *Journal of Infection*. **51**(5): 383–9. (RS-200)

30 Peralta G, Padron E, Roiz MP, De Benito I, *et al*. (2006) Risk factors for bacteremia in patients with limb cellulitis. *European Journal of Clinical Microbiology and Infectious Diseases*. **25**(10): 619–26. (RS-308)

31 Damstra RJ, van Steensel MA, Boomsma JH, Nelemans P, Veraart JC. (2008) Erysipelas as a sign of subclinical primary lymphoedema: a prospective quantitative scintigraphic study of 40 patients with unilateral erysipelas of the leg. *British Journal of Dermatology*. **158**(6): 1210–15. (OS-40)

32 Vignes S, Dupuy A. (2006) Recurrence of lymphoedema-associated cellulitis (erysipelas) under prophylactic antibiotherapy: a retrospective cohort study. *Journal of the European Academy of Dermatology and Venereology*. **20**(7): 818–22. (RS-43)

33 Bray T, Barrett J. (2000) Pneumatic compression therapy. In: Twycross R, Jenns K, Todd J, eds. *Lymphoedema*. Oxford: Radcliffe Medical Press. pp. 236–43. (Ch)

34 Twycross R. (2000) Drug treatment for lymphoedema. In: Twycross R, Jenns K, Todd J, eds. *Lymphoedema*. Oxford: Radcliffe Medical Press. pp. 244–70. (Ch)

35 Keeley V. (2008) Pharmacological treatment for chronic oedema. *British Journal of Community Nursing*. **13**(4): S4, S6, S8–10. (R, 15 refs)

36 Badger C, Preston N, Seers K, Mortimer P. (2004) Benzo-pyrones for reducing and controlling lymphoedema of the limbs. *Cochrane Database of Systematic Reviews*. **2**: CD003140. (R, 80 refs)

37 Bruns F, Micke O, Bremer M. (2003) Current status of selenium and other treatments for secondary lymphedema. *Journal of Supportive Oncology*. **1**: 121–30.

38 Waller A, Bercovitch M. (2000) Novel treatments: transcutaneous electrical nerve stimulation. In: Twycross R, Jenns K, Todd J, eds. *Lymphoedema*. Oxford: Radcliffe Medical Press. pp. 271–84. (Ch)

39 Clein LJ, Pugachev E. (2004) Reduction of edema of lower extremities by subcutaneous, controlled drainage: eight cases. *American Journal of Hospice and Palliative Care*. **21**(3): 228–32. (CS-8)

40 Faily J, de Kock I, Mirhosseini M, Fainsinger R. (2007) The use of subcutaneous drainage for the management of lower limb edema in cancer patients. *Journal of Palliative Care*. **23**: 185–7. (CS-1)

41 Sant K. (2007) Reduction of oedema by subcutaneous drainage. *BLS (British Lymphology Society) News and Views*. **63**: 8. (R)

NOTES

Fatigue, drowsiness, lethargy and weakness

CLINICAL DECISION AND ACTION CHECKLIST

1 Is the prognosis very short (day-by-day deterioration)?
2 Has the patient's alertness reduced rapidly?
3 Has the patient's alertness reduced slowly?
4 Is postural hypotension present?
5 Is the weakness, lethargy, or fatigue all over the body?
6 Is the weakness localized?
7 Is the problem persisting?

KEY POINTS

- Fatigue is the commonest symptom in advanced disease.
- Drowsiness, tiredness, lethargy, fatigue, and weakness have different meanings for different patients.
- Consider reversible causes, but fatigue, drowsiness, lethargy, and weakness are also a part of the natural dying process.
- Dexamethasone is not first-line treatment.

INTRODUCTION

Fatigue is the commonest symptom in advanced disease and is reported in up to 80% of patients. Although it is as common as pain,[1] patients often view it as more troublesome than pain, nausea, or vomiting.[2–5] The effects of fatigue can be profound, including a negative effect on hope.[6] It occurs as commonly in AIDS, heart disease, rheumatic disease, pulmonary disease, and renal disease as in cancer.[7,8] Although many patients use a common set of words, patients use them to describe different symptoms that range from drowsiness to paralysis. Consequently, some additional exploration of the complaint is needed.

THE WORDS PATIENTS USE

Drowsiness, reduced alertness, tiredness, fatigue, lethargy, and weakness have different meanings for different patients and their carers:[3]

Drowsiness: patients usually link this to a sensation of wanting to sleep.

Reduced alertness may be due to drowsiness but can be due to causes that make patients less aware of their surroundings.

Tiredness is often linked to mild energy loss, although some patients use the term to describe drowsiness.

Lethargy can be used to describe low mood or depression, but may also be used to describe fatigue or weakness.

Weakness is usually used to describe a loss of physical strength, but patients and carers can use the terms fatigue and weakness interchangeably.[9] When due to fatigue, the weakness is usually perceived as generalized, but the profound muscle loss that can occur in cachexia also will cause a generalized muscle weakness. Localized weakness is invariably due to neurological lesions.

Fatigue: in contrast, fatigue is perceived by patients as more severe and persistent than tiredness.[10] It can be accompanied by a lack of energy, exhaustion, restlessness, boredom, lack of interest in activities, weakness, dyspnea, pain, altered taste, and itching.[10,11] The concept of fatigue seems to be a combination of physical sensations (e.g. slowing up), affective sensations (e.g. irritability, loss of interest) and cognitive sensations (e.g. loss of concentration).[12,13] Although fatigue is different to drowsiness (since it does not improve with sleep)[14] or weakness (since there is no reduction in muscle strength), many of these conditions coexist.

CAUSES

Dying

Patients deteriorating day-by-day because of their underlying disease often have fatigue, drowsiness, lethargy, or weakness. This is a natural part of dying, but can be an important opportunity to open discussions with the patient and family about what is happening.

Reduced alertness

Rapid onset: reduced alertness occurring in minutes or hours needs urgent review. Drugs are a common cause of sudden drowsiness, especially if they are given parenterally, or their rate of elimination alters rapidly (e.g. the onset of acute renal failure in a patient on morphine). Other possible causes are severe infection, hypoglycemia, hypercalcemia, hemorrhage, hypoadrenalism (adrenal insufficiency or steroid withdrawal), hypercapnia (due to chronic respiratory failure), and metabolic crises (especially in children with congenital metabolic disease). Delirium is associated with altered alertness, usually a reduction.

Slow onset: reduced alertness occurring over days or weeks may be due to drug accumulation (e.g. diazepam), hyperglycemia, organ failure (liver or kidney), endocrine problems such as hypothyroidism, or chronic hypercapnia. Disturbed sleep is associated with fatigue.[14] Sleep may be disturbed by many problems such as physical symptoms (e.g. pain, sleep apnea), depression, and anxiety. Depression and anxiety are associated with fatigue.[15]

Hypotension

A number of problems can reduce blood pressure and many are associated with fatigue, drowsiness, and lethargy. Autonomic failure is common in advanced disease[16–18] and symptoms include hypotension (causing dizziness on standing or associated with eating),

Clinical decision	If YES carry out the action below
1 Is the prognosis very short?	e.g. day-by-day deterioration due to an irreversible cause. • Any Fatigue, drowsiness, lethargy and weakness is likely to be a natural part of the dying process and no action will be needed.
2 Has the patient's alertness reduced rapidly? (i.e. drowsiness or reduced awareness over minutes or hours)	• **Bleeding:** *see Bleeding*, p. 93. • **Drugs:** many drugs may cause this, not just opioids. If the sedation is unwanted by the patient, reduce or change the drug. If the sedation was rapid, consider partial reversal if an antagonist is available, e.g. naloxone for opioids (for correct procedure *see* cd-3b in *Emergencies*, p. 333) or flumazenil for benzodiazepines. Antagonists are short-acting and often need repeated doses or infusions. • **Epilepsy:** minor or major seizures. If the cause is known, start sodium valproate 300 mg q12h (for children 20 mg/kg in divided doses) and titrate to control the symptoms (unlike phenytoin, valproate treats major and minor seizures, has few drug interactions and is easier to titrate). • **Hypercapnia:** if due to inappropriately high inhaled oxygen concentration then reduce oxygen to 24% and aim for S_pO_2 of 88–90%.[19] • **Hypoadrenalism** (adrenal insufficiency, steroid withdrawal): hydrocortisone 100 mg IV, then continue with oral hydrocortisone (20 mg on waking, 10 mg at 4pm) and fludrocortisone (100–200 microg on waking). • **Hypoglycemia** (e.g. treated diabetic on little or no diet): *see* cd-7d in *Emergencies*, p. 341. • **Raised intracranial pressure due to tumor:** try high-dose dexamethasone (16 mg daily) and consider referral for cranial irradiation. Consider an MRI scan to exclude hydrocephalus. • **Respiratory depression:** *see* cd-3b in *Emergencies*, p. 333. • **Severe infection:** take cultures if possible and start IV antibiotics according to local policies.
3 Has the patient's alertness reduced slowly? (i.e. drowsiness or reduced awareness over days or weeks)	• **Delirium:** *see Confusional states*, p. 245. • **Hypercalcemia:** *see* cd-7b in *Emergencies*, p. 341. • **Accumulation of drugs with a long half-life** (e.g. diazepam, amitriptyline): it takes 5 half-lives to reach a steady state. Tolerance to the sedative effect may occur, but otherwise reduce the daily dose or change the drug. • **Hyperglycemia** (e.g. corticosteroids): *see* cd-7c in *Emergencies*, p. 341. • **Organ failure** (renal, hepatic): refer for specialist care if the prognosis allows. • **Poor quality sleep:** treat any physical symptom that wakes the patient. Exclude sleep apnea, depression, and anxiety. Treat the cause if possible. Avoid late-night caffeine. Consider temazepam 10–30 mg or similar at night. • **Tumor load** (*see* p. 152): dexamethasone PO 2–4 mg once daily. • **Hypercapnia:** refer to respiratory physician for advice, especially if non-invasive ventilation is an option (*see Respiratory problems*, p. 192). • **Frequent partial (minor) seizures:** check for exacerbating factors and review anticonvulsants. • **Hypothyroidism/hypoadrenalism:** evaluate and treat as appropriate.

Adapted from Regnard and Mannix[20]
cd = clinical decision

fatigue, syncope, inability to sweat, impotence, bladder symptoms (including incontinence), and gastric stasis. If the cause cannot be treated, simple measures or the use of midodrine to increase blood pressure can help (*see* cd-4 opposite).[21–23] However, some of the other symptoms such as sexual dysfunction will need additional help (*see Urinary problems and sexual difficulties*, p. 223).[24]

Generalized fatigue and lethargy

The possibilities include infection, anemia, breathlessness, cachexia, depression, drugs, low sodium (SIADH-syndrome of inappropriate ADH, chest infection, diuretics), hypercapnia, low potassium (diuretics, corticosteroids, vomiting and/or diarrhea), high calcium (due to cancer), low magnesium[25,26] (poor nutrition or chemotherapy), low oxygen levels (chest infection, pleural effusion, lung metastases), nutritional deficiency, psychological causes (severe anxiety, clinical depression), or recent surgery.[27] In advanced cancer fatigue may be related to low cortisol levels.[28] Anemia, unless severe, is not a major cause of fatigue or lethargy in palliative care patients.[29] Chemotherapy and radiotherapy both cause generalized fatigue which peaks 1–2 weeks after chemotherapy,[30] and at the end of a course of radiotherapy,[30,31] diminishing after 3 weeks.[32]

Pro-inflammatory cytokines such as tumor necrosis factor (TNFα) and interleukin 1 and 6 may partly mediate fatigue.[33–35] These mediators play a major role in the pathophysiology of cachexia, fever, anemia and infection, all of which aggravate fatigue. Corticosteroids can suppress their production[36] and produce a temporary but worthwhile increase in well-being.[37]

Localized weakness

Proximal weakness (weakness of muscles closest to the trunk) can be caused by corticosteroids, low potassium, thyroid abnormalities, amyotrophic lateral sclerosis (ALS), and osteomalacia. The Lambert–Eaton myasthenic syndrome (LEMS) is an autoimmune disease that causes a proximal weakness (legs worse than arms) which improves after sustained contraction or with cold.[38,39] Patients can have a waddling type of gait when walking, dysphagia, and features of autonomic failure. Treatment is under the advice and care of immunologists and/or neurologists.[40,41]

Localized muscle weakness: possibilities are intracerebral causes (CVA, brain metastases), localized nerve compression or damage, spinal cord compression, or peripheral neuropathy.

FINDING THE CAUSE

A screening checklist is useful:

If the reduced alertness is sudden check for hypoxia, hypercapnia, bleeding, cardiac arrhythmia, respiratory depression, and recently administered drugs.

Enquire about
- sleep patterns and mood
- recent treatment (radiotherapy, chemotherapy, surgery, drugs started or withdrawn).

Assess for depression and anxiety.

Examine for
- chest or urinary infection
- local weakness
- postural hypotension.

Take blood for
hemoglobin, calcium, liver function, renal function and electrolytes.

Screening checklist for fatigue, drowsiness, lethargy and weakness

Clinical decision	If YES carry out the action below
4 Is postural hypotension present? (i.e. feeling faint on standing)	i.e. after lying supine for 2 min, a drop in blood pressure on standing of 20 mmHg systolic or 10 mmHg diastolic. • **Possible causes:** *Drugs:* ACE inhibitors, amitriptyline, beta-blockers, chemotherapy (e.g. cisplatinum, vincristine), diuretics, methotrimeprazine (Canada only). *Autonomic failure* (*see* text for the symptoms): causes include chronic alcohol abuse, diabetes, cancer (paraneoplastic effect), prolonged bed-rest, Lambert–Eaton myasthenic syndrome (*see* cd-6 on p. 155), multiple system atrophy, Parkinson's disease, and spinal cord compression. *Cardiopulmonary:* arrhythmia (atrial fibrillation, bradycardia), cardiac tamponade, myocardial infarction, pulmonary emboli. *Endocrine:* adrenocortical insufficiency (primary or due to steroid withdrawal). *Intravascular volume loss:* dehydration, blood loss. *Procedures:* intraspinal local anesthetic, rapid paracentesis in cirrhosis. • **Treat the cause if possible** • **If hypotension persists** consider treatments that may give short-term benefit: — increase salt and caffeine intake — graduated compression stockings, e.g. 20–30 mmHg — fludrocortisone 50–100 microg q12h — α_1-adrenergic agonist midodrine (Pro Amantine) 5 mg q8h and titrated up to 15 mg q8h.
5 Is the weakness, fatigue, or lethargy all over the body? (i.e. a sensation of getting persistently tired without an obvious cause and which does not improve after sleep)	Screening question for fatigue: *"Do you get tired for no reason for a good part of the time?"*[12] • **Anemia:** transfuse if the hemoglobin <100 g/L (full benefit takes 72 hours). Aim for 110–120 g/L. If ventricular failure is present give 20 mg furosemide with each unit, transfuse over 4 hours and give no more than two units/24 hr. • **Cardiac failure:** ACE inhibitor. • **Chronic infection despite antimicrobials** (e.g. persistent mycobacteria in AIDS): consider low-dose corticosteroids in addition to antimicrobials. • **Depression or anxiety:** *see Anxiety*, p. 239 and *Withdrawal and depression*, p. 253. • **Drugs** (many drugs – check the current product monograph): reduce the dose or change the drug. • **Electrolyte abnormalities:** low Na^+ (SIADH, hypoadrenalism, chest infection, diuretics), low K^+ (diuretics, corticosteroids, vomiting, diarrhea) or low Mg^{++}. Treat the cause. • **Infection** (viral, bacterial): treat with appropriate antimicrobial. • **Nutritional deficiency** (iron, magnesium, vitamin B, D): there is no evidence that one nutritional supplement is better than any other, so consult a dietician. • **Radiotherapy or chemotherapy:** exclude bone marrow suppression. • **Recent surgery:** ensure adequate nutrition. • **Severe dyspnea:** *see Respiratory problems*, p. 191. • **Tumor load** (*see* text): dexamethasone PO 2–4 mg once daily.

Adapted from Regnard and Mannix[20]
cd = clinical decision

TREATING THE CAUSE

This is possible in a wide range of conditions. In a patient with advanced disease such as cancer or AIDS it is important not to assume that the fatigue is due to the primary condition. Such patients can develop unrelated treatable conditions, or a treatable condition indirectly caused by the primary condition (e.g. recurrent infection), or an adverse effect of treatment (e.g. corticosteroid-induced diabetes).

Nutrition

This is important in the earlier stages of any disease, and it is important to ensure that good food presentation encourages sufficient nutritional intake. The advice of a dietician can be useful.[42] In the late stages of disease, nutrition becomes more important for pleasure and comfort. *See Nutrition and hydration problems*, p. 175.

Persisting problems

It is common for fatigue, drowsiness, lethargy, or weakness to persist as part of the underlying condition.

Modifying activities that cause fatigue: although counter-intuitive, graded and planned aerobic exercise can help patients cope more effectively with fatigue.[43–50] Activities are changed by using rest periods between activities, re-timing activities to a time of day when energy is highest, planning regular gentle exercise, arranging help for low-priority activities, and reviewing sleep behaviors and sleep environment.[51]

Drugs: In fatigue related to advanced disease without a clear cause, there is little evidence that drugs have any long-term benefit.[52] However, corticosteroids remain an option for short-term use,[53,54] and dexamethasone 2–4 mg daily can give a short-term improvement for up to 4 weeks. Corticosteroids are sometimes used with long-term antimicrobials to suppress the symptoms of chronic, persistent infection (e.g. candida, mycobacteria) in conditions such as AIDS.[55,56] Psychostimulants are occasionally used to achieve a rapid effect when this is needed for a special event, but can cause a wide range of adverse effects at higher doses such as anxiety, anorexia, and insomnia. Examples are methylphenidate and modafinil.[57–66] In contrast, dexamphetamine does not improve fatigue or quality of life.[67] An alternative is bupropion, an antidepressant that may be useful when fatigue and depression are combined.[68]

Helping the patient and family adjust: if the problems cannot be changed by treatment or altered activities, much can be done to enable the patient, partner and family adjust to the change through support, and by altering the environment. There is limited evidence for the role of psychosocial interventions in fatigue.[69] Cognitive behavioral therapy is ineffective in fatigued patients not suffering from advanced disease,[70] but a brief behavior-oriented intervention has been shown to help cancer-related fatigue.[71]

Complementary therapy: this can help with the impact of fatigue on mood and hope and enable patients to cope more effectively.[72]

Clinical decision	If YES carry out the action below
6 Is the weakness localized? (i.e. a local loss of strength)	• **If this is a proximal motor weakness** consider the following as possible causes: *Corticosteroids:* reduce the dose and consider stopping (the weakness may persist despite stopping). *Hypokalemia:*[73] correct the cause if possible (e.g. loop diuretic and corticosteroid-induced loss). Increase dietary potassium (fruit drinks, bananas, or oral potassium medication). Correct with IV potassium only if the condition is life threatening and treatment is appropriate. *Hypothyroidism or hyperthyroidism:* check thyroid function and treat. *Lambert–Eaton myasthenic syndrome (LEMS):* see text for symptoms. If LEMS is suspected refer to the immunologists or neurologists for diagnosis (voltage-gated calcium channel antibodies) and treatment. *ALS:* involve the occupational therapist. *Osteomalacia:* confirm the diagnosis (X-rays, alkaline phosphatase), find the cause (consider anticonvulsants, malabsorption) and treat. *Polymyositis:* check creatinine kinase serum levels. Prednisolone may help (or methylprednisolone in children).[74] Muscle strengthening exercises can be helpful.[75] Consider referral to rheumatologists for advice on further treatment. • **If this is a localized motor weakness** consider: *Cord compression: see* cd-9a in *Emergencies*, p. 345 *Intracerebral cause* (cerebrovascular accident, metastases): if metastases are present consider high-dose dexamethasone (8–16 mg daily) and referral for cranial irradiation. *Nerve compression:* dexamethasone PO 6 mg daily. *Neuropathy:* assess the cause and treat if appropriate (e.g. B_{12} deficiency).
7 Is the problem persisting?	• **Treat coexisting physical symptoms** (e.g. pain, dyspnea, nausea, vomiting) • **Exclude an anxiety state or depression:** *see Anxiety*, p. 239 and *Withdrawal and Depression*, p. 253. • **Modify activities:** — use rest periods between activities — re-schedule activities to a time of day when energy is highest — plan regular, gentle exercise — arrange help for low-priority activities — review sleep behaviors and sleep environment. • **Ensure food presentation encourages sufficient nutritional intake** (*see Nutrition and hydration problems*, p. 175). • **If a rapid response would help** (e.g. for a special event): consider — methylphenidate 2.5–5 mg in the morning, increasing in stages if necessary to 10–15 mg. A second dose can be given, but no later than lunchtime to avoid insomnia. Some patients can tolerate higher doses (up to 60 mg/24 hr) in divided doses — bupropion 100–300 mg PO daily may help depression and fatigue (increased risk of seizures) — modafinil in low doses (50–200 mg/24 hr) for fatigue, up to 400 mg/24 hr for drowsiness, but wide range of adverse effects at higher doses. Avoid in hypertension or left ventricular failure.

Adapted from Regnard and Mannix[20]
cd = clinical decision

REFERENCES: FATIGUE, DROWSINESS, LETHARGY, AND WEAKNESS

B = book; C = comment; Ch = chapter; CS-n = case study-no. of cases; CT-n = controlled trial-no. of cases; E = editorial; GC = group consensus; I-n = interviews-no. of cases; Let = Letter; LS = laboratory study; MC = multicenter; OS-n = open study-no. of cases; Q = questionnaire; R = review; RCT-n = randomized controlled trial-no. of cases; RS-n = retrospective survey-no. of cases; SA-n = systematic or meta analysis-no. of studies.

1 Higginson IJ, Costantini M. (2008) Dying with cancer, living well with advanced cancer. *European Journal of Cancer*. **44**(10): 1414–24. (SA, RS)

2 Stone P, Richardson A, Ream E, Smith AG, Kerr DJ, Kearney N. (2000) Cancer-related fatigue: inevitable, unimportant and untreatable? Results of a multi-centre patient survey. Cancer Fatigue Forum. *Annals of Oncology*. **11**(8): 971–5. (MC, Q-576)

3 Håvard Loge J. Unpacking fatigue. (2003) *European Journal of Palliative Care*. **10**(Suppl. 2): 14–20. (R, 88 refs)

4 Jhamb M, Weisbord SD, Steel JL, Unruh M. (2008) Fatigue in patients receiving maintenance dialysis: a review of definitions, measures, and contributing factors. *American Journal of Kidney Diseases*. **52**(2): 353–65. (R, 130 refs)

5 Radbruch L, Strasser F, Elsner F, Goncalves JF, *et al.* (2008) Research Steering Committee of the European Association for Palliative Care (EAPC). Fatigue in palliative care patients: an EAPC approach. *Palliative Medicine*. **22**(1): 13–32. (R, 181 refs)

6 Benzein EG, Berg AC. (2005) The level of and relation between hope, hopelessness and fatigue in patients and family members in palliative care. *Palliative Medicine*. **19**(3): 234–40. (OS-85)

7 Solano JP, Gomes B, Higginson IJ. (2006) A comparison of symptom prevalence in far advanced cancer, AIDS, heart disease, chronic obstructive pulmonary disease and renal disease. *Journal of Pain and Symptom Management*. **31**(1): 58–69. (SA-64)

8 Thombs BD, Bassel M, McGuire L, Smith MT, Hudson M, Haythornthwaite JA. (2008) A systematic comparison of fatigue levels in systemic sclerosis with general population, cancer and rheumatic disease samples. *Rheumatology*. **47**(10): 1559–63. (R, 63 refs)

9 Richardson A. (1995) Fatigue in cancer patients: a review of the literature. *European Journal of Cancer Care*. **4**: 20–32. (R, 93 refs)

10 Richardson A, Ream E. (1996) The experience of fatigue and other symptoms in patients receiving chemotherapy. *European Journal of Cancer Care*. **5**: 24–30. (OS-100)

11 Gall H. (1996) The basis of fatigue: where does it come from? *European Journal of Cancer Care*. **5**: 31–4. (R, 24 refs)

12 Kirsh KL, Passik S, Holtsclaw E, Donaghy K, Theobald D. (2001) I get tired for no reason: a single item screening for cancer-related fatigue. *Journal of Pain and Symptom Management*. **22**(5): 931–7. (OS-52)

13 Okuyama T, Akechi T, Shima Y, Sugahara Y, *et al.* (2008) Factors correlated with fatigue in terminally ill cancer patients: a longitudinal study. *Journal of Pain and Symptom Management*. **35**(5): 515–23. (OS-402)

14 Ancoli-Israel S, Moore PJ, Jones V. (2001) The relationship between fatigue and sleep in cancer patients: a review. *European Journal of Cancer Care*. **10**(4): 245–55. (R, 66 refs)

15 Yennurajalingam S, Palmer JL, Zhang T, Poulter V, Bruera E. (2008) Association between fatigue and other cancer-related symptoms in patients with advanced cancer. *Supportive Care in Cancer*. **16**(10): 1125–30. (RS-268)

16 Goldstein DS, Holmes CS, Dendi R, Bruce SR, Li ST. (2002) Orthostatic hypotension from sympathetic denervation in Parkinson's disease. *Neurology*. **58**(8): 1247–55. (CT-57)

17 Bruera E. (1989) Autonomic failure in patients with advanced cancer. *Journal of Pain and Symptom Management*. **4**(3): 163–6. (CS)

18 Bruera E, Chadwick S, Fox R, Hanson J, MacDonald N. (1986) Study of cardiovascular autonomic insufficiency in advanced cancer patients. *Cancer Treatment Reports*. **70**(12): 1383–7. (CT-63)

19 O'Driscoll BR, Howard LS, Davison AG. (2008) British Thoracic Society guideline for emergency oxygen use in adults. *Thorax*. **63**(Suppl. 6): vi, 1–68. (GS)

20 Regnard C, Mannix K. (1995) Weakness and fatigue. In: *Flow Diagrams in Advanced Cancer and Other Diseases*. London: Edward Arnold. pp. 64–7. (Ch)

21 Perez-Lugones A, Schweikert R, Pavia S, Sra J, *et al.* (2001) Usefulness of midodrine in patients with severely symptomatic neurocardiogenic syncope: a randomized control study. *Journal of Cardiovascular Electrophysiology*. **12**(8): 935–8. (RCT-61)

22 Wright RA, Kaufmann HC, Perera R, Opfer-Gehrking TL, *et al.* (1998) A double-blind, dose-response study of midodrine in neurogenic orthostatic hypotension. *Neurology*. **51**(1): 120–4. (CT-25)

23 Kaufmann H, Saadia D, Voustianiouk A. (2002) Midodrine in neurally mediated syncope: a double-blind, randomized, crossover study. *Annals of Neurology*. **52**(3): 342–5. (RCT-12)

24 Strasser F, Palmer JL, Schover LR, Yusuf SW, *et al.* (2006) The impact of hypogonadism and autonomic dysfunction on fatigue, emotional function, and sexual desire in male patients with advanced cancer: a pilot study. *Cancer*. **107**(12): 2949–57. (OS-48)

25 Brogan G, Exton L, Kurowska A, Tookman A. (2000) The importance of low magnesium levels in palliative care: two case reports. *Palliative Medicine*. **14**: 59–61. (CS-2)

26 Crosby V, Wilcock A, Lawson N, Corcoran R. (2000) The importance of low magnesium in palliative care. *Palliative Medicine*. **14**(6): 544. (Let)

27 Hwang SS, Chang VT, Rue M, Kasimis B. (2003)

Multidimensional independent predictors of cancer-related fatigue. *Journal of Pain and Symptom Management*. **26**: 604–14.

28 Lundström S, Fürst CJ. (2003) Symptoms in advanced cancer: relationship to endogenous cortisol levels. *Palliative Medicine*. **17**: 503–8. (OS-23)

29 Munch TN, Zhang T, Willey J, Palmer JL, Bruera E. (2005) The association between anemia and fatigue in patients with advanced cancer receiving palliative care. *Journal of Palliative Medicine*. **8**(6): 1144–9. (RS-177)

30 Irvine D, Vincent L, Graydon JE, Bubela N, Thompson L. (1994) The prevalence and correlates of fatigue in patients receiving treatment with chemotherapy and radiotherapy: a comparison with the fatigue experienced by healthy individuals. *Cancer Nursing*. **17**: 367–78. (CT-101)

31 Hickok JT, Morrow GR, McDonald S, Bellg AJ. (1996) Frequency and correlates of fatigue in lung cancer patients receiving radiation therapy: implications for management. *Journal of Pain and Symptom Management*. **11**: 370–7. (RS-50)

32 Greenberg DB, Sawicka J, Eisenthal S, *et al.* (1992) Fatigue syndromes due to localized radiation. *Journal of Pain and Symptom Management*. **7**: 38–45.

33 Cicoira M, Bolger AP, Doehner W, Rauchhaus M, *et al.* (2001) High tumour necrosis factor-alpha levels are associated with exercise intolerance and neurohormonal activation in chronic heart failure patients. *Cytokine*. **5**(2): 80–6. (OS)

34 Tisdale MJ. (2008) Catabolic mediators of cancer cachexia. *Current Opinion in Supportive and Palliative Care*. **2**(4): 256–61. (R, 52 refs)

35 Stephens NA, Skipworth RJ, Fearon KC. (2008) Cachexia, survival and the acute phase response. *Current Opinion in Supportive and Palliative Care*. **2**(4): 267–74. (R, 75 refs)

36 Chikanza IC. (2002) Mechanisms of corticosteroid resistance in rheumatoid arthritis: a putative role for the corticosteroid receptor beta isoform. *Annals of the New York Academy of Sciences*. **966**: 39–48. (R, 60 refs)

37 Mercadante S, Fulfaro F, Casuccio A. (2001) The use of corticosteroids in home palliative care. *Supportive Care in Cancer.* **9**(5): 386–9. (OS-376)

38 Maddison P, Lang B, Mills K, Newsom-Davis J. (2001) Long term outcome in Lambert–Eaton myasthenic syndrome without lung cancer. *Journal of Neurology, Neurosurgery and Psychiatry*. **70**(2): 212–7. (RS-47)

39 Elrington G. (1992) The Lambert–Eaton myaesthenic syndromes. *Palliative Medicine*. **6**: 9–17. (R)

40 Mahadeva B, Phillips LH 2nd, Juel VC. (2008) Autoimmune disorders of neuromuscular transmission. *Seminars in Neurology*. **28**(2): 212–27. (R, 136 refs)

41 Newsom-Davis J. (2001) Lambert–Eaton myasthenic syndrome. *Current Treatment Options in Neurology*. **3**(2): 127–31. (R)

42 Stratton RJ, Elia M. (2000) Are oral nutritional supplements of benefit to patients in the community? Findings from a systematic review. *Current Opinion in Clinical Nutrition and Metabolic Care*. **3**(4): 311–15. (SA)

43 Nail LM. (2002) Fatigue in patients with cancer. *Oncology Nursing Forum*. **29**(3): 537–46. (R, 92 refs)

44 Mock V, Dow KH, Meares CJ, Grimm PM, *et al.* (1997) Effects of exercise on fatigue, physical functioning, and emotional distress during radiation therapy for breast cancer. *Oncology Nursing Forum*. **24** (6): 991–1000. (CT-46)

45 MacVicar MG, Winningham ML, Nickel JL. (1989) Effects of aerobic interval training on cancer patients' functional capacity. *Nursing Research*. **38**(6): 348–51. (RCT–50)

46 Schwartz AL, Mori M, Gao R, Nail LM, King ME. (2001) Exercise reduces daily fatigue in women with breast cancer receiving chemotherapy. *Medicine and Science in Sports and Exercise*. **33**(5): 718–23. (OS-61)

47 Porock D, Kristjanson LJ, Tinelly K, Duke T, Blight J. (2000) An exercise intervention for advanced cancer patients experiencing fatigue: a pilot study. *Journal of Palliative Care*. **16**(3): 30–6. (OS-11)

48 Cramp F, Daniel J. (2008) Exercise for the management of cancer-related fatigue in adults. *Cochrane Database of Systematic Reviews*. **2**: CD006145. (SA-28)

49 Fillion L, Gagnon P, Leblond F, Gelinas C, *et al.* (2008) A brief intervention for fatigue management in breast cancer survivors. *Cancer Nursing*. **31**(2): 145–59. (RCT-87)

50 Kangas M, Bovbjerg DH, Montgomery GH. (2008) Cancer-related fatigue: a systematic and meta-analytic review of non-pharmacological therapies for cancer patients. *Psychological Bulletin*. **134**(5): 700–41. (SA-119)

51 Johnston MP, Coward DD. (2001) Cancer-related fatigue: nursing assessment and management: increasing awareness of the effect of cancer-related fatigue. *American Journal of Nursing*. **101**(Suppl.): S19–22. (R, 24 refs)

52 Stone P. (2002) The measurement, causes and effective management of cancer-related fatigue. *International Journal of Palliative Nursing*. **8**(3): 120–8. (R, 77 refs)

53 Carroll JK, Kohli S, Mustian KM, Roscoe JA, Morrow GR. (2007) Pharmacologic treatment of cancer-related fatigue. *Oncologist*. **12**(Suppl. 1): S43–51. (SA, 75 refs)

54 Lundstrom SH, Furst CJ. (2006) The use of corticosteroids in Swedish palliative care. *Acta Oncologica*. **45**(4): 430–7. (I-1594)

55 Castro M. (1998) Treatment and prophylaxis of Pneumocystis carinii pneumonia. *Seminars in Respiratory Infections*. **13**(4): 296–303. (R, 65 refs)

56 Dorman SE, Heller HM, Basgoz NO, Sax PE. (1998) Adjunctive corticosteroid therapy for patients whose treatment for disseminated Mycobacterium avium complex infection has failed. *Clinical Infectious Diseases*. **26**(3): 682–6. (OS-12)

57 Homsi J, Walsh D, Nelson K. (2000) Psychostimulants in supportive care. *Supportive Care in Cancer*. **8**: 385–97.

58 Sugawara Y, Akechi T, Shima Y, Okuyama T.

(2002) Efficacy of methylphenidate for fatigue in advanced cancer patients: a preliminary study. *Palliative Medicine*. **16**: 261–3. (OS-14)

59 Breitbart W, Rosenfeld B, Kaim M, Funesti-Esch J. (2001) A randomized, double-blind, placebo-controlled trial of psychostimulants for the treatment of fatigue in ambulatory patients with human immunodeficiency virus disease. *Archives of Internal Medicine*. **161**(3): 411–20. (RCT-144)

60 Dein S, George R. (2002) A place for psychostimulants in palliative care? *Journal of Palliative Care*. **18**(3): 196–9. (R, 27 refs)

61 Wilwerding MB, Loprinzi CL, Mailliard JA, O'Fallon JR, *et al.* (1995) A randomized, crossover evaluation of methylphenidate in cancer patients receiving strong narcotics. *Supportive Care in Cancer.* **3**(2): 135–8. (RCT)

62 Bruera E, Valero V, Driver L, Shen L, Willey J, Zhang T, Palmer JL. (2006) Patient-controlled methylphenidate for cancer fatigue: a double-blind, randomized, placebo-controlled trial. *Journal of Clinical Oncology*. **24**(13): 2073–8. (RCT-112)

63 Minton O, Richardson A, Sharpe M, Hotopf M, Stone P. (2008) A systematic review and meta-analysis of the pharmacological treatment of cancer-related fatigue. *Journal of the National Cancer Institute*. **100**(16): 1155–66. (SA-27, 70 refs)

64 Lower EE, Harman S, Baughman RP. (2008) Double-blind, randomized trial of dexmethylphenidate hydrochloride for the treatment of sarcoidosis-associated fatigue. *Chest.* **133**(5): 1189–95. (RCT-10)

65 Rao AV, Cohen HJ. (2008) Fatigue in older cancer patients: etiology, assessment, and treatment. *Seminars in Oncology*. **35**(6): 633–42. (R, 56 refs)

66 Minton O, Stone P, Richardson A, Sharpe M, Hotopf M. (2008) Drug therapy for the management of cancer related fatigue. *Cochrane Database of Systematic Reviews.* **1**: CD006704. (SA-27, 91 refs)

67 Auret K, Schug SA, Bremner AP, Bulsara M. (2009) A randomized, double-blind, placebo-controlled trial assessing the impact of dexamphetamine on fatigue in patients with advanced cancer. *Journal of Pain and Symptom Management*. **37**(4): 613–21. (RCT-50)

68 Harris JD. (2008) Fatigue in chronically ill patients. *Current Opinion in Supportive and Palliative Care*. **2**(3): 180–6. (R, 63 refs)

69 Goedendorp MM, Gielissen MF, Verhagen CA, Bleijenberg G. (2009) Psychosocial interventions for reducing fatigue during cancer treatment in adults. *Cochrane Database of Systematic Reviews.* **1**: CD006953. (SA-27, 127 refs)

70 Leone SS, Huibers MJ, Kant I, van Amelsvoort LG, *et al.* (2006) Long-term efficacy of cognitive-behavioral therapy by general practitioners for fatigue: a 4-year follow-up study. *Journal of Psychosomatic Research*. **61**(5): 601–7. (RCT)

71 Armes J, Chalder T, Addington-Hall J, Richardson A, Hotopf M. (2007) A randomized controlled trial to evaluate the effectiveness of a brief, behaviorally oriented intervention for cancer-related fatigue. *Cancer.* **110**(6): 1385–95. (RCT-60)

72 Kohara H, Miyauchi T, Suehiro Y, Ueoka H, Takeyama H, Morita T. (2004) Combined modality treatment of aromatherapy, footsoak, and reflexology relieves fatigue in patients with cancer. *Journal of Palliative Medicine*. **7**(6): 791–6. (OS-20)

73 Rastergar A, Soleimani M. (2001) Hypokalaemia and hyperkalaemia. *Postgraduate Medical Journal.* **77**(914): 759–64. (R, 21 refs)

74 Reed AM. (2001) Myositis in children. *Current Opinion in Rheumatology*. **13**(5): 428–33. (R, 60 refs)

75 Lawson Mahowald M. (2001) The benefits and limitations of a physical training program in patients with inflammatory myositis. *Current Rheumatology Reports.* **3**(4): 317–24. (R, 50 refs)

Malignant ulcers and fistulae

CLINICAL DECISION AND ACTION CHECKLIST

1 Can the local malignancy be treated?
2 Is the wound bleeding?
3 Is the wound causing psychosocial effects?
4 Is the exudate or discharge troublesome?
5 Is the odor troublesome?
6 Is the wound painful?
7 Is the wound itchy?

KEY POINTS

- Each malignant ulcer requires individual assessment.
- Healing may be possible, but comfort is the primary aim.
- Malignant ulcers can have a major impact on body image and the ability to cope.

INTRODUCTION

A malignant ulcer can cause disfigurement, altered function, discharge, and odor. Common physical symptoms are pain, discharge, odor, itching, and bleeding, with 22% having two or more symptoms, especially in perineal and genital wounds.[1] The psychosocial effects of such wounds are at least as great as their physical effects.[2–6] They can have a profound effect on how the patient perceives themselves, causing anxiety, depression, and social isolation. Sexuality can be seriously affected,[7] but this is not often elicited by professionals.[8] Social relationships can suffer so that reduced contact worsens the low self-esteem. The fact that many malignant ulcers cannot be removed or healed adds to the despair.

MANAGING THE EFFECTS OF AN ULCER

Treating a malignancy

If the area has not previously received a maximum radiation dose, more radiotherapy may be possible. Chemotherapy or hormone therapy can be useful in sensitive tumors.[9,10] Surgery has a limited role for localized lesions.[11]

Managing exudate and discharge

This may be exudate from a wound, discharge caused by infection, or leakage from a fistula.

Wound exudates: unlike acute wounds which need to be kept moist, exudate from chronic wounds needs to be removed.[12] The key is well-fitting dressings that can absorb fluid and allow its evaporation.[13] The ability of alginates to absorb fluid is limited, but polyurethane foam dressings (e.g. Lyofoam Extra, Allevyn) allow evaporation and the removal of more fluid.[14] If an exudate is severe, plastic food wrap can be used over dressings to protect clothes. Use barrier preparations to protect the surrounding skin (*see* cd-4 opposite). There are reports of use of vacuum-assisted closure therapy to control pain and malodorous exudate from a malignant wound,[15,16] but this is expensive, and should be used very selectively.

Vaginal and rectal discharges: these can be due to local ulcerating carcinomas. They may become less offensive with antiseptic douches/lavage, e.g. povidone-iodine. Topical corticosteroids will reduce local inflammation and pain. Regularly changed tampons can control vaginal discharges if there is no discomfort on insertion. Perineal and perianal skin often needs protection from the continual moisture with barrier preparations (*see* cd-4 opposite).

Fistulae: some malignant ulcers are associated with an enterocutaneous fistula (an abnormal link between a hollow organ and the skin). They occur most commonly with Crohn's disease, but also occur with abdominal cancers.[17] Colostomy bags can be fitted over the fistula if the surrounding area is flat – the pediatric types are easier to fit because of a softer flange. If the area around the wound is uneven, the irregularities can be made smooth with fillers such as Orabase paste, allowed to dry and covered with a hydrocolloid dressing (e.g. Comfeel, Duoderm, Signal).[18]

Fistulae with the oral cavity: silicone foam dressing (e.g. Cavi-Care) is helpful when it is desirable to block an external fistula connecting with the oral cavity. It forms a close fitting, comfortable, and washable dressing that reduces fluid loss.[19,20] Less readily available alternatives include a latex mold,[21] or self-polymerizing silicone materials normally reserved for dentistry. Silicone materials are more versatile and longer lasting and a local dentist or a dental school would advise.[22]

Rectovaginal fistulae may cause stool to pass vaginally. A firmer stool is less likely to enter the fistula, and stopping softening laxatives while starting a low dose of stimulant laxative will produce a firmer stool. If necessary, a low dose of loperamide will produce a firmer stool.

Octreotide is helpful in patients with bowel fistulae,[23–26] and may be useful in other fistulae. There may be a delay of 2–3 days before the output reduces.

Clinical decision	If YES carry out the action below
1 Can the local malignancy be treated?	• **Refer to an oncologist for advice.** *If the tumor is radiosensitive and further local radiation is possible:* discuss the option of radiotherapy with the patient. Do not use metal-containing topical agents (e.g. silver sulfadiazine – Flamazine) during treatment. *If the tumor is chemosensitive:* discuss the option of chemotherapy with the patient. • **Consider surgery** if the tumor is localized, the patient agrees, and the patient is fit for surgery.
2 Is the wound bleeding?	• *See* cd-3 in *Bleeding*, p. 95.
3 Is the wound causing psychosocial effects?	• **Improve the cosmetic appearance if possible:** treat any odor (*see* cd-5 on p. 163), fill the defect with dressings. Consider using self-polymerizing silicone materials (a dentist or dental school can advise).[22] • **Elicit the problems:** e.g. adjustment issues, social isolation, relationships, sexual issues. • **Enable the patient to cope with altered image** through active listening. Consider referral for cognitive behavioral therapy. • ***See also*** *Anger*, p. 235, *Anxiety*, p. 239, *Withdrawal and depression*, p. 253, and *Urinary problems and sexual difficulties*, p. 223.
4 Is the exudate or discharge troublesome?	• **If the exudate or discharge is from the wound:** *Absorb the discharge:* use conformable polyurethane foam dressing (e.g. Lyofoam Extra, Allevyn). If exudate soaks through, cover the dressing with plastic food wrap to protect the patient's clothes. *Protect the surrounding skin:* use a barrier preparation (e.g. zinc ointments or simethicone cream) or a barrier application (e.g. Critic Aid). *Reduce any inflammation:* topical corticosteroid (e.g. Dermovate (Canada) or Temovate (clobetasol) or Cutivate (fluticasone) (US)) once daily for one week. If the area is too sensitive to apply cream, reduce the local pain by applying beclomethasone inhaler (400 microg/spray) sprayed directly onto the skin for a few days. *Rectal or vaginal discharge:* if infection is present treat with topical antimicrobials (systemic if necessary) and antiseptic douches or lavage (e.g. povidone-iodine). • **If a fistula is present:** reduce the volume of the discharge: — for a distal small bowel fistula try loperamide 8–24 mg/24 hours in divided doses — for a more proximal gastrointestinal fistula try hyoscine butylbromide 60–120 mg/24 hours by SC infusion. In the US use hyoscyamine (Levsin) 0.25–0.5 mg IV/SC q4h PRN or 0.125–0.25 mg SL q4h PRN. • **If the discharge volume is large**, e.g. more than 300 mL/24 hours: *Octreotide* 100–200 microg q8h or 300–600 microg/24 hours by SC infusion. Alternatively, and if the prognosis is 4 weeks or more, try lanreotide 30 mg IM q2 weeks or Sandostatin LAR Depot (long-acting octreotide) given as 20 mg q4 weeks. *Divert the discharge:* use a collecting bag (stoma bag for a flat surface, or a fecal collecting bag for rectal fluid – *see Diarrhea*, p. 118). *Block the discharge:* consider a soft rectal plug rectally or vaginally (*see Diarrhea*, p. 120). *Consider surgical diversion*, e.g. colostomy, urostomy.

Adapted from Saunders and Regnard[27]
cd = clinical decision

Pain

This is a common problem in malignant ulcers.

Skin inflammation: this occurs if the skin is wet from wound exudates or irritated by urine, stool, or bowel fistula contents. Local infection such as candida needs to be excluded. Even if the cause can be managed, it is helpful to resolve painful skin inflammation with topical steroids. Sometimes the area is too sensitive to apply any cream and using an inhaler-type steroid spray will apply steroid with little discomfort, allowing cream to be applied after 1–2 days.

Dressings: it is important to avoid dressings that are difficult to remove, such as hydrocolloids or adhesive dressings, and replace these with non-adherent types.[28–31] Protecting the surrounding skin with barrier preparations is important to prevent damage to normal skin.

Analgesia: there is some evidence that topical opioids reduce pain in areas of tissue damage.[32–36] Topical NSAIDs may also have a role.[37] However, some patients with deeper wounds need systemic opioids.

Removing debris

The concept of physical debridement has been superseded by the concept of encouraging debridement through the correct use of dressings. Washing clears loose debris but does not promote healing or reduce infection.[38]

Larval therapy: debridement using larvae is now well established and has been used in malignant ulcers with good effect.[39,40] The larvae (*Phaenicia (=Lucilia) sericata*) cannot pupate into flies and will clear any non-viable tissue within 1–3 days. They can be applied in a sealed mesh pouch (e.g. Creature Comforts[41]) and covered in an air-permeable dressing. Surrounding skin must be protected with a barrier preparation. Larvae may be less effective in older patients and those with ischemic ulcers. They are contraindicated in the presence of exposed major vessels, severe wound pain, anticoagulant therapy, troublesome bleeding, and hard eschars. In addition, a quarter of patients find the concept unacceptable.[42,43] (There is no source of medical larvae in Canada. They can be ordered from the US,[41] but import licenses, etc. are required).

Ultrasound at a low frequency (25 Hz) is an alternative that has been used to debride chronic leg ulcers and may have a role in malignant ulcers.[44]

Odor

Treating the odor: malignant ulcers are colonized by anaerobic bacteria.[45] Systemic metronidazole can be effective and reactions with alcohol are rare.[46] Topical metronidazole gel or cream can help,[47–49] but is expensive, may make a wound too wet, and can be ineffective on large wounds.[50] It is useful when systemic metronidazole is not tolerated or is ineffective, but a better alternative is to crush a metronidazole tablet and apply this directly to the wound since this gives a higher local concentration without making the wound wetter.[51]

Attempts to mask a smell with room perfumes or aromatic oils often fail as the patient associates the new odor with the unpleasant one. This effect may be lessened by using essential oil blended in tea-tree oil and applied in a water-based cream, or using oils intermittently.[52,53] Honey has often been suggested as being helpful[54] but, apart from partial thickness burns, trials have shown no advantages and some disadvantages compared with standard agents.[55,56]

Clinical decision	If YES carry out the action below
5 Is the odor troublesome?	• **Start metronidazole** 400 mg PO q8h (or 500 mg PR q12h) for 5 days, then continue with 400–500 mg once daily. If adverse effects are a problem, use crushed tablets applied directly to the wound, or topical metronidazole gel/cream. • **Use hydrogels** (e.g. Intrasite) or polyurethane foam dressings (e.g. Lyofoam Extra, Allevyn) to help clear debris. • **Mask the odor:** charcoal dressings may help for a few hours. Perfumes and aromatic oils are only temporary solutions, but can be helpful during dressing changes. If the odor persists, cover the dressings with a layer of plastic food wrap to trap the odor.
6 Is the wound painful?	• **If pain is only present at dressing changes:** *If this is infection (e.g. candida):* treat infection. *If this is skin inflammation: see* cd-5 on p. 51. *Change the type of dressing:* stop using hydrocolloid dressings or dressings with adhesive. Change to non-adherent, soft silicone net dressings next to the ulcer (e.g. Mepitel). *Add extra breakthrough analgesia:* buccal fentanyl or alfentanil prior to changing the dressing. *See* cd-2 in *Diagnosing and treating pain*, p. 45, for more information on breakthrough pain. *Protect the surrounding skin* with a barrier cream (e.g. simethicone-containing cream) or a barrier application (e.g. Critic-Aid). • **Persistent pain:** Consider topical morphine or review the systemic analgesia and consider ketamine or spinal analgesia.
7 Is the wound itchy?	• **Remove allergen:** exclude allergy to dressing or topical agent. • **Reduce inflammation:** NSAID or use topical steroid. *See* cd-5 on p. 51. • **Consider using TENS** on intact skin between the wound and the spine.

Adapted from Saunders and Regnard[27]
cd = clinical decision

Isolating the odor may be possible with specific dressings.[57] Charcoal dressings are only effective for a few hours. Colostomy bags can be used for fistulae. Dressings that absorb exudate can help, such as hydrogels and polyurethane foam dressings.[58] Plastic food wrap can be placed over dressings to provide an additional barrier to odor.

REFERENCES: MALIGNANT ULCERS AND FISTULAE

B = book; C = comment; Ch = chapter; CS-n = case study-no. of cases; CT-n = controlled trial-no. of cases; E = editorial; GC = group consensus; I = interviews; LS = laboratory study; MC = multi-center; OS-n = open study-no. of cases; Q-n = questionnaire-no. of respondents; R = review; RCT-n = randomized controlled trial-no. of cases; RS-n = retrospective survey-no. of cases; SA = systematic or meta analysis.

1 Maida V, Ennis M, Kuziemsky C, Trozzolo L. (2009) Symptoms associated with malignant wounds: a prospective case series. *Journal of Pain and Symptom Management.* **37**(2): 206–11. (OS-67)

2 Ivetic O, Lyne PA. (1990) Fungating and ulcerating malignant lesions: a review of the literature. *Journal of Advanced Nursing.* **15**(1): 83–8. (R, 42 refs)

3 Bird C. (2000) Managing malignant fungating wounds. *Professional Nurse.* **15**(4): 253–6. (R, 28 refs)

4 Schulz V, Triska OH, Tonkin K. (2002) Malignant wounds: caregiver-determined clinical problems. *Journal of Pain and Symptom Management.* **24**(6): 572–7. (Q-136)

5 Piggin C, Jones V. (2007) Malignant fungating wounds: an analysis of the lived experience. *International Journal of Palliative Nursing.* **13**(8): 384–91. (I-5)

6 Lindahl E, Norberg A, Soderberg A. (2007) The meaning of living with malodorous exuding ulcers. *Journal of Clinical Nursing.* **16**(3A): 68–75. (I-9)

7 Lund-Nielsen B, Muller K, Adamsen L. (2005) Malignant wounds in women with breast cancer: feminine and sexual perspectives. *Journal of Clinical Nursing.* **14**(1): 56–64. (OS-12)

8 Rice AM. (2000) Sexuality in cancer and palliative care 1: effects of disease and treatment. *International Journal of Palliative Nursing.* **6**(8): 392–7. (R, 49 refs)

9 Dauphin S, Katz S, el Tamer M, Wait R, Sohn C, Braverman AS. (1997) Chemotherapy is a safe and effective initial therapy for infected malignant breast and chest wall ulcers. *Journal of Surgical Oncology.* **66**(Suppl. 3): 186–8. (OS-33)

10 Heirler F, de la Motte S, Popp W. (1995) Influence of metronidazole and tamoxifen in a case of otherwise untreated ulcerous breast carcinoma. *European Journal of Gynaecological Oncology.* **16**(6): 448–52. (CS-1)

11 Sanders R, Goodacre TE. (1989) When radiotherapy offers no more: the surgical management of advanced breast malignancy. *Annals of the Royal College of Surgeons of England.* **71**(6): 349–53. (RS-47)

12 Parnham A. (2002) Moist wound healing: does the same theory apply to chronic wounds? *Journal of Wound Care* **11**(4): 143–6. (R, 36 refs)

13 Grocott P. (1998) Exudative management in fungating wounds. *Journal of Wound Care.* **7**(9): 445–8. (CS-3)

14 Grocott P. (2000) The palliative management of fungating malignant wounds. *Journal of Wound Care.* **9**(1): 4–9. (OS-45)

15 Ford-Dunn S. (2006) Use of vacuum assisted closure therapy in the palliation of a malignant wound. *Palliative Medicine.* **20**(4): 477–8. (CS-1)

16 Draus JM Jr., Huss SA, Harty NJ, Cheadle WG, Larson GM. (2006) Enterocutaneous fistula: are treatments improving? *Surgery.* **140**(4): 570–6. (MC, RS-106)

17 Metcalf C. (1999) Enterocutaneous fistulae. *Journal of Wound Care.* **8**: 141–2. (R, 10 refs)

18 Pringle WK. (1995) The management of patients with enterocutaneous fistulae. *Journal of Wound Care.* **4**: 211–13. (R, 6 refs)

19 Regnard C, Meehan S. (1982) The use of a silicone foam dressing in the management of malignant oral-cutaneous fistula. *British Journal of Clinical Practice.* **36**: 243–5. (CS-1)

20 Regnard C, Ruckley R. (1985) Silastic foam dressing: an appraisal. *Annals of the Royal College of Surgeons of England.* **67**: 271. (R)

21 Grocott P. (1992) The latest on latex. *Nursing Times.* **88**: 61–2. (R, 6 refs)

22 Walls AWG, Regnard CFB, Mannix KA. (1994) The closure of an abdominal fistula using self-polymerising silicone rubbers: a case study. *Palliative Medicine.* **8**: 59–62. (CS-1)

23 Alivizatos V, Felekis D, Zorbalas A. (2002) Evaluation of the effectiveness of octreotide in the conservative treatment of postoperative enterocutaneous fistulas. *Hepato-Gastroenterology.* **49**(46): 1010–12. (RS-39)

24 Gonzalez-Pinto I, Gonzalez EM. (2001) Optimising the treatment of upper gastrointestinal fistulae. *Gut.* **49**(Suppl. 4): 22–31. (R, 81 refs)

25 Yeo CJ, Cameron JL, Lillemoe KD, Sauter PK, *et al.* (2000) Does prophylactic octreotide decrease the rates of pancreatic fistula and other complications after pancreaticoduodenectomy? Results of a prospective randomized placebo-controlled trial. *Annals of Surgery.* **232**(3): 419–29. (RCT, 211)

26 Mercadante S. (1994) The role of octreotide in palliative care. *Journal of Pain and Symptom Management.* **9**(6): 406–11. (R, 37 refs)

27 Saunders J, Regnard C. (1995) Malignant ulcers. In: *Flow Diagrams in Advanced Cancer and Other Diseases.* London: Edward Arnold. pp. 57–9. (Ch)

28 Jones V, Milton T. (2000) When and how to use hydrocolloid dressings. *Nursing Times Plus.* **96**: 5–7. (R)

29 Collier M. (2000) Tissue viability: management of patients with fungating wounds. *Nursing Standard.* **15**(11): 46–52. (CS-1)

30 Gotschall CS, Morrison MI, Eichelberger MR. (1998) Prospective randomized study of the efficacy of Mepitel on partial thickness scalds in children. *Journal of Burn Care Rehabilitation.* **19**: 279–83. (RCT)

31 Taylor R. (1999) Use of a silicone net dressing in severe mycosis fungoides. *Journal of Wound Care.* **8**(9): 429–30. (CS-1)

32 Back IN, Finlay I. (1995) Analgesic effect of topical opioids on painful skin ulcers. *Journal of Pain and Symptom Management.* **10**: 493. (Let)

33 Krajnik M, Zylicz Z. (1997) Topical morphine for cutaneous cancer pain. *Palliative Medicine*. **11**: 325–6. (CS-6)
34 Twillman RK, Long TD, Cathers TA, Mueller DW. (1999) Treatment of painful skin ulcers with topical opioids. *Journal of Pain and Symptom Management*. **17**(4): 288–92. (CS-9)
35 Briggs M, Nelson EA. (2003) Topical agents or dressings for pain in venous leg ulcers (Cochrane review). In: *The Cochrane Library, Issue 3*. Oxford: Update Software (also on www.update-software.com/abstracts/ab001177.htm).
36 Zeppetella G, Porzio G, Aielli F. (2007) Opioids applied topically to painful cutaneous malignant ulcers in a palliative care setting. *Journal of Opioid Management*. **3**(3): 161–6. (CS-4)
37 Palao i Domenech R, Romanelli M, Tsiftsis DD, *et al.* (2008) Effect of an ibuprofen-releasing foam dressing on wound pain: a real-life RCT. *Journal of Wound Care*. **17**(8): 342, 344–8. (MC, RCT-853)
38 Fernandez R, Griffiths R. (2008) Water for wound cleansing. *Cochrane Database of Systematic Reviews*. **1**: CD003861. (SA-11, 59 refs)
39 Sealby N. (2004) The use of maggot therapy in the treatment of a malignant foot wound. *British Journal of Community Nursing*. **9**(3): S16–9. (CS-1)
40 Steenvoorde P, van Doorn LP, Jacobi CE, Oskam J. (2007) Maggot debridement therapy in the palliative setting. *American Journal of Hospice and Palliative Care*. **24**(4): 308–10. (CS-1)
41 See www.monarchlabs.com (accessed 28 January 2010).
42 Petherick ES, O'Meara S, Spilsbury K, Iglesias CP, Nelson EA, Torgerson DJ. (2006) Patient acceptability of larval therapy for leg ulcer treatment: a randomised survey to inform the sample size calculation of a randomised trial. *BMC Medical Research Methodology*. **6**: 43. (CT-35)
43 Steenvoorde P, Jacobi CE, Van Doorn L, Oskam J. (2007) Maggot debridement therapy of infected ulcers: patient and wound factors influencing outcome: a study on 101 patients with 117 wounds. *Annals of the Royal College of Surgeons of England*. **89**(6): 596–602. (OS-101)
44 Tan J, Abisi S, Smith A, Burnand KG. (2007) A painless method of ultrasonically assisted debridement of chronic leg ulcers: a pilot study. *European Journal of Vascular and Endovascular Surgery*. **33**(2): 234–8. (OS-19)
45 Rotimi VO, Durosinmi-Etti FA. (1984) The bacteriology of infected malignant ulcers. *Journal of Clinical Pathology*. **37**(5): 592–5. (OS-70)
46 Visapaa JP, Tillonen JS, Kaihovaara PS, Salaspuro MP. (2002) Lack of disulfram-like reaction with metronidazole and ethanol. *Annals of Pharmacotherapy*. **36**(6): 971–4.
47 Newman V, Allwood M, Oakes RA. (1989) The use of metronidazole gel to control the smell of malodorous lesions. *Palliative Medicine*. **3**: 303–5.
48 Finlay IG, Bowszyc J, Ramlau C, Gwiezdzinski Z. (1996) The effect of topical 0.75% metronidazole gel on malodorous cutaneous ulcers. *Journal of Pain and Symptom Management*. **11**(3): 158–62. (OS-47)
49 Paul JC, Pieper BA. (2008) Topical metronidazole for the treatment of wound odor: a review of the literature. *Ostomy Wound Management*. **54**(3): 18–27. (R, 39 refs)
50 Grocott P. (1999) The management of fungating wounds. *Journal of Wound Care*. **8**(5): 232–4. (R, 24 refs)
51 Twycross R, Wilcock A, Dean M, Kennedy B, eds. (2010) *Palliative Care Formulary*, Canadian ed. Nottingham: palliativedrugs.com. p. 356. (Ch); and Twycross R, Wilcock A. eds. (2008) *Hospice and Palliative Care Formulary USA, 2nd ed.* Nottingham: palliativedrugs.com. p. 348. (Ch)
52 Kane FM, Brodie EE, Coull A, Coyne L, *et al.* (2004) The analgesic effect of odour and music upon dressing change. *British Journal of Nursing*. **13**(19): S4–12. (RCT-8)
53 Mercier D, Knevitt A. (2005) Using topical aromatherapy for the management of fungating wounds in a palliative care unit. *Journal of Wound Care*. **14**(10): 497–501. (CS-4)
54 Dunford CE, Hanano R. (2004) Acceptability to patients of a honey dressing for non-healing venous leg ulcers. *Journal of Wound Care*. **13**(5): 193–7. (OS-40)
55 Jull A, Walker N, Parag V, Molan P, Rodgers A. (2008) Honey as Adjuvant Leg Ulcer Therapy trial collaborators. Randomized clinical trial of honey-impregnated dressings for venous leg ulcers. *British Journal of Surgery*. **95**(2): 175–82. (MC, RCT-368)
56 Jull AB, Rodgers A, Walker N. (2008) Honey as a topical treatment for wounds. *Cochrane Database of Systematic Reviews*. **4**: CD005083. (SA-19, 93 refs)
57 Grocott P. (1995) The palliative management of fungating malignant wounds. *Journal of Wound Care*. **4**(5): 240–2. (R, 36 refs)
58 Kelly N. (2002) Malodorous fungating wounds: a review of current literature. *Professional Nurse*. **17**(5): 323–6. (R, 40 refs)

NOTES

Nausea and vomiting

CLINICAL DECISION AND ACTION CHECKLIST

1 If vomiting, make available a large bowl, tissues, and water.
2 Is the patient troubled mainly by vomiting?
3 Is constipation present?
4 Could the cause be drugs, toxins, or biochemical?
5 Is the nausea or vomiting worse on movement?
6 Is gastritis present?
7 Could fear or anxiety be contributing?
8 Is the nausea or vomiting persisting?

KEY POINTS

- Antiemetic choice depends on the cause.
- A single antiemetic is sufficient in two-thirds of patients.[1]
- Any added antiemetics should have a different action.[2]
- Gastric motility disorders have specific signs and symptoms.

INTRODUCTION

Nausea and vomiting occur in up to 50% of patients with cancer,[3,4] and both are common in AIDS,[5] end-stage heart failure,[6,7] and in children at the end of life.[8] Most patients find it very distressing.[9] Assessment of the cause will depend on knowledge of the underlying disease, history, and examination. Commonly overlooked causes are hypercalcemia,[10] pharyngeal stimulation by copious sputum, gastric stasis, constipation, and drugs other than opioids. In one-third of patients there is more than one cause of emesis.[2]

ASSESSMENT

There are no clinically useful tools for assessing nausea and vomiting in palliative care.[11] Therefore the assessment should be based firstly on the patient's description of the symptoms such as its onset, precipitating factors, pattern of nausea and vomiting, relieving factors, and the presence of constipation. Secondly, observation is important (context of the nausea or vomiting, content of any vomited products, the hydration status of the patient, and the psychological impact of persistent nausea or vomiting).

TREATMENT

The principles of treatment

1 Start metoclopramide.
2 Is this gastric stasis?
If yes, give metoclopramide SC.
3 Is there a chemical cause?
If yes, start haloperidol.
4 For other causes use a third-line antiemetic.

Basic decisions

The principles of treatment are based on the current knowledge of the emetic pathway (*see* figure). At least 17 neurotransmitters or receptors have been identified, but at present six receptors are routinely targeted by five antiemetic drugs. When these are applied to specific causes, vomiting can be reduced by 89% in the first week and nausea by 56%.[12] Most causes have a non-specific pattern, but some can be identified on history:

Gastric stasis is the commonest cause of vomiting in advanced disease.[12,13] It is suggested by large-volume vomiting with esophageal reflux, epigastric fullness, early satiation or hiccups, usually without dehydration. The causes are not clear but include opioids, antimuscarinic drugs, causes of autonomic neuropathy (e.g. diabetes, paraneoplastic), and celiac axis damage or compression.[14]

Total outflow obstruction produces a similar picture to gastric stasis but with rapid dehydration.

"Squashed stomach syndrome": this occurs when the gastric cavity is reduced by gastric tumor or by external compression. Symptoms are similar to gastric stasis but with low-volume vomiting.

"Floppy stomach syndrome": here gastric tone is absent, resulting in a distended stomach, discomfort, and small-volume vomits.

Regurgitation produces vomits of undigested material that test negative to acid.

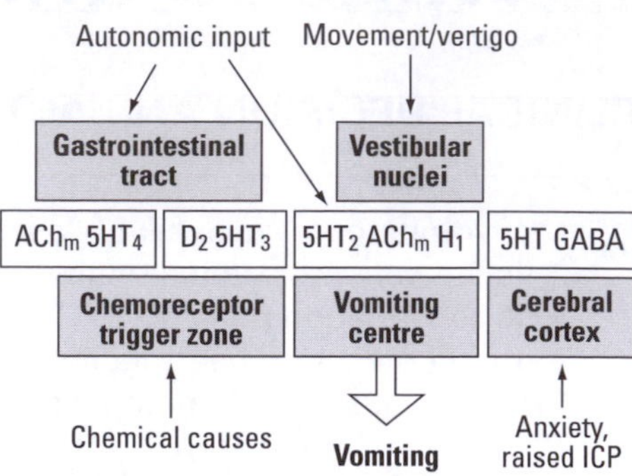

dimenhydrinate/diphenhydramine block H_1 receptors and reduce ACh_m tone
haloperidol blocks D_2 receptors
methotrimeprazine (Canada only) blocks D_2, H_1 and $5HT_2$ receptors and reduces ACh_m tone
metoclopramide blocks D_2 and stimulates $5HT_4$ receptors
domperidone (from compounding pharmacy in US) blocks D_2 receptors
ondansetron blocks $5HT_3$ receptors
olanzapine blocks D_2, H_2, $5HT_2$, and weakly reduces ACh_m tone

Receptor basis for treating nausea and vomiting[15–18]

Choosing an antiemetic

Five key antiemetics: these are dimenhydrinate (Canada) or diphenhydramine (US), haloperidol,[19,20] metoclopramide,[21,22] domperidone,[23–25] and methotrimeprazine (Canada only).[26–28] The receptors likely to be involved dictate the choice of antiemetic[15] (*see* figure above and clinical decisions opposite). Most are available in parenteral and oral preparations. In some parts of North America it is common practice to use metoclopramide as a first-line antiemetic. When maintaining a patient on oral prokinetic therapy, domperidone is preferred to metoclopramide since the risk of extrapyramidal adverse effects is reduced, especially if a second drug with the same risk is added later.

Clinical decision	If YES carry out the action below
1 If vomiting, make available a large bowl, tissues, and water. Start metoclopramide 10 mg PO or SC q8h	
2 Is the patient troubled mainly by vomiting? (i.e. no nausea or brief nausea relieved by vomiting)	a. **Large-volume vomiting** (with heartburn, hiccups, fullness, or early satiation) *If dehydrating rapidly consider total gastric outflow obstruction:* will need NG tube and IV hydration for comfort. If tumor is the cause, high-dose dexamethasone SC or IV (16 mg daily) may help clear the obstruction, but if persisting refer for consideration of stenting, or a venting gastrostomy. *If not dehydrating rapidly:* this is probably *gastric stasis* due to drugs (*see* text), partial outflow obstruction (local tumor, hepatomegaly, ascites, disordered motility of duodenum), or autonomic failure; start metoclopramide 10 mg SC q6h or 40–100 mg SC infusion per 24 hours. For children use domperidone (*see Drugs in children: starting doses*, p. 303). Maintain adults on oral domperidone 10–20 mg q6h (available in US from compounding pharmacy). *If gastric stasis is still a problem:* consider erythromycin 100–250 mg q12h. b. **Regurgitation** (unaltered food or drink vomited within minutes of ingestion, litmus test is negative to acid): *See* cd-2 in *Dysphagia*, p. 133. c. **Distended stomach** ("floppy stomach syndrome"): may contain fluid, air or both. Brief nasogastric suction will bring rapid relief, even in unconscious patients. d. **Compressed stomach** ("squashed stomach syndrome"): the features are the same as gastric stasis but vomits are small. Treat as for gastric stasis in cd-2a above. e. **Raised intracranial pressure:** dimenhydrinate or diphenhydramine 25–50 mg PO, SC or PR q8h, or 75–150 mg SC infusion per 24 hours. *If due to intracranial tumor:* start high-dose dexamethasone and refer to clinical oncologist for possible cranial irradiation.
3 Is constipation present?	• **Exclude bowel obstruction:** *see Bowel obstruction*, p. 99. • **If constipation is present:** *see Constipation*, p. 107.
4 Could the cause be drugs, toxins, or biochemical?	• **Chemoreceptor trigger zone (CTZ) stimulation** (bacterial toxins, most drugs, hypercalcemia, uremia): low-dose haloperidol 1.5–3 mg PO or SC once at night. For hypercalcemia *see* cd-7b in *Emergencies*, p. 341. • **$5HT_3$ receptor stimulation** (e.g. antibiotics, cytotoxic drugs, SSRI antidepressants): ondansetron 4–8 mg q8h SC or PO. • **Gastrointestinal mucosal irritation** (antibiotics, blood, cytotoxic drugs, iron supplements, NSAIDs, tranexamic acid): change drug if possible. For gastritis *see* cd-6, p. 171. For bleeding *see* cd-4 in *Bleeding*, p. 95. • **Gastric stasis** (antimuscarinic drugs including amitriptyline, hyoscine, and opioids): change drug or treat as in cd-2a above.

Adapted from Regnard and Comiskey[29]
cd = clinical decision

Other antiemetics: $5HT_3$ antagonists are important in radiotherapy and chemotherapy,[30] are often given with dexamethasone, and sometimes with aprepitant (Emend).[31,32] Cannabinoids have been used[33] such as dronabinol for GI metastases[34] and nabilone for chemotherapy.[35] $5HT_3$ antagonists have sometimes been helpful in emesis due to bowel obstruction,[36] AIDS and cancer,[37] and in multiple sclerosis,[38] but are rarely of benefit outside chemotherapy-induced emesis.[39,40] Olanzapine may have a role in refractory nausea but parenterally can only be given IV or IM.[41] Erythromycin has gastric stimulant actions since it has a motilin-agonist action. Mirtazapine may improve resistant gastric stasis,[42] and may have a role in other causes of nausea,[43] but can cause nausea if it is abruptly withdrawn, and is not available in injectable form.

ASSOCIATED MANAGEMENT

Bucket, tissues and water: a decent-sized bowl is essential to avoid the distress to patients of soiling their clothes and bedsheets. Also available should be tissues to wipe the mouth and water or juice to rinse the mouth.

Parenteral hydration: 500–1000 mL/24 hours may help to reduce persistent nausea,[44,45] but this should be done with careful attention to electrolyte levels and avoiding fluid overload.

Nasogastric tube and suction has no role to play in most causes of nausea and vomiting.[46–50] There are three exceptions where it may help:

a. Gastric outflow or duodenal obstruction to reduce high-volume vomiting.[51]
b. Gastric atony ("floppy stomach") where a nasogastric tube can be passed easily (even in semiconscious or unconscious patients) and removed once all the fluid and air has been aspirated.
c. Feculant vomiting to reduce odor (*see* p. 100).

Acupuncture has good evidence for efficacy in nausea and vomiting,[52–56] but acupuncture-like TENS has not been shown to help.[57]

Acupressure at the P6 acupuncture point on the wrist may have a role in some patients.[58–61]

Chemotherapy is only helpful in treating nausea and vomiting if there is likely to be a good tumor response.[62]

Hypnosis and behavioral therapy: Anxiety and fear can cause nausea and vomiting[63] especially prior to chemotherapy. Hypnosis has been used to good effect in anticipatory emesis.[64–66] Behavioral therapy may have a role by resetting the triggers that usually set off a cycle of fear, anxiety, and emesis.[67]

PERSISTENT NAUSEA AND VOMITING

Chemotherapy: a $5HT_3$ antagonist is more effective when combined with dexamethasone.[68]

Dexamethasone can help in persistent nausea due to other causes.[69,70]

Stenting: this is an option in persistent gastric outflow or duodenal obstruction.[71,72]

Gastrostomy is usually a means of giving enteral nutrition and hydration when oral feeding is not possible (*see* p. 134), but can be useful in cases of inoperable small bowel or gastric outflow obstruction when it is known as a "venting gastrostomy."[73–75]

Thalidomide (Special Access category) may have a role in persistent emesis.[76]

Clinical decision	If YES carry out the action below
5 Is the nausea or vomiting worse on movement?	• **Mechanical distortion of a distended stomach or bowel:** for gastric stasis treat as in cd-2a on p. 169. For vomiting secondary to bowel or liver distension use dimenhydrinate or diphenhydramine 25–50 mg PO or 50–100 mg PR q8h, or 25 mg SC q6-8h. • **Motion sickness:** hyoscine hydrobromide (scopolamine) transdermally 1 mg/72 hr (more than one patch may be needed). • **Other causes** (e.g. middle ear infection, vestibular viral neuronitis such as zoster infection, ototoxic drugs, tumor at cerebellopontine angle, Ménière's disease): dimenhydrinate or promethazine 25–50 mg PO or 50–100 mg PR q8h or 25 mg SC q6-8h.
6 Is gastritis present?	• **If on an NSAID:** start PPI cover. Do not use ranitidine or cimetidine since these are less effective at protecting against gastric NSAID damage.[77] If there is no response, stop the NSAID and start sucralfate PO 2g q6h. • **If not on ulcer healing drug:** start ranitidine 300 mg q12h or PPI (omeprazole in children). • **If nausea or vomiting persists**, start metoclopramide 10 mg SC q6h or 40–100 mg SC infusion per 24 hours. Maintain on oral route 10–20 mg q6h. For children use domperidone (available from compounding pharmacy in US) (*see Drugs in children: starting doses*, p. 307). Maintain adults on oral domperidone 10–20 mg q6h. • **If anxiety is contributing:** *see* cd-7 below.
7 Could fear or anxiety be contributing?	• *See Anxiety*, p. 239. • Consider lorazepam 0.5 mg SL 2–4 hours prior to chemotherapy. • Persistent emesis may respond to hypnosis, or behavioral therapy.
8 Is the nausea or vomiting persisting?	• Start methotrimeprazine (Canada only) 3–6 mg PO or 2.5–5 mg SC at bedtime. This can be used instead of dimenhydrinate or diphenhydramine. If this is ineffective, replace with olanzapine 2.5 mg 12 hourly PO, IV or IM. • If dehydrated, moderate rehydration of 500–1000 mL/24 hours may help. • Other antiemetics: consider adding *one* of the following: — ondansetron 4 mg q8h PO or SC — dexamethasone 4 mg once daily PO or SC — mirtazapine 15 mg daily PO.

Adapted from Regnard and Comiskey[29]
cd = clinical decision

REFERENCES: NAUSEA AND VOMITING

B = book; C = comment; Ch = chapter; CS-n = case study-no. of cases; CT-n = controlled trial-no. of cases; E = editorial; GC = group consensus; I-n = interviews-no. of cases; LS = laboratory study; MC = multi-center; OS-n = open study-no. of cases; R, refs = review, no. of references; RCT-n = randomized controlled trial-no. of cases; RS-n = retrospective survey-no. of cases; SA-n = systematic or meta analysis-no. of studies.

1 Hanks GW. (1982) Antiemetics for terminal cancer patients. *Lancet.* **1**(8286): 1410.
2 Lichter I. (1993) Which antiemetic? *Journal of Palliative Care.* **9**: 42–50.
3 Morita T, Tsunoda J, Inoue S, Chihara S. (1999) Contributing factors to physical symptoms in terminally-ill cancer patients. *Journal of Pain and Symptom Management.* **18**(5): 338–46. (OS-350)
4 Vainio A, Auvinen A. (1996) Prevalence of symptoms among patients with advanced cancer: an international collaborative study. *Journal of Pain and Symptom Management.* **12**(1): 3–10. (OS-1840)
5 Newshan G, Sherman DW. (1999) Palliative care: pain and symptom management in persons with HIV/AIDS. *Nursing Clinics of North America.* **34**(1): 131–45.
6 Davies N, Curtis M. (2000) Providing palliative care in end-stage heart failure. *Professional Nurse.* **15**(6): 389–92. (R, 31 refs)
7 McCarthy M, Lay M, Addington-Hall J. (1996) Dying from heart disease. *Journal of the Royal College of Physicians of London.* **30**(4): 325–8. (I-600)
8 Santucci G, Mack JW. (2007) Common gastrointestinal symptoms in pediatric palliative care: nausea, vomiting, constipation, anorexia, cachexia. *Pediatric Clinics of North America.* **54**(5): 673–89. (R, 43 refs)
9 Addington-Hall J, Altmann D. (2000) Which terminally ill cancer patients in the United Kingdom receive care from community specialist palliative care nurses? *Journal of Advanced Nursing.* **32**(4): 799–806. (I-2074)
10 Lamy O, Jenzer-Closuit A, Burckhardt P. (2001) Hypercalcaemia of malignancy: an undiagnosed and undertreated disease. *Journal of Internal Medicine.* **250**(1): 73–9. (OS-71)
11 Saxby C, Ackroyd R, Callin S, Mayland C, Kite S. (2007) How should we measure emesis in palliative care? *Journal of Palliative Medicine.* **21**(5): 369–83. (R, 62 refs)
12 Stephenson J, Davies A. (2006) An assessment of aetiology-based guidelines for the management of nausea and vomiting in patients with advanced cancer. *Supportive Care in Cancer.* **14**(4): 348–53. (OS-121)
13 Bentley A, Boyd K. (2001) Use of clinical pictures in the management of nausea and vomiting: a prospective audit. *Palliative Medicine.* **15**(3): 247–53. (OS-40)
14 Trinidad-Hernandez M, Keith P, Habib I, White JV. (2006) Reversible gastroparesis: functional documentation of celiac axis compression syndrome and postoperative improvement. *American Surgeon.* **72**(4): 339–44. (CS-3)
15 Peroutka SJ, Snyder SH. (1982) Antiemetics: Neurotransmitter receptor binding predicts therapeutic actions. *Lancet.* **1**(8273): 658–9. (R)
16 Sanger GJ. (1993) The pharmacology of anti-emetic agents. In: *Emesis in Anti-cancer Therapy: mechanisms and treatment.* London: Chapman and Hall. pp. 179–210. (Ch)
17 Twycross R, Wilcock A, Dean M, Kennedy B, eds. (2010) *Palliative Care Formulary*, Canadian ed. Nottingham: palliativedrugs.com. (B); and Twycross R, Wilcock A. eds. (2008) *Hospice and Palliative Care Formulary USA, 2nd ed.* Nottingham: palliativedrugs.com. (B)
18 Mannix KA. (2009) Palliation of nausea and vomiting. In: Hanks G, Cherney NI, Christakis NA, Fallon M, Kaasa S, Portenoy RK. *The Oxford Textbook of Palliative Medicine, 4th ed.* Oxford: Oxford University Press. (Ch)
19 Vella-Brincat J, Macleod AD. (2004) Haloperidol in palliative care. *Palliative Medicine.* **18**(3): 195–201. (R, 34 refs)
20 Buttner M, Walder B, von Elm E, Tramer MR. (2004) Is low-dose haloperidol a useful antiemetic? A meta-analysis of published and unpublished randomized trials. *Anesthesiology.* **101**(6): 1454–63. (RCT-1468)
21 Wilson J, Plourde JY, Marshall D, Yoshida S, *et al.* (2002) Long-term safety and clinical effectiveness of controlled-release metoclopramide in cancer-associated dyspepsia syndrome: a multicentre evaluation. *Journal of Palliative Care.* **18**(2): 84–91. (OS-48)
22 Bruera E, Belzile M, Neumann C, Harsanyi Z, Babul N, Darke A. (2000) A double-blind, crossover study of controlled-release metoclopramide and placebo for the chronic nausea and dyspepsia of advanced cancer. *Journal of Pain and Symptom Management.* **19**(6): 427–35. (RCT-26)
23 Hiyama T, Yoshihara M, Tanaka S, Haruma K, Chayama K. (2009) Effectiveness of prokinetic agents against diseases external to the gastrointestinal tract. *Journal of Gastroenterology and Hepatology.* **24**(4): 537–46. (R, 149 refs)
24 Dailly E, Drouineau MH, Gournay V, Roze JC, Jolliet P. (2008) Population pharmacokinetics of domperidone in preterm neonates. *European Journal of Clinical Pharmacology.* **64**(12): 1197–200. (OS-34)
25 Pfeil N, Uhlig U, Kostev K, Carius R, *et al.* (2008) Antiemetic medications in children with presumed infectious gastroenteritis: pharmacoepidemiology in Europe and Northern America. *Journal of Pediatrics.* **153**(5): 659–62. (RS)
26 Twycross RG, Barkby GD, Hallwood PM. (1997) The use of low dose levomepromazine (methotrimeprazine) in the management of nausea and vomiting. *Progress in Palliative Care.* **5**(2): 49–53.
27 Eisenchlas JH, Garrigue N, Junin M, De Simone GG. (2005) Low-dose levomepromazine in refractory emesis in advanced cancer patients: an

open-label study. *Palliative Medicine*. **19**(1): 71–5. (OS-70)

28 Kennett A, Hardy J, Shah S, A'Hern R. (2005) An open study of methotrimeprazine in the management of nausea and vomiting in patients with advanced cancer. *Supportive Care in Cancer*. **13**(9): 715–21. (OS-65)

29 Regnard C, Comiskey M. (1995) Nausea and vomiting. In: *Flow Diagrams in Advanced Cancer and Other Diseases*. London: Edward Arnold. pp. 14–18. (Ch)

30 Priestman TJ. (1996) Controlling the toxicity of palliative radiotherapy: the role of 5-HT3 antagonists. *Canadian Journal of Oncology*. **1**(Suppl.): 17–22. (R)

31 Gralla RJ, de Wit R, Herrstedt J, Carides AD, *et al*. (2005) Antiemetic efficacy of the neurokinin-1 antagonist, aprepitant, plus a 5HT3 antagonist and a corticosteroid in patients receiving anthracyclines or cyclophosphamide in addition to high-dose cisplatin: analysis of combined data from two phase III randomized clinical trials *Cancer*. **15**: 864–8. (RCT-1043)

32 Massaro AM, Lenz KL. (2005) Aprepitant: a novel antiemetic for chemotherapy-induced vomiting. *Annals of Pharmacotherapy*. **39**(1): 77–85. (R)

33 Hall W, Christie M, Currow D. (2005) Cannabinoids and cancer: causation, remediation, and palliation. *Lancet Oncology*. **6**(1): 35–42. (R, 70 refs)

34 Gonzales-Rosales F, Walsh D. (1997) Palliative care rounds: intractable nausea and vomiting due to gastrointestinal mucosal metastases relieved by tetrahydrocannabinol (dronabinol). *Journal of Pain and Symptom Management*. **14**(5): 311–14. (CS-1)

35 Tramer MR, Carroll D, Campbell FA, Reynolds DJ, Moore RA, McQuay HJ. (2001) Cannabinoids for control of chemotherapy induced nausea and vomiting: quantitative systematic review. *British Medical Journal*. **323**(7303): 16–21. (R, 38 refs)

36 Tuca A, Roca R, Porta J, Serrano G, Gonzalez-Barboteo J, Gomez-Batiste X. (2009) Efficacy of granisetron in the antiemetic control of non-surgical intestinal obstruction in advanced cancer: a phase II clinical trial. *Journal of Pain and Symptom Management*. **37**(2): 259–70. (MC, OS-24)

37 Currow DC, Coughlan M, Fardell B, Cooney NJ. (1997) Clinical note: use of ondansetron in palliative medicine. *Journal of Pain and Symptom Management*. **13**(5): 302–7. (RS-16)

38 Macleod AD. (2000) Ondansetron in multiple sclerosis. *Journal of Pain and Symptom Management*. **20**(5): 388–91. (CS-2)

39 Warden CR, Moreno R, Daya M. (2008) Prospective evaluation of ondansetron for undifferentiated nausea and vomiting in the prehospital setting. *Prehospital Emergency Care*. **12**(1): 87–91. (OS-952)

40 Braude D, Crandall C. (2008) Ondansetron versus promethazine to treat acute undifferentiated nausea in the emergency department: a randomized, double-blind, noninferiority trial. *Academic Emergency Medicine*. **15**(3): 209–15. (RCT-120)

41 Passik SD, Lundberg J, Kirsh KL, Theobald D, *et al*. (2002) A pilot exploration of the antiemetic activity of olanzapine for the relief of nausea in patients with advanced cancer and pain. *Journal of Pain and Symptom Management*. **23**(6): 526–32. (OS-15)

42 Kim SW, Shin IS, Kim JM, Kang HC, *et al*. (2006) Mirtazapine for severe gastroparesis unresponsive to conventional prokinetic treatment. *Psychosomatics*. **47**(5): 440–2. (CS-1)

43 Kim SW, Shin IS, Kim JM, Kim YC, *et al*. (2008) Effectiveness of mirtazapine for nausea and insomnia in cancer patients with depression. *Psychiatry and Clinical Neurosciences*. **62**(1): 75–83. (OS-28)

44 Ripamonti C, Mercadante S, Groff L, Zecca E, De Conno F, Casuccio A. (2000) Role of octreotide, scopolamine butylbromide, and hydration in symptom control of patients with inoperable bowel obstruction and nasogastric tubes: a prospective randomized trial. *Journal of Pain and Symptom Management*. **19**(1): 23–34. (CT-17)

45 Cerchietti L, Navigante A, Sauri A, Palazzo F. (2000) Clinical trial: hypodermoclysis for control of dehydration in terminal-stage cancer. *International Journal of Palliative Nursing*. **6**(8): 370–4. (CT-42)

46 Ripamonti C, Panzeri C, Groff L, Galeazzi G, Boffi R. (2001) The role of somatostatin and octreotide in bowel obstruction: pre-clinical and clinical results. *Tumori*. **87**(1): 1–9. (R, 82 refs)

47 Ripamonti C, Twycross R, Baines M, Bozzetti F, *et al*. (2001) Working Group of the European Association for Palliative Care. Clinical-practice recommendations for the management of bowel obstruction in patients with end-stage cancer. *Supportive Care in Cancer*. **9**(4): 223–33. (R)

48 Nelson R, Edwards S, Tse B. (2005) Prophylactic nasogastric decompression after abdominal surgery. *Cochrane Database of Systematic Reviews*. **1**: CD004929. (R, 39 refs)

49 Cheatham ML, Chapman WC, Key SP, Sawyers JL. (1995) A meta-analysis of selective versus routine nasogastric decompression after elective laparotomy. *Annals of Surgery*. **221**(5): 469–76; discussion 476–8. (SA)

50 Koukouras D, Mastronikolis NS, Tzoracoleftherakis E, Angelopoulou E, *et al*. (2001) The role of nasogastric tube after elective abdominal surgery. *Clinica Terapeutica*. **152**(4): 241–4. (RCT-100)

51 Upadhyay V, Sakalkale R, Parashar K, Mitra SK, *et al*. (1996) Duodenal atresia: a comparison of three modes of treatment. *European Journal of Pediatric Surgery*. **6**(2): 75–7. (RS-33)

52 Wang SM, Kain ZN. (2002) P6 acupoint injections are as effective as droperidol in controlling early postoperative nausea and vomiting in children. *Anesthesiology*. **97**(2): 359–66. (CT-186)

53 Kaptchuk TJ. (2002) Acupuncture: theory, efficacy, and practice. *Annals of Internal Medicine*. **136**(5): 374–83. (R, 113 refs)

54 Ezzo J, Streitberger K, Schneider A. (2006) Cochrane systematic reviews examine P6 acupuncture-point stimulation for nausea and

vomiting. *Journal of Alternative and Complementary Medicine*. **12**(5): 489–95. (R, 23 refs)

55 Johnstone PA, Polston GR, Niemtzow RC, Martin PJ. (2002) Integration of acupuncture into the oncology clinic. *Palliative Medicine*. **16**(3): 235–9. (OS-123)

56 Nystrom E, Ridderstrom G, Leffler AS. (2008) Manual acupuncture as an adjunctive treatment of nausea in patients with cancer in palliative care: a prospective, observational pilot study. *Acupuncture in Medicine*. **26**(1): 27–32. (OS-12)

57 Gadsby JG, Franks A, Jarvis P, Dewhurst F. (1997) Acupuncture-like transcutaneous electrical nerve stimulation within palliative care: a pilot study. *Complementary Therapies in Medicine*. **5**(1): 13–18. (RCT-15)

58 Can Gurkan O, Arslan H. (2008) Effect of acupressure on nausea and vomiting during pregnancy. *Complementary Therapies in Clinical Practice*. **14**(1): 46–52. (OS-75)

59 Stern RM, Jokerst MD, Muth ER, Hollis C. (2001) Acupressure relieves the symptoms of motion sickness and reduces abnormal gastric activity. *Alternative Therapies in Health and Medicine*. **7**(4): 91–4. (RCT-25)

60 Gardani G, Cerrone R, Biella C, Galbiati G, *et al*. (2007) A progress study of 100 cancer patients treated by acupressure for chemotherapy-induced vomiting after failure with the pharmacological approach. *Minerva Medica*. **98**(6): 665–8. (OS-100)

61 Roscoe JA, Jean-Peirre P, Heckler CE, Purnell JQ, *et al*. (2009) Acupressure bands are effective in reducing radiation therapy-related nausea. *Journal of Pain and Symptom Management*. **38**(3): 381–9. (RCT-148)

62 Geels P, Eisenhauer E, Bezjak A, Zee B, Day A. (2000) Palliative effect of chemotherapy: objective tumor response is associated with symptom improvement in patients with metastatic breast cancer. *Journal of Clinical Oncology*. **18**(12): 2395–405. (RCT-300)

63 Watson M, Meyer L, Thomson A, Osofsky S. (1998) Psychological factors predicting nausea and vomiting in breast cancer patients on chemotherapy. *European Journal of Cancer*. **34**(6): 831–7. (OS-100)

64 Richardson J, Smith JE, McCall G, *et al*. (2007) Hypnosis for nausea and vomiting in cancer chemotherapy: a systematic review of the research evidence. *European Journal of Cancer Care*. **16**(5): 402–12. (R, 47 refs)

65 Eckert RM. (2001) Understanding anticipatory nausea. *Oncology Nursing Forum*. **28**(10): 1553–8; quiz 1559–60. (R, 44 refs)

66 Marchioro G, Azzarello G, Viviani F, Barbato F, *et al*. (2000) Hypnosis in the treatment of anticipatory nausea and vomiting in patients receiving cancer chemotherapy. *Oncology*. **59**(2): 100–4. (OS-16)

67 Redd WH, Montgomery GH, DuHamel KN. (2001) Behavioral intervention for cancer treatment side effects. *Journal of the National Cancer Institute*. **93**(11): 810–23. (R, 106 refs)

68 Fabi A, Ciccarese M, Metro G, Savarese A, *et al*. (2008) Oral ondansetron is highly active as rescue antiemetic treatment for moderately emetogenic chemotherapy: results of a randomized phase II study. *Supportive Care in Cancer*. **16**(12): 1375–80. (RCT-89)

69 Bruera E, Seifert L, Watanabe S, Babul N, *et al*. (1996) Chronic nausea in advanced cancer patients: a retrospective assessment of a metoclopramide-based antiemetic regimen. *Journal of Pain and Symptom Management*. **11**(3): 147–53. (RS-100)

70 Hardy JR, Rees E, Ling J, Burman R, *et al*. (2001) A prospective survey of the use of dexamethasone on a palliative care unit. *Palliative Medicine*. **15**(1): 3–8. (OS-106)

71 Seo EH, Jung MK, Park MJ, Park KS, *et al*. (2008) Covered expandable nitinol stents for malignant gastroduodenal obstructions. *Journal of Gastroenterology and Hepatology*. **23**(7 Pt. 1): 1056–62. (OS-68)

72 Uthappa MC, Ho SM, Boardman P. (2003) Role of metallic stents in palliative care. *Progress in Palliative Care*. **11**(1): 3–9. (R, 29 refs)

73 Meyer L, Pothuri B. (2006) Decompressive percutaneous gastrostomy tube use in gynecologic malignancies. *Current Treatment Options in Oncology*. **7**(2): 111–20. (R, 30 refs)

74 Watson JP, Mannix KA, Matthewson K. (1997) Percutaneous endoscopic gastroenterostomy and jejunal extension for gastric stasis in pancreatic carcinoma. *Palliative Medicine*. 11: 407–10.

75 Holm AN, Baron TH. (2007) Palliative use of percutaneous endoscopic gastrostomy and percutaneous endoscopic cecostomy tubes. *Gastrointestinal Endoscopy Clinics of North America*. **17**(4): 795–803. (R, 38 refs)

76 Peuckmann V, Fisch M, Bruera E. (2000) Potential novel uses of thalidomide: focus on palliative care. *Drugs*. **60**(2): 273–92. (R, 120 refs)

77 Graham DY, Agrawal NM, Campbell DR, Haber MM, *et al*. (2002) NSAID-Associated Gastric Ulcer Prevention Study Group. Ulcer prevention in long-term users of nonsteroidal anti-inflammatory drugs: results of a double-blind, randomized, multicenter, active- and placebo-controlled study of misoprostol vs lansoprazole. *Archives of Internal Medicine*. **162**(2): 169–75. (MC, RCT-537)

Nutrition and hydration problems

CLINICAL DECISION AND ACTION CHECKLIST

1 Is the prognosis short (day-by-day deterioration)?
2 Is there a request to withdraw hydration or feeding?
3 Are physical symptoms present?
4 Is the feeding tube blocked?
5 Could drugs be the cause?
6 Is the food presentation or environment a problem?
7 Is anorexia persisting?
8 Is thirst still present?

KEY POINTS

- Consider reversible causes before starting an appetite stimulant.
- Reduced intake is normal at the end of life.

INTRODUCTION

Hunger and thirst make us eat and drink for survival. But we also eat out of habit, boredom, pleasure, satisfaction or comfort, and because we choose to make it a social activity. Advanced disease can severely reduce our ability, need, or desire to eat and drink, which has a major impact on quality of life for two main reasons.[1]

Firstly, deficiencies of hydration and nutrition are common in advanced disease in both adults and children.[2–4] This becomes obvious when weight starts to decrease in an adult or a child fails to thrive.[5] However, long before weight loss develops there can be deficiencies in micronutrients such as vitamins, minerals, and essential fats. The impact of this malnutrition on function is poorly understood, but it may contribute to symptoms such as fatigue, and impair recovery from treatment and infection.[6]

Secondly, there is a large psychosocial impact in the way that problems with hydration and nutrition impact a patient's quality of life and their relationships with partners and relatives.[7,8]

DECISIONS

Palliative care doctors and nurses believe that non-oral routes rarely benefit patients at the end of life.[9] In contrast, partners and relatives may believe that withholding fluid or nutrition will cause distress.[10] The truth lies in assessing each individual since some will not need hydration or nutrition, while in others reversing dehydration can be important in symptom control, and in the earlier stages of illness non-oral nutrition can bring important benefits.

The decision lies with the patient, and sometimes with the advice of carers. Every situation is different and fixed policies are indefensible,[11] especially as data on the advantages or disadvantages of hydration are lacking.[12,13] In Canada, the US and UK, non-oral feeding falls into the category of medical treatment and, depending on the medical condition, the legal obligation to provide (artificial) nutrition and hydration is not always clear.[14] As with any treatment decisions, consent of the patient (or of the legally authorized substitute decision maker/ health care proxy) must be considered. In cases of patients lacking capacity for this decision and where no prior wishes have been expressed or are known, the best interests of the patient (including a weighing of the burdens and benefits to the patient) must be taken into account (*see Making ethical choices*, p. 263, and *Decisions around capacity*, p. 267).

As patients near end of life there is a gradual decline in oral intake, and with good mouth care patients do not suffer ill-effects, although partners and relatives may not understand this. In patients who are comatose and comfortable, dehydration causes few symptoms,[12] but dehydration can cause or contribute to a delirium in some patients,[15,16] (*see also Confusional states*, p. 245). Thirst may only need sips of water or may need parenteral rehydration.[17] Hunger is not usually a problem in the terminal stages,[18] and unwanted feeding by any route may increase distress.[19] Partners, relatives, friends, or staff may feel a need to continue hydration or feeding and they will need explanation and support.[20] Occasionally, the relatives or parents persist with the request for hydration or feeding in a dying adult or child, even though the patient is comfortable. In such circumstances it is reasonable to provide some hydration since a low rate subcutaneous (e.g. 1 litre/24 hr) or fluids through an existing PEG tube is unlikely to cause discomfort while refusing their request may complicate their bereavement.

MANAGING REDUCED HYDRATION AND FEEDING

Oral hydration and feeding

Environment: when healthy we have the choice of eating when, what, where, and with whom we choose. Illness greatly reduces that choice. Problems will result from inflexible mealtimes or crowded eating areas.

Food presentation is a key factor.[21] There should be a pleasant atmosphere, and food should be attractive, varied, at the correct temperature, and in appropriately sized portions for the patient. An alcoholic drink before meals is more effective poured from bottle to glass rather than dispensed in calibrated plastic pots. Patients may develop taste abnormalities and may prefer sweeter, colder, and spicier foods, while others cannot tolerate the bitterness of urea in red meats.[22,23] The skills of an enthusiastic chef and the advice of a dietician can be invaluable.

Clinical decision	If YES carry out the action below
1 Is the prognosis short? i.e. day-by-day deterioration due to an irreversible cause	• **If hydration or feeding would help** (e.g. thirst, hunger, or confusion due to dehydration): hydrate and feed for comfort or pleasure (may include IV or SC hydration). • **If hydration or feeding is unnecessary** (e.g. comatose and comfortable): ensure the partner, family, and staff understand the situation. If the family or partner feel a need to continue hydration and/or feeding, the family will need help to understand the situation. If they remain firm in their belief, try to negotiate maintenance hydration IV or SC or by PEG if this is already present (*see* text opposite).
2 Is there a request to withdraw hydration or feeding?	• **If this is from a person who has capacity for this decision:** — ensure good oral hygiene (*see Oral problems*, p. 183) — prevent skin pressure damage (*see Skin problems*, p. 203) • **If this is about an adult or child who does not have capacity for this decision:** — *see Decisions around capacity*, p. 267.
3 Are physical symptoms present?	• **Swallowing problems:** *see Dysphagia*, p. 131, *Oral problems*, p. 183. • **Constipation:** *see Constipation*, p. 107. • **Nausea and vomiting:** *see Nausea and vomiting*, p. 167. • **Infection:** treat infection with appropriate antibiotics. • **Odor:** *see* cd-5 in *Malignant ulcers and fistulae*, p. 163. • **Breathlessness:** *see Respiratory problems*, p. 191. • **Weakness:** exclude reversible causes of weakness (*see Fatigue, drowsiness, lethargy and weakness*, p. 149). • **Disability:** regular help with feeding and drinking (ask occupational therapist for advice).
4 Is the feeding tube blocked?	• **Check the tube** is in the correct position. • **Flush the tube** with 30 mL of warm water, followed if necessary by 30 mL of carbonated water. If still blocked put in 30 mL of pineapple juice and leave for 1 hour before flushing again (ananase will dissolve any protein material). • **Avoid drugs that interact with feeds** (*see Drug interactions*, p. 292).
5 Could drugs be the cause?	Consider drugs that cause nausea (e.g. opioids, metronidazole, trimethoprim), mucosal irritation (e.g. antibiotics, chemotherapy, NSAIDs, SSRIs), delayed gastric emptying (e.g. opioids, amitriptyline) or drugs with a central appetite suppressant effect (e.g. opioids, amphetamines): • Reduce the dose, change the drug, or stop.

Adapted from Regnard and Mannix[24]
cd = clinical decision

Equipment: if necessary the patient should be assessed by a physiotherapist and occupational therapist for seating and advice on utensils.

Communication: mealtimes are a time for communication, especially if the carer pays attention, is responsive, is at face to face level, gives eye contact, asks simple questions, creates choices, uses simple language about the meal, and allows the patient to use all sensory information such as looking, smelling, and touching.

Enriching the diet: this can be done in many ways, but there is no evidence that one type of supplement is better than any other.[25] Neutral flavor types are most versatile since they can be added to many different foods. Some nutritional deficiencies such as zinc may themselves alter taste,[24] and there is some evidence that replacing zinc improves salt taste.[26–28]

Non-oral hydration and nutrition

Parenteral hydration: this is most conveniently given subcutaneously (hypodermoclysis).[29] The suprascapular area is safe, convenient, and up to 100 mL/hr can be infused. Other sites can be used but can cause problems with SC hydration: sites in arms can become swollen and sites in the pectoral region can cause breast swelling. It is not necessary to add hyaluronidase to infusions.[30–32] Unlike the intravenous route, subcutaneous cannulae can be left in place for 7–10 days without problems. It is safe to use 5% dextrose solutions for SC hydration.[30] Other non-oral routes are discussed in *Dysphagia*, p. 131.

Parenteral nutrition: it is unusual to use total parenteral nutrition (TPN) in palliative care.[33] However, some patients may benefit, especially those with short-bowel syndromes or severe malabsorption.[34] In the last days of life, non-oral feeding offers no advantages.

Tube hydration and nutrition: although nasogastric tubes can be useful as a short-term measure, they have several disadvantages. Gastrostomies are a longer-term solution. More detail is given in *Dysphagia* (*see* p. 134).

Refeeding syndrome

This is a risk when a malnourished patient is given carbohydrates early in their feeding regime.[35] It results in low levels of phosphate, potassium, and magnesium, which can be life threatening. It is prevented by keeping carbohydrates (e.g. glucose) to a minimum initially and increasing them gradually. The advice of a dietician is essential.

PERSISTENT ANOREXIA

Gastric stasis: this is common in advanced disease (*see* cd-2a, *Nausea and vomiting*, p. 169).

Cachexia: this is a syndrome of weight loss (fat and skeletal muscle), anorexia, anemia, fatigue, and edema that reduces survival.[36] It is caused by the triggering of a cytokine-mediated systemic inflammatory response to the underlying illness, is metabolically distinct from starvation, and cannot be reversed with nutrition alone.[37–41] It is seen in cancer, AIDS, heart failure, rheumatoid arthritis, chronic infection, chronic respiratory disease, and liver cirrhosis.[42–46] In contrast, there is no evidence that the cachexia syndrome is a feature of degenerative neurological or neuromuscular diseases such as dementia, ALS or muscular dystrophy. When weight loss occurs in these conditions it is inevitably due to dysphagia (*see Dysphagia*, p. 131).

Clinical decision	If YES carry out the action below
6 Is the food presentation or environment a problem?	• **Food:** — ensure the food is presented attractively on small plates. — keep portions small, have snacks available, use calorie and protein additives that add little bulk (e.g. Ensure, Casilan). Vary food consistency, temperature, and taste. — add "neutral flavor" supplements to soups, potatoes, or desserts. — ask advice from a dietician and from catering staff. • **Environment:** ensure a pleasant atmosphere (coffee or baking smells, company, attractive table cover, alcohol before meals, avoid frying smells and overcrowding). *If the patient is embarrassed* (e.g. unavoidable dribbling): ensure privacy. *If cultural food is required* (e.g. kosher food): ensure this is available.
7 Is anorexia persisting?	• **Exclude gastric stasis:** *see* cd-2a in *Nausea and vomiting*, p. 169. • **Consider central suppression of appetite** due to pain (*see Diagnosing and treating pain*, p. 43), depression (*see Withdrawal and depression*, p. 253) or anxiety (*see Anxiety*, p. 239). • **Consider altered taste** due to: *Nutritional deficiency* (zinc, vitamin B complex): zinc and vitamin supplements might help. *Drugs* (phenytoin, flurazepam). *Dry mouth* (dyspnea, drugs, radiotherapy, chemotherapy) *see* cd-4 in *Oral problems*, p. 187. *Related conditions* (diabetes, chronic infection, renal failure). • **If all else is inappropriate or fails to improve appetite:** treat empirically with appetite stimulant, e.g. dexamethasone PO 2–4 mg once daily *or* prednisolone PO 20–30 mg once daily, *or* medroxyprogesterone 400 mg daily *or* megestrol acetate 160–480 mg/day. • **If cachexia is present:** consider adding EPA up to 6 g/day (found in omega-3 concentrated fish oil) possibly along with an NSAID plus PPI.
9 Is thirst still present?	• **Moisten mouth** frequently. • **Consider non-oral hydration:** use IV route or subcutaneous infusion into the suprascapular area (*see* text). The nasogastric route is a less well tolerated alternative. If needed for 1 month or more: consider percutaneous gastrostomy. *See also Dysphagia*, p. 134.

Adapted from Regnard and Mannix[24]
cd = clinical decision

Drug treatments: anorexia may be linked to low cortisol levels,[47] and dexamethasone or prednisolone can improve anorexia,[48–50] although any weight gain may be due to fluid retention.[51] Progestins are effective,[52] and megestrol acetate 800 mg daily has comparable benefits in terms of weight gain, appetite stimulation, and sense of well-being as 3 mg dexamethasone daily,[53] but is much more expensive.[54] However, one study suggests that there is benefit at even 160 mg/day, although benefit increases as the dose increases.[55] The majority of weight gain is due to the formation of adipose tissue,[56] not lean body tissue. Two studies have found a 5% incidence of thrombosis.[53,55] Cachexia in cancer can be modified by 1–3 g daily of the fatty acid eicosapentaenoic acid (EPA).[57] Concentrated omega-3 fish oils are widely available and contain 15–20% EPA, but can cause diarrhea in some patients especially at higher doses. More recently an improved outcome (increased body weight and muscle strength as well as better appetite and less fatigue) has been shown when fish-oil (6 g/day) capsules are taken along with a COX-2 NSAID.[58,59] Thalidomide may also have a role.[60,61] A combination of approaches may offer the best response.[62]

Support and reassurance: in many patients, the anorexia is part of the advanced illness and is more of a concern to carers.[63] It is helpful to support the patient to adapt to their reduced intake, and so reduce their anxiety, as well as to reassure the partner and family it is not due to a failure in their care.

REFERENCES: NUTRITION AND HYDRATION PROBLEMS

B = book; C = comment; CC = Court case; Ch = chapter; CS-n = case study-no. of cases; CT-n = controlled trial-no. of cases; E = editorial; GC = group consensus; I = interviews; Let = letter; LS = laboratory study; MC = multi-center; OS-n = open study-no. of cases; R = review; Rep = report; RCT-n = randomized controlled trial-no. of cases; RS-n = retrospective survey-no. of cases; SA = systematic or meta analysis; Th = thesis.

1 Marin Caro MM, Laviano A, Pichard C. (2007) Impact of nutrition on quality of life during cancer. *Current Opinion in Clinical Nutrition and Metabolic Care*. **10**(4): 480–7. (R, 60 refs)

2 Kubrak C, Jensen L. (2007) Critical evaluation of nutrition screening tools recommended for oncology patients. *Cancer Nursing*. **30**(5): E1–6. (R, 36 refs)

3 Argiles JM. (2005) Cancer-associated malnutrition. *European Journal of Oncology Nursing*. **9**(Suppl. 2): S39–50. (R, 112 refs)

4 Sala A, Pencharz P, Barr RD. (2004) Children, cancer, and nutrition: a dynamic triangle in review. *Cancer*. **100**(4): 677–87. (R, 100 refs)

5 Sarhill N, Mahmoud FA, Christie R, Tahir A. (2003) Assessment of nutritional status and fluid deficits in advanced cancer. *American Journal of Hospice and Palliative Medicine*. **20**(6): 465–73. (R, 75 refs)

6 Marin Caro MM, Laviano A, Pichard C. (2007) Impact of nutrition on quality of life during cancer. *Current Opinion in Clinical Nutrition and Metabolic Care*. **10**(4): 480–7. (R, 60 refs)

7 Strasser F, Binswanger J, Cerny T, Kesselring A. (2007) Fighting a losing battle: eating-related distress of men with advanced cancer and their female partners: a mixed-methods study. *Palliative Medicine*. **21**(2): 129–37. (I-19)

8 Shragge JE, Wismer WV, Olson KL, Baracos VE. (2006) The management of anorexia by patients with advanced cancer: a critical review of the literature. *Palliative Medicine*. **20**(6): 623–9. (R, 52 refs)

9 van der Riet P, Good P, Higgins I, Sneesby L. (2008) Palliative care professionals' perceptions of nutrition and hydration at the end of life. *International Journal of Palliative Nursing*. **14**(3): 145–51. (I)

10 Van der Riet P, Brooks D, Ashby M. (2006) Nutrition and hydration at the end of life: pilot study of a palliative care experience. *Journal of Law and Medicine*. **14**(2): 182–98. (I)

11 Joint working party of the National Council for Hospice and Palliative Care Services and the ethics committee of the Association for Palliative Medicine of Great Britain and Ireland. (1997) Artificial hydration (AH) for people who are terminally ill. *European Journal of Palliative Care*. **4**: 124. (Rep)

12 Dunphy K, Finlay I, Rathbone G, Gilbert J, Hicks F. (1995) Rehydration in palliative and terminal

care: if not – why not? *Palliative Medicine*. **9**(3): 221–8. (R, 32 refs)

13 Burge FI. (1996) Dehydration and provision of fluids in palliative care: what is the evidence? *Canadian Family Physician*. **42**: 2383–8. (SA, 14 refs)

14 Greer George W, Circuit Judge (2005-02-25). "In re: The guardianship of Theresa Marie Schiavo, Incapacitated. Michael Schiavo, Petitioner, v. Robert Schindler and Mary Schindler, Respondents, File No. 90-2908-GD-003". [Florida Sixth Judicial Circuit]. Retrieved 2006-06-26. p. 3. (CC)

15 Fainsinger RL, Bruera E. (1997) When to treat dehydration in a terminally ill patient? *Supportive Care in Cancer*. **5**: 205–11. (R, 54 refs)

16 Lawlor PG, Gagnon B, Mancini IL, Pereira JL, *et al.* (2000) Occurrence, causes, and outcome of delirium in patients with advanced cancer: a prospective study. *Archives of Internal Medicine*. **160**(6): 786–94. (OS-104)

17 Morita T, Tei Y, Tsunoda J, Inoue S, Chihara S. (2001) Determinants of the sensation of thirst in terminally ill cancer patients. *Supportive Care in Cancer.* **9**(3): 177–86. (OS-88)

18 McCann RM, Hall WJ, Groth-Juncker A. (1994) Comfort care for terminally ill patients: the appropriate use of nutrition and hydration. *Journal of the American Medical Association*. **272**(16): 1263–6. (OS-32)

19 Winter SM. (2000) Terminal nutrition: framing the debate for the withdrawal of nutritional support in terminally ill patients. *American Journal of Medicine*. **109**(9): 723–6. (R, 30 refs)

20 Parkash R, Burge F. (1997) The family's perspective on issues of hydration in terminal care. *Journal of Palliative Care*. **13**(4): 23–7. (I)

21 Williams J, Copp G. (1990) Food presentation and the terminally ill. *Nursing Standard*. **4**: 29–32.

22 DeWys D. (1978) Changes in taste sensation and feeding behaviour in cancer patients: a review. *Journal of Human Nutrition*. **32**: 447–53. (R, 16 refs)

23 Moody C. (1997) Taste acuity, appetite and zinc status in patients with terminal cancer: BSc thesis in Food and Human Nutrition. Newcastle: University of Newcastle upon Tyne (Department of Biological and Nutritional Sciences). (Thesis)

24 Regnard C, Mannix K. (1995) Reduced hydration and feeding. *Flow Diagrams in Advanced Cancer and Other Diseases*. London: Edward Arnold. pp. 25–8. (Ch)

25 Stratton RJ, Elia M. (2000) Are oral nutritional supplements of benefit to patients in the community? Findings from a systematic review. *Current Opinion in Clinical Nutrition and Metabolic Care*. **3**(4): 311–15. (R, 37 refs)

26 Ikeda M, Ikui A, Komiyama A, Kobayashi D, Tanaka M. (2008) Causative factors of taste disorders in the elderly, and therapeutic effects of zinc. *Journal of Laryngology and Otology*. **122**(2): 155–60. (OS-408)

27 Polito A, Intorre F, Andriollo Sanchez M, *et al.* (2008) Taste acuity in response to zinc supplementation in older Europeans. *British Journal of Nutrition*. **99**(1): 129–36. (OS–199)

28 Stewart-Knox BJ, Simpson EE, Parr H, Rae G, *et al.* (2005) Zinc status and taste acuity in older Europeans: the ZENITH study. *European Journal of Clinical Nutrition*. **59**(Suppl. 2): S31–6. (OS-387)

29 Fainsinger RL, MacEachern T, Miller MJ, Bruera E, *et al.* (1994) The use of hypodermoclysis for rehydration in terminally ill cancer patients. *Journal of Pain and Symptom Management*. **9**: 298–302. (CT-100)

30 Bruera E, Neumann CM, Pituskin E, Calder K, Hanson J. (1999) A randomized controlled trial of local injections of hyaluronidase versus placebo in cancer patients receiving subcutaneous hydration. *Annals of Oncology*. **10**(10): 1255–8. (RCT-21)

31 Regnard CFB. (1996) Comparison of concentrations of hyaluronidase. *Journal of Pain and Symptom Management*. **12**: 147. (Let)

32 Bruera E. (1996) Comparison of concentrations of hyaluronidase: author's response. *Journal of Pain and Symptom Management*. **12**: 148. (Let)

33 Bozzetti F. (2007) Total parenteral nutrition in cancer patients. *Current Opinion in Supportive and Palliative Care*. **1**(4): 281–6. (R, 49 refs)

34 Soo I, Gramlich L. (2008) Use of parenteral nutrition in patients with advanced cancer. *Applied Physiology, Nutrition, and Metabolism (Physiologie Appliquee, Nutrition et Metabolisme)*. **33**(1): 102–6. (OS-38)

35 Marinella MA. (2008) Refeeding syndrome in cancer patients. *International Journal of Clinical Practice*. **62**(3): 460–5. (R, 38 refs)

36 Bachmann J, Heiligensetzer M, Krakowski-Roosen H, Buchler MW, Friess H, Martignoni ME. (2008) Cachexia worsens prognosis in patients with resectable pancreatic cancer. *Journal of Gastrointestinal Surgery*. **12**(7): 1193–201. (OS-227)

37 Fearon KC. (2008) Cancer cachexia: developing multimodal therapy for a multidimensional problem. *European Journal of Cancer.* **44**(8): 1124–32. (R)

38 Strasser F, Bruera E. (2002) Mechanism of cancer cachexia: progress on disentangling a complex problem. *Progress in Palliative Care*. **10**(4): 161–7. (R, 55refs)

39 Bosaeus I. (2008) Nutritional support in multimodal therapy for cancer cachexia. *Supportive Care in Cancer*. **16**(5): 447–51. (R, 34 refs)

40 Stephens NA, Skipworth RJ, Fearon KC. (2008) Cachexia, survival and the acute phase response. *Current Opinion in Supportive and Palliative Care*. **2**(4): 267–74. (R, 75 refs)

41 Evans WJ, Morley JE, Argiles J, Bales C, *et al.* (2008) Cachexia: a new definition. *Clinical Nutrition*. **27**(6): 793–9. (GC)

42 Anker S, Sharma R. (2002) The syndrome of cardiac cachexia. *International Journal of Cardiology*. **85**(1): 51. (R)

43 Berry C, Clark AL. (2000) Catabolism in chronic heart failure. *European Heart Journal*. **21**(7): 521–32. (R, 187 refs)

44 Summers GD, Deighton CM, Rennie MJ, Booth AH. (2008) Rheumatoid cachexia: a clinical perspective. *Rheumatology*. **47**(8): 1124–31. (R, 123 refs)

45 Plauth M, Schütz E. (2002) Cachexia in liver cirrhosis. *International Journal of Cardiology*. **85**(1): 83. (R)
46 Schols A. (2002) Pulmonary cachexia. *International Journal of Cardiology*. **85**(1): 101. (R)
47 Lundström S, Fürst CJ. (2003) Symptoms in advanced cancer: relationship to endogenous cortisol levels. *Palliative Medicine*. **17**: 503–8. (OS-23)
48 Willox JC, Corr J, Shaw J, Richardson M, Calman KC, Drennan M. (1984) Prednisolone as an appetite stimulant in patients with cancer. *British Medical Journal*. **288**: 27. (RCT)
49 Mercadante S, Fulfaro F, Casuccio A. (2001) The use of corticosteroids in home palliative care. *Supportive Care in Cancer*. **9**(5): 386–9. (OS-376)
50 Hardy JR, Rees E, Ling J, Burman R, *et al.* (2001). A prospective survey of the use of dexamethasone on a palliative care unit. *Palliative Medicine*. **15**(1): 3–8. (OS-106)
51 Loprinzi CL, Goldberg RM, Burnham NL. (1992) Cancer-associated anorexia and cachexia: implications for drug therapy. *Drugs*. **43**(4): 499–506. (R)
52 Maltoni M, Nanni O, Scarpi E, Rossi D, Serra P, Amadori D. (2001) High-dose progestins for the treatment of cancer anorexia-cachexia syndrome: a systematic review of randomised clinical trials. *Annals of Oncology*. **12**(3): 289–300. (SA, 50 refs)
53 Loprinzi CL, Kugler JW, Sloan JA, Mailliard JA, *et al.* (1999) Randomized comparison of megestrol acetate versus dexamethasone versus fluoxymesterone for the treatment of cancer anorexia/cachexia. *Journal of Clinical Oncology*. **17**(10): 3299–306. (RCT)
54 Alimentary symptoms. In: Twycross R, Wilcock A, Stark Toller C. (2009) *Symptom Management in Advanced Cancer*. Nottingham: palliativedrugs.com. pp. 61–144. (Ch)
55 Gebbia V, Testa A, Gebbia N. (1996) Prospective randomised trial of two dose levels of megestrol acetate in the management of anorexia-cachexia syndrome in patients with metastatic cancer. *British Journal of Cancer*. **73**: 1576–80. (RCT-122)
56 Loprinzi CL, Schaid DJ, Dose AM, Burnham NL, Jensen MD. (1993) Body-composition changes in patients who gain weight while receiving megestrol acetate. *Journal of Clinical Oncology*. **11**: 152–4. (RCT-12)
57 Barber MD, Fearon KC, Tisdale MJ, McMillan DC, Ross JA. (2001) Effect of a fish oil-enriched nutritional supplement on metabolic mediators in patients with pancreatic cancer cachexia. *Nutrition and Cancer*. **40**(2): 118–24. (OS-20)
58 Cerchietti LC, Navigante AH, Castro MA. (2007) Effects of eicosapentaenoic and docosahexaenoic n-3 fatty acids from fish oil and preferential Cox-2 inhibition on systemic syndromes in patients with advanced lung cancer. *Nutrition and Cancer*. **59**(1): 14–20. (RCT-22)
59 Mantovani G, Madeddu C. (2008) Cyclooxygenase-2 inhibitors and antioxidants in the treatment of cachexia. *Current Opinion in Supportive and Palliative Care*. **2**(4): 275–81. (R, 47 refs)
60 Davis MP, Dickerson ED. (2001) Thalidomide: dual benefits in palliative medicine and oncology. *American Journal of Hospice and Palliative Care*. **18**(5): 347–51. (R, 56 refs)
61 Jatoi A, Loprinzi CL. (2001) An update: cancer-associated anorexia as a treatment target. *Current Opinion in Clinical Nutrition and Metabolic Care*. **4**(3): 179–82. (R, 17 refs)
62 Mantovani G, Maccio A, Madeddu C, Gramignano G, *et al.* (2008) Randomized phase III clinical trial of five different arms of treatment for patients with cancer cachexia: interim results. *Nutrition*. **24**(4): 305–13. (RCT-125)
63 Poole K, Froggatt K. (2002) Loss of weight and loss of appetite in advanced cancer: a problem for the patient, the carer or the health professional? *Palliative Medicine*. **16**(6): 499–506. (SA, 53 refs)

Oral problems

CLINICAL DECISION AND ACTION CHECKLIST

1 Is oral health at risk?
2 Is an ulcer present?
3 Is the mouth dirty?
4 Is the mouth dry?
5 Is the mouth painful?
6 Is there too much saliva?

KEY POINTS

- A healthy mouth has an intact mucosa and is clean, moist, and pain-free.
- Regular mouth care will prevent many oral problems.
- Candidiasis and dry mouth are the two commonest problems.

INTRODUCTION

Poor oral hygiene may be due to a reduced fluid intake, mouth breathing when asleep and reduced host immunity. Maintaining oral hygiene is very important to reduce infections and treatment-induced mucositis,[1–3] but standards of mouth care vary considerably.[4] A soft toothbrush will gently clean coated tongues and teeth, but foam sticks or gauze are less effective.[5,6] Irrigation with warm water or 0.9% saline will help removal of oral debris, and is soothing and non-traumatic.[7] Some other solutions have problems such as an unpleasant taste, exhausting the salivary glands, or causing damage to the teeth or the mucosa.[6–8] The frequency of oral care depends on the circumstances (*see* cd-1 in the table).

MANAGING ORAL PROBLEMS

Aphthous ulcers

These painful, shallow ulcers are common and can be associated with autoimmune diseases, immunodeficiency, and deficiency of iron, zinc, folate, or vitamin B_{12}.[9] Topical corticosteroids[10–12] or a tetracycline can help.[13–16] Thalidomide (Special Access category in N. America) has a role in treating persistent ulceration in adults and children, but can have serious adverse effects such as neuropathy and venous thrombosis, while its potential for causing birth defects remains.[17–20]

Candidiasis

This may present as white semi-adherent plaques, a red tongue, hyperplastic candidiasis, angular cheilitis, or a denture-associated stomatitis.[21,22] The type of candidiasis depends on the candida species and local immunity.[23] Candida is in the mouths of up to two-thirds of cancer and AIDS patients, especially those with a dry mouth and dentures,[24–27] but there is no association with systemic steroids and antibiotics.[28] Cross-infection does not easily occur by way of cups and cutlery but may occur by way of carers' hands.[29] Prophylactic nystatin does not reduce the incidence of positive mouth swabs,[29] but in AIDS patients long-term therapy with systemic antifungals may be necessary.

Antifungals: all candida species are sensitive to nystatin or amphotericin, but to be effective patients must take these in high doses, e.g. nystatin 500 000 units (i.e. 1 tablet or 5 mL suspension) q6h for up to 10 days, and avoid eating or drinking for 30 minutes afterwards.[30] Up to 72% of some candida strains are resistant to fluconazole and itraconazole,[31] but this may due to inadequate dosing.[32] The risk of resistance developing to systemic antifungals may be reduced if short courses are used.[33]

Ketoconazole 200 mg once daily rapidly clears candidal plaques,[34] is more convenient to the patient, and cheaper than one week with nystatin. Serious adverse effects with ketoconazole are rare,[35] and low-dose ketoconazole long term is well tolerated.[36] Fluconazole is effective in a single dose[34] making it useful in patients with a short prognosis. Fluconazole is used for longer term prophylaxis in AIDS patients with itraconazole as second line.[37] Systemic antifungals interact with several drugs used in palliative care (*see Drug interactions*, p. 294). Chlorhexidine also has antifungal activity[38] but it inactivates nystatin if used together.[39]

Dentures are associated with a higher incidence of candidiasis, but only in the elderly.[28,40,41] Cleaner dentures are associated with less candidiasis.[42] Microwave energy has been studied as an effective sterilization method of dentures.[43,44] Microwaving was most effective when done in 200 mL water for 6 min at 650 W,[43] which suggests regular boiling may be as effective.

Diet: taking regular probiotics may reduce candida overgrowth in elderly patients.[45]

Children: with topical antifungals in babies it is usual to treat both the mouth and perineum at the same time. In older children, single dose fluconazole is often used.

Dry mouth

This is very common in advanced cancer and drugs are a common cause.[46–49]

Artificial salivas: glycerin dehydrates the mucosa and should be avoided.[50] All acidic salivas, i.e. pH 5.5 or less, should not be used long term.[51] A well-tolerated alternative is a salivary enzyme-based product, e.g. Oral Balance. This and other artificial salivas such as Moi-Stir, Salivart

Clinical decision	If YES carry out the action below
1 Is oral health at risk?	• **Twice daily:** brush the teeth with fluoride-containing toothpaste and rinse with a fluoride mouthwash. • **Throughout the day:** rinse the mouth regularly with water or 0.9% saline, and provide adequate hydration. Clear debris from teeth and tongue with a soft toothbrush. *Frequency of oral care:*[52] — general care: q4-6h (after meals) — prevention of oral problems: q2h — patients at high risk or with severe problems (e.g. oxygen therapy, oral infections, coma, severe mucositis, dehydration, immunosuppression, diabetes): hourly.
2 Is an ulcer present?	• **Viral** (zoster or herpes simplex): oral acyclovir 200 mg q4h for 1 week (400 mg if immunosuppressed). • **Aphthous ulcers:** exclude deficiencies of iron, folate, and B_{12}. Try topical corticosteroid (triamcinolone in Orabase, or betamethasone tablets) or dispersible doxycycline dissolved in water and used as a mouthwash. *For persistent and severe ulcers:* these may respond to thalidomide 50–300 mg/day (Special Access category N. America). Thalidomide has been used in children, but ask for specialist advice regarding doses. • **Malignant ulcers:** anaerobic infection causing halitosis: *see* cd-3 below. For bleeding use sucralfate suspension 1 g (5 mL) diluted with 5 mL water as a mouthwash (*see also Bleeding*, p. 93).
3 Is the mouth dirty?	• **Clean the tongue:** gently brush with a soft toothbrush. Chewing pineapple (fresh or tinned, unsweetened) or cleaning the mouth with pineapple juice may help remove debris. • **Clean the mucosa:** helped by rinsing frequently with water or 0.9% saline. • **If candidiasis is the cause** (white patches, thick debris): try nystatin or amphotericin suspension or lozenges/pastilles. Treat any dryness if present (*see* cd-4 on p. 187). In babies, treat the mouth and perineum simultaneously. *If topical antifungals are not tolerated or there is no response:* start ketoconazole 200 mg once daily for 5 days. For a longer course use fluconazole 50 mg daily. If systemic antifungals are not tolerated consider ketoconazole 40 mg q12h as a mouthwash. If compliance is difficult give fluconazole 150 mg as a single dose. For children *see Drugs for children: starting doses*, p. 307. • **If halitosis is due to local tumor:** start metronidazole 400 mg PO q8h (or 500 mg PR q12h) for 5 days, then continue with 400–500 mg once daily. If adverse effects are a problem, rinse the mouth with metronidazole suspension 400 mg (10 mL) and spit out.

Adapted from Regnard and Fitton[53]
cd = clinical decision

(US only), or Saliva Substitute (US only) only last 10–15 minutes and may be little better than placebo.[54] Frequent sprays with water may be just as effective.

Chewing gum is as effective as artificial salivas[55] but sugarless gum (Trident, Extra, Biotene) should be used to avoid the risk of caries.[56]

Salivary stimulants: acidic solutions should be avoided. Pilocarpine in low doses is as effective as artificial saliva in cancer patients, but it can cause sweating, dizziness, and rhinorrhea,[57] and should be used with caution in patients with hepatic or renal impairment.[58] The evidence for pilocarpine with radiotherapy is conflicting, but it seems more effective after treatment has ended than during treatment.[59–63] Pilocarpine 4% eye drops taken orally are one-tenth the cost of pilocarpine tablets,[64] and lower doses can be used. Bethanechol may be a better tolerated and cheaper alternative.[58]

Acupuncture may help in resistant cases.[65,66]

Oral pain relief

There is no evidence that the following ease oral pain: benzydamine, sucralfate, chlorhexidine, or diphenhydramine.[67–69] Mucosal protection can be offered by some topical agents. Carmellose (carboxymethylcellulose) paste (Orabase Protective Paste) is an effective protective agent for local lesions. Choline salicylate gel (US only, from a compounding pharmacy) can help but can cause pain on application. Lidocaine (cream, gel, or spray) can help acutely painful lesions at the expense of numbness, but toxicity has been reported with frequent use.[70] Topical doxepin can reduce the pain of mucositis.[71] In very severe pain, topical opioids may provide some relief in the same way as they do for painful skin ulcers.[72–74] Loperamide is a potent opioid with no central action and can be used topically.[64] The cherry-flavoured syrup (not Canada) contains alcohol so may cause stinging initially – an alternative is quick-dissolve (buccal) loperamide tablets (not US). However, systemic opioids are often required, but may have to be given by a non-oral route.[75] Topical ketamine may have a useful role in extensive, painful mucositis.[76]

In persistent cases of mucositis, dietary supplementation with zinc and the use of topical vitamin E may help speed healing.[77,78] In chemotherapy-induced mucositis the keratinocyte growth factor palifermin (US only) can help.[79]

Excessive saliva

This is usually due to an impairment of controlling or swallowing saliva (*see Dysphagia*, p. 131). Some drugs can cause salivation (*see* cd-6 opposite).[80] Sometimes excessive respiratory secretions are the cause. Anticholinergic medications are often first-line treatment, but these are often only effective at doses that cause adverse effects, especially a dry mouth. Longer-term control can be achieved with radiotherapy or botulinum injection to the salivary glands.[81] Radiotherapy can cause a permanently dry mouth and using low doses in two or more fractions at 4-week intervals is a wise precaution. Botulinum toxin doses should be low and there have been concerns that it may cause more distant neuromuscular problems in patients who already have bulbar symptoms.[81] In addition, it should not be injected into salivary ducts as this can cause a painful parotitis.[81]

Neurologically impaired children

Teething can present in unusual ways in these children, such as an increase in seizures. Dental caries is also common in this population and regular oral hygiene and checks are important.

Clinical decision	If YES carry out the action below
4 Is the mouth dry? (dry mucosa, difficulty swallowing and talking)	• **Treat the cause if possible** (e.g. drugs, dehydration, anxiety). • **Use local measures** such as frequent sprays or sips of cold water, or sucking ice cubes and petroleum jelly to lips. Avoid acidic solutions (e.g. fruit juices). Chewing gum may help. • **Consider:** — artificial salivas, e.g. Moi-Stir, Mouth-Kote, Salivart (US only), Oral Balance (US only) — Pilocarpine 4% eye drop solution, 2–3 drops or 5 mg tablets PO q8h. Use bethanechol 10–25 mg PO q8h if side-effects are a problem. Do not use pilocarpine or bethanechol in patients with bowel obstruction, asthma, glaucoma, cardiovascular disease, or COPD.
5 Is the mouth painful?	• **If the pain is localized:** *Topical analgesia:* benzocaine products (e.g. Orajel, Anbesol) *Protection:* carboxymethylcellulose (Carmellose) paste (Orabase Protective paste). • **If the pain is extensive:** *Exclude infection:* a red, painful mouth may be caused by acute or chronic erythematous candidiasis in the absence of white patches. Blisters suggest herpes (simplex or zoster). *Topical analgesia:* benzocaine lozenges, lidocaine spray, gel or cream, or acetaminophen suspension as a mouthwash. Topical doxepin as a mouthwash may help (mix the contents of one capsule in 10 mL water). *Protection:* try Gelclair (US only),[82] but it is unlikely to help the pain of extensive mucositis. *Consider:* topical opioids such as morphine (5 mg morphine in hydrogel), or loperamide (as quick-dissolve tablets (Canada only)). A compounding pharmacy may be able to make up a metered spray of hydromorphone or morphine. Alternatives are to start or increase systemic oral morphine, or to use a ketamine mouthwash (20 mg in 5 mL artificial saliva swish and spit q3h). • **If this is radiotherapy- or chemotherapy-induced mucositis:** Use pain-relieving measures above *If due to methotrexate:* ensure folic acid replacement is being given. *If the mucositis persists consider:* — regular topical mouthwash with vitamin E suspension 100 mg (1 mL) in 5 mL water — zinc oral supplementation as effervescent zinc tablets 125 mg q8h — palifermin IV 60 microg/kg once daily (US only) (on the advice of an oncologist).
6 Is there too much saliva? (leakage from the mouth)	• **If there is difficulty clearing saliva:** *see Dysphagia*, p. 131. • **Review drug causes:** e.g. buprenorphine, clonazepam, haloperidol, ketamine, risperidone, venlafaxine. • **Reduce salivary production:** *For thick respiratory secretions: see* cd-4 in *Respiratory problems*, p. 193. *Consider:* hyoscine hydrobromide 75–150 microg sublingually q8–12h, or hyoscine hydrobromide transdermal patch (scopolamine patch) (delivers approx. 1.5 mg per 72 hours). For doses in children *see Drugs in children: starting doses*, p. 308. *If problems persist* consider — a CSCI of hyoscine butylbromide 30–120 mg/24 hr (hyoscyamine in US 0.125–0.25 mg SC/IV q4h). More sedating alternatives are glycopyrrolate or hyoscine hydrobromide — radiotherapy to salivary glands, 2–6 Gy to the parotids only, followed if needed 4 weeks later by a further 2–6 Gy — botulinum toxin injection 10–15 MU into parotid gland (not into salivary ducts).

Adapted from Regnard and Fitton[53]
cd = clinical decision

REFERENCES: ORAL PROBLEMS

B = book; C = comment; Ch = chapter; CS-n = case study-no. of cases; CT-n = controlled trial-no. of cases; E = editorial; GC = group consensus; I = interviews; Let = letter; LS = laboratory study; MC = multi-center; OS-n = open study-no. of cases; R = review; RCT-n = randomized controlled trial-no. of cases; RS-n = retrospective survey-no. of cases; SA = systematic or meta analysis.

1 Chen KK, Molassiotis A, Chang AM, Wai WC, Cheung SS. (2001) Evaluation of an oral care protocol intervention in the prevention of chemotherapy-induced oral mucositis in paediatric cancer patients. *European Journal of Cancer*. **37**(16): 2056–63. (CT-42)
2 Larson PJ, Miaskowski C, MacPhail L, Dodd MJ, *et al.* (1998) The PRO-SELF Mouth Aware program: an effective approach for reducing chemotherapy-induced mucositis. *Cancer Nursing*. **21**(4): 263–8. (R, 44 refs)
3 Xavier G. (2000) The importance of mouth care in preventing infection. *Nursing Standard*. **14**(18): 47–51. (R, 16 refs)
4 Gillam JL, Gillam DG. (2006) The assessment and implementation of mouth care in palliative care: a review. *Journal of the Royal Society of Health*. **126**(1): 33–7. (R, 18 refs)
5 Sammon P, Page C, Shepherd G. (1987) Oral hygiene. *Nursing Times*. **83**: 25–27.
6 Evans G. A rationale for oral care. (2001) *Nursing Standard*. **15**(43): 33–6. (R, 43 refs)
7 Miller M, Kearney N. (2001) Oral care for patients with cancer: a review of the literature. *Cancer Nursing*. **24**(4): 241–54. (R, 100 refs)
8 Davis W, Winter P. (1980) The effect of abrasion on enamel and dentine after exposure to dietary acid. *British Dental Journal*. **148**: 11–12, 253–256. (OS)
9 Scully C, Shotts R. (2000) ABC of oral health: mouth ulcers and other causes of orofacial soreness and pain. *British Medical Journal*. **321**: 162–5. (R)
10 Zegarelli EV, Kutscher AH, Silvers HF, *et al.* (1960) Triamcinolone acetonide in the treatment of acute and chronic lesions of the oral mucous membranes. *Oral Surgery, Oral Medicine, and Oral Pathology*. **13**: 170–5.
11 Miles DA, Bricker SL, Razmus TF, Potter RH. (1993) Triamcinolone acetonide versus chlorhexidine for treatment of recurrent stomatitis. *Oral Surgery, Oral Medicine, and Oral Pathology*. **75**(3): 397–402. (RCT-20)
12 Merchant HW, Gangarosa LP, Glassman AB, Sobel RE. (1978) Betamethasone-17-benzoate in the treatment of recurrent aphthous ulcers. *Oral Surgery*. **45**: 870–5. (CT)
13 Graykowski EA, Kingman A. (1978) Double blind trial of tetracycline in recurrent aphthous ulceration. *Journal of Oral Pathology*. **7**: 376–82. (CT-25)
14 Preshaw PM, Grainger P, Bradshaw MH, Mohammad AR, *et al.* (2007) Subantimicrobial dose doxycycline in the treatment of recurrent oral aphthous ulceration: a pilot study. *Journal of Oral Pathology and Medicine*. **36**(4): 236–40. (RCT-50)
15 Gorsky M, Epstein J, Rabenstein S, Elishoov H, Yarom N. (2007) Topical minocycline and tetracycline rinses in treatment of recurrent aphthous stomatitis: a randomized cross-over study. *Dermatology Online Journal*. **13**(2): 1. (RCT-17)
16 Gorsky M, Epstein J, Raviv A, Yaniv R, Truelove E. (2008) Topical minocycline for managing symptoms of recurrent aphthous stomatitis. *Special Care in Dentistry*. **28**(1): 27–31. (RCT-33)
17 Shetty K. (2007) Current role of thalidomide in HIV-positive patients with recurrent aphthous ulcerations. *General Dentistry*. **55**(6): 537–42. (R)
18 Peuckmann V, Fisch M, Bruera E. (2000) Potential novel uses of thalidomide: focus on palliative care. *Drugs*. **60**: 273–93. (R)
19 Sharma NL, Sharma VC, Mahajan VK, Shanker V, *et al.* (2007) Thalidomide: an experience in therapeutic outcome and adverse reactions. *Journal of Dermatological Treatment*. **18**(6): 335–40. (OS-25)
20 Twycross R, Wilcock A, Dean M, Kennedy B, eds. (2010) *Palliative Care Formulary*, Canadian ed. Nottingham: palliativedrugs.com. (B); and Twycross R, Wilcock A. eds. (2008) *Hospice and Palliative Care Formulary USA, 2nd ed.* Nottingham: palliativedrugs.com. (B)
21 Dorko E, Jenca A, Pilipcinec E, Danko J, *et al.* (2001). Candida-associated denture stomatitis. *Folia Microbiologica*. **46**(5): 443–6. (OS-240)
22 Bagg J. (2003) Oral candidosis: how to treat a common problem. *European Journal of Palliative Care*. **10**(2): 54–6. (R, 23 refs)
23 Reichart PA, Samaranayake LP, Philipsen HP. (2000) Pathology and clinical correlates in oral candidiasis and its variants: a review. *Oral Diseases*. **6**(2): 85–91. (R, 51 refs)
24 Davies AN, Brailsford S, Broadley K, Beighton D. (2002) Oral yeast carriage in patients with advanced cancer. *Oral Microbiology and Immunology*. **17**(2): 79–84. (OS-120)
25 Campisi G, Pizzo G, Milici ME, Mancuso S, Margiotta V. (2002) Candidal carriage in the oral cavity of human immunodeficiency virus-infected subjects. *Oral Surgery, Oral Medicine, Oral Pathology, Oral Radiology, and Endodontics*. **93**(3): 281–6. (OS-83)
26 Finlay IG. (1986) Oral symptoms and candida in the terminally ill. *British Medical Journal*. **292**: 592–3. (OS)
27 Torres SR, Peixoto CB, Caldas DM, Silva EB, *et al.* (2002) Relationship between salivary flow rates and Candida counts in subjects with xerostomia. *Oral Surgery, Oral Medicine, Oral Pathology, Oral Radiology, and Endodontics*. **93**(2): 149–54.
28 Davies AN, Brailsford SR, Beighton D. (2006) Oral candidosis in patients with advanced cancer. *Oral Oncology*. **42**(7): 698–702. (OS-120)
29 Burnie JP, Odds FC, Lee W, Webster C, Williams JD. (1985) Outbreak of systemic Candida albicans in intensive care unit caused by cross-infection. *British Medical Journal*. **290**: 746–8. (OS-55)
30 Butticaz G, Zulian GB, Preumont M, Budtz-Jorgensen E. (2003) Evaluation of a nystatin-

containing mouth rinse for terminally ill patients in palliative care. *Journal of Palliative Care*. **19**(2): 95–9. (OS-52)

31 Bagg J, Sweeney MP, Lewis MA, Jackson MS, *et al.* (2003) High prevalence of non-albicans yeasts and detection of anti-fungal resistance in the oral flora of patients with advanced cancer. *Palliative Medicine*. **17**(6): 477–81. (OS-207)

32 Garey KW, Pai MP, Suda KJ, Turpin RS, *et al.* (2007) Inadequacy of fluconazole dosing in patients with candidemia based on Infectious Diseases Society of America (IDSA) guidelines. *Pharmacoepidemiology and Drug Safety*. **16**(8): 919–27. (OS-206)

33 Davies A, Brailsford S, Broadley K, Beighton D. (2002) Resistance amongst yeasts isolated from the oral cavities of patients with advanced cancer. *Palliative Medicine*. **16**(3): 527–31. (OS-70)

34 Regnard CFB. (1994) Single dose fluconazole versus five day ketoconazole in oral candidiasis. *Palliative Medicine*. **8**: 72–3. (OS-100)

35 Hay RJ. (1985) Ketoconazole: a reappraisal. *British Medical Journal*. **290**: 260–1. (E)

36 Harris KA, Weinberg V, Bok RA, Kakefuda M, Small EJ. (2002) Low dose ketoconazole with replacement doses of hydrocortisone in patients with progressive androgen independent prostate cancer. *Journal of Urology*. **168**(2): 542–5. (OS-28)

37 Ball K, Sweeney MP, Baxter WP, Bagg J. (1998) Fluconazole sensitivities of Candida species isolated from the mouths of terminally ill cancer patients. *American Journal of Hospice and Palliative Care*. **15**(6): 315–9. (OS-30)

38 Ellepola AN, Samaranayake LP. (2001) Adjunctive use of chlorhexidine in oral candidoses: a review. *Oral Diseases*. **7**(1): 11–7. (R, 74 refs)

39 Barkvoll P, Attramadal A. (1989) Effect of nystatin and chlorhexidine digluconate on Candida albicans. *Oral Surgery, Oral medicine and Oral Pathology*. **67**(3): 279–81. (OS)

40 Pentenero M, Broccoletti R, Carbone M, Conrotto D, Gandolfo S. (2008) The prevalence of oral mucosal lesions in adults from the Turin area. *Oral Diseases*. **14**(4): 356–66. (RS-4098)

41 Zaremba ML, Daniluk T, Rozkiewicz D, Cylwik-Rokicka D, *et al.* (2006) Incidence rate of Candida species in the oral cavity of middle-aged and elderly subjects. *Advances in Medical Sciences*. **51**(Suppl. 1): 233–6. (OS-103)

42 Kanli A, Demirel F, Sezgin Y. (2005) Oral candidosis, denture cleanliness and hygiene habits in an elderly population. *Aging-Clinical and Experimental Research*. **17**(6): 502–7. (OS-42)

43 Silva MM, Vergani CE, Giampaolo ET, Neppelenbroek KH, *et al.* (2006) Effectiveness of microwave irradiation on the disinfection of complete dentures. *International Journal of Prosthodontics*. **19**(3): 288–93. (LS)

44 Webb BC, Thomas CJ, Harty DW, Willcox MD. (1998) Effectiveness of two methods of denture sterilization. *Journal of Oral Rehabilitation*. **25**(6): 416–23. (LS)

45 Hatakka K, Ahola AJ, Yli-Knuuttila H, Richardson M. (2007) Probiotics reduce the prevalence of oral candida in the elderly: a randomized controlled trial. *Journal of Dental Research*. **86**(2): 125–30. (RCT-276)

46 Sweeney MP, Bagg J, Baxter WP, Aitchison TC. (1998) Oral disease in terminally ill cancer patients with xerostomia. *Oral Oncology*. **34**(2): 123–6. (OS-70)

47 Mercadante S. (2002) Dry mouth and palliative care. *European Journal of Palliative Care*. **9**(5): 182–5. (R, 10 refs)

48 Davies AN, Broadley K, Beighton D. (2002) Salivary gland hypofunction in patients with advanced cancer. *Oral Oncology*. **38**(7): 680–5. (OS-120)

49 Davies AN, Broadley K, Beighton D. (2001) Xerostomia in patients with advanced cancer. *Journal of Pain and Symptom Management*. **22**(4): 820–5. (OS-120)

50 Van Drimmelen J, Rollins HF. (1969) Evaluation of a commonly used oral hygiene agent. *Nursing Research*. **18**: 327–32.

51 Kielbassa AM, Shohadai SP, Schulte-Monting J. (2001) Effect of saliva substitutes on mineral content of demineralised and sound dental enamel. *Supportive Care in Cancer*. **9**(1): 40–7. (LS)

52 Krishnasamy M. (1995) Oral problems in advanced cancer. *European Journal of Cancer Care*. **4**: 173–7. (R, 100 refs)

53 Regnard C, Fitton S. (1995) Mouth care. In: *Flow Diagrams in Advanced Cancer and Other Diseases*. London: Edward Arnold. pp. 22–4. (Ch)

54 Sweeney MP, Bagg J, Baxter WP, Aitchison TC. (1997) Clinical trial of a mucin-containing oral spray for treatment of xerostomia in hospice patients. *Palliative Medicine*. **11**: 225–32. (RCT-31)

55 Oneschuk D, Hanson J, Bruera E. (2000) A survey of mouth pain and dryness in patients with advanced cancer. *Supportive Care in Cancer*. **8**(5): 372–6. (RCT)

56 Birkhed D, Edwardsson S, Wikesjo U, Ahlden ML, Ainamo J. (1983) Effect of 4 days consumption of chewing gum containing sorbitol or a mixture of sorbitol and xylitol on dental plaque and saliva. *Caries Research*. **17**: 76–8.

57 Davies AN, Daniels C, Pugh R, Sharma K. (1998) A comparison of artificial saliva and pilocarpine in the management of xerostomia in patients with advanced cancer. *Palliative Medicine*. **12**(2): 105–11. (MC, RCT)

58 BNF (British National Formulary), see www.bnf.org (UK edition).

59 Haddad P, Karimi M. (2002) A randomized, double-blind, placebo-controlled trial of concomitant pilocarpine with head and neck irradiation for prevention of radiation-induced xerostomia. *Radiotherapy and Oncology*. **64**(1): 29. (RCT-60)

60 Warde P, O'Sullivan B, Aslanidis J, Kroll B, *et al.* (2002) A phase III placebo-controlled trial of oral pilocarpine in patients undergoing radiotherapy for head-and-neck cancer. *International Journal of Radiation Oncology, Biology, Physics*. **54**(1): 9–13. (RCT-130)

61 Nyarady Z, Nemeth A, Ban A, Mukics A, *et*

al. (2006) A randomized study to assess the effectiveness of orally administered pilocarpine during and after radiotherapy of head and neck cancer. *Anticancer Research*. **26**(2B): 1557–62. (CT-66)

62 Scarantino C, LeVeque F, Swann RS, White R, *et al.* (2006) Effect of pilocarpine during radiation therapy: results of RTOG 97-09, a phase III randomized study in head and neck cancer patients. *The Journal of Supportive Oncology*. **4**(5): 252–8. (RCT-245)

63 Berk L. (2008) Systemic pilocarpine for treatment of xerostomia. *Expert Opinion On Drug Metabolism and Toxicology*. **4**(10): 1333–40. (R, 44 refs)

64 See www.palliativedrugs.com.

65 Johnstone PA, Peng YP, May BC, Inouye WS, Niemtzow RC. (2001) Acupuncture for pilocarpine-resistant xerostomia following radiotherapy for head and neck malignancies. *International Journal of Radiation Oncology, Biology, Physics*. **50**(2): 353–7. (OS-18)

66 Cho JH, Chung WK, Kang W, Choi SM, Cho CK, Son CG. (2008) Manual acupuncture improved quality of life in cancer patients with radiation-induced xerostomia. *Journal of Alternative and Complementary Medicine*. **14**(5): 523–6. (RCT-12)

67 Chiara S, Nobile MT, Vincenti M, Gozza A, *et al.* (2001). Sucralfate in the treatment of chemotherapy-induced stomatitis: a double-blind, placebo-controlled pilot study. *Anticancer Research*. **21**(5): 3707–10. (RCT-40)

68 Loprinzi CL, Ghosh C, Camoriano J, Sloan J, *et al.* (1997) Phase III controlled evaluation of sucralfate to alleviate stomatitis in patients receiving fluorouracil-based chemotherapy. *Journal of Clinical Oncology*. **15**(3): 1235–8. (RCT-131)

69 Clarkson JE, Worthington HV, Eden OB. (2007) Interventions for treating oral mucositis for patients with cancer receiving treatment. (Update of *Cochrane Database of Systematic Reviews*. 2004; **2**: CD001973; *Cochrane Database of Systematic Reviews*. **2**: CD001973. (SA, R-113 refs)

70 Yamashita S, Sat S, Kakiuchi Y, Miyabe M, Yamaguchi H. (2002) Lidocaine toxicity during frequent viscous lidocaine use for painful tongue ulcer. *Journal of Pain and Symptom Management*. **24**(6): 543–5. (CS-1)

71 Epstein JB, Epstein JD, Epstein MS, Oien H, Truelove EL. (2006) Oral doxepin rinse: the analgesic effect and duration of pain reduction in patients with oral mucositis due to cancer therapy. *Anesthesia and Analgesia*. **103**(2): 465–70. (OS-51)

72 Back IN, Finlay I. (1995) Analgesic effect of topical opioids on painful skin ulcers. *Journal of Pain and Symptom Management*. **10**: 493. (Let)

73 Krajnik M, Zylicz Z. (1997) Topical morphine for cutaneous cancer pain. *Palliative Medicine*. **11**: 325–6. (CS-6)

74 Twillman RK, Long TD, Cathers TA, Mueller DW. (1999) Treatment of painful skin ulcers with topical opioids. *Journal of Pain and Symptom Management*. **17**(4): 288–92. (CS-9)

75 Shaiova L, Mori M, Anderson K, Loewen G, *et al.* (2007) Administration of morphine sulfate extended-release capsules via gastrostomy: dissolution study and case reports. *Journal of Palliative Medicine*. **10**(5): 1063–7. (OS)

76 Slatkin NE, Rhiner M. (2003) Topical ketamine in the treatment of mucositis pain. *Pain Medicine*. **4**(3): 298–303.

77 Lin LC, Que J, Lin LK, Lin FC. (2006) Zinc supplementation to improve mucositis and dermatitis in patients after radiotherapy for head-and-neck cancers: a double-blind, randomized study. *International Journal of Radiation Oncology, Biology, Physics*. **65**(3): 745–50. (RCT-100)

78 El-Housseiny AA, Saleh SM, El-Masry AA, Allam AA. (2007) The effectiveness of vitamin "E" in the treatment of oral mucositis in children receiving chemotherapy. *Journal of Clinical Pediatric Dentistry*. **31**(3): 167–70. (RCT-80)

79 Horsley P, Bauer JD, Mazkowiack R, Gardner R, Bashford J. (2007) Palifermin improves severe mucositis, swallowing problems, nutrition impact symptoms, and length of stay in patients undergoing hematopoietic stem cell transplantation. *Supportive Care in Cancer*. **15**(1): 105–9. (OS-59)

80 Scully C, Bagan JV. (2004) Adverse drug reactions in the orofacial region. *Critical Reviews in Oral Biology and Medicine*. **15**(4): 221–39. (R, 324 refs)

81 Stone CA, O'Leary N. (2009) Systematic review of the effectiveness of botulinum toxin or radiotherapy for sialorrhoea in patients with amyotrophic lateral sclerosis. *Journal of Pain and Symptom Management*. **37**(2): 246–58. (SA-5, 29 refs)

82 Smith T. (2001) Gelclair: managing the symptoms of oral mucositis. *Hospital Medicine (London)*. **62**(10): 623–6. (R, 21 refs)

Respiratory problems

CLINICAL DECISION AND ACTION CHECKLIST

1 If the patient is breathless, call for help and start simple measures.
2 Is the patient hypoxic or hypercapnic?
3 Has the problem developed rapidly?
4 Are airway secretions causing distress?
5 Is infection present?
6 Are hiccups present?
7 Has the breathlessness developed slowly?
8 Is a cough present?
9 Is the breathlessness persisting?

KEY POINTS

- Breathlessness is what the patient says it is.
- Breathlessness is often frightening, and managing the fear is essential.
- Simple measures are often helpful for breathlessness.
- Most treatments are conventional and logical.
- Other symptoms such as cough, secretions, and hiccups can be eased.

INTRODUCTION

Breathlessness is the commonest respiratory problem. It is common in advanced disease, being present in 94% of chronic lung disease, 83% of heart failure patients, and up to 70% of cancer patients, but it is also common in dementia, multiple sclerosis and AIDS.[1–8] Helping the breathless patient needs a whole person approach, especially when breathlessness is persistent and distressing.[9] Other respiratory problems include airway secretions, cough and hiccups.

ASSESSMENT

For many respiratory problems a clear history and bedside examination provide most of the information. Standard breathlessness assessments and tests such as spirometry do not reflect the effect of breathlessness on the patient.[10–14] Patients describe breathlessness in their own way, and individual assessment tools are of little value.[15,16] Like pain, breathlessness is what the patient says it is. Apart from emergencies, much of the evaluation is about eliciting the patient's concerns since fear, anxiety, and low mood are common companions to breathlessness. (*See Helping the person to share their problems*, p. 15).

URGENT MANAGEMENT

Managing sudden breathlessness

See cd-6 in ***Emergencies***, p. 337.

First aid for breathlessness: simple measures can be offered by any carer (*see* cd-1 opposite).[17–20] It needs a minimum of two carers, one to ensure that the assessment of the cause begins, and the other to start the simple measures to help the patient. Mild facial cooling reduces breathlessness and discomfort.[21,22] Sitting upright increases peak ventilation and reduces airway obstruction.[23–25] If it is known that a patient has a compromised lung, e.g. collapse, lobectomy, pleural effusion, ensure that the patient is not lying on the uncompromised lung. Relaxing and dropping the shoulders improves ventilation by reducing the "hunching" that occurs with anxiety. This can be helped by a carer gently massaging the shoulders while standing behind or to one side. This gives the carer a helpful role, is comforting to the patient, and avoids the increase in anxiety caused by eye-to-eye contact. Being with a patient is essential to ease the fear of breathlessness.

Hypoxia is not always accompanied by cyanosis and a pulse oximeter is invaluable to confirm hypoxia in the absence of cyanosis.[26] Nocturnal hypoxia is present in a third of advanced cancer patients, especially those with lung cancer.[27] Oxygen can help if hypoxia is present and gas exchange is sufficient to allow the increased oxygen to be transferred to the blood. The aim is an oxygen saturation (S_pO_2) of 94–98% (unless the patient is also hypercapnic when the target should be lower – *see* below). Some patients with persistent breathlessness report finding that oxygen is helpful,[28] but this is probably as much due to the movement of air across the face.[29]

Hypercapnia: this is most commonly seen in chronic respiratory failure due to conditions such as neuromuscular disease (e.g. motor neurone disease/ ALS, muscular dystrophy) or primary lung disease (e.g. chronic obstructive pulmonary disease – COPD). Some of these patients are dependent on hypoxia to stimulate respiration. If they are given oxygen above 24% their hypercapnia will worsen and they will go into rapid respiratory failure. Since a pulse oximeter does not measure carbon dioxide levels, a hypercapnic patient can have normal O_2 saturation readings. Therefore, it is best to restrict oxygen in these patients to 24% and aim for a target oxygen saturation (S_pO_2) of 88–92%.[30] Some will need support with non-invasive ventilation.[31]

Excess secretions

Thick airway secretions need to be loosened. Nebulized saline is often helpful. Nebulized Dornase alpha has a role in cystic fibrosis and may help with infected secretions.[32,33]

Clinical decision	If YES carry out the action below
1 If the patient is breathless, call for help and start simple measures: — sit the patient upright and increase air movement over the patient's face (fan, open window) — encourage the patient to relax and lower the shoulders since this reduces the "hunching" caused by anxiety — explain what is happening and stay with the patient.	
2 Is the patient hypoxic or hypercapnic?	• **Confirm hypoxia** with a pulse oximeter if available (the absence of cyanosis does not exclude hypoxia). If S_pO_2 is <90% start oxygen (24% on 4L/min). Continue working through the clinical decisions. • **If hypercapnia is present** (flushed skin, full pulse, muscle twitches, hand flap tremor, delirium, hyperventilation, drowsiness, coma): exclude ventilatory failure due to drugs (*see* cd-3b in *Emergencies*, p. 333). If symptoms are distressing, consider referral for investigation and possibility of non-invasive ventilation (*see* text p. 196).
3 Has the problem developed rapidly? (minutes to hours)	**For sudden breathlessness *see* cd-6 in *Emergencies*, p. 337.**
4 Are airway secretions causing distress?	• **Start respiratory exercises** with a physiotherapist if the patient is well enough. • **If the sputum is thick and difficult to cough up** use hypertonic saline 6% 4 mL nebulized q12h. Alternatively, try Dornase alfa 2500 U by jet nebulizer once daily. • **If the sputum is thin and loose** *If this is bronchorrhea due to alveolar cell carcinoma:* try inhaled beclomethasone 400–800 microg 8–12 hourly. If this fails try erythromycin PO 500–1000 mg 12 hourly, *or* nebulized indomethacin 25 mg in 2 mL with the pH corrected to 7.4 with sodium bicarbonate. *For other secretions:* try hyoscine hydrobromide (scopolamine) 400 microg SC or as a transdermal patch. If the problem persists, try nebulized terbutaline. • **If secretions continue to be a problem** consider these causes: ventricular (heart) failure, aspiration (*see Dysphagia*, p. 131), chest infection, tracheoesophageal fistula. • **If there are retained secretions at the end of life:** give glycopyrrolate 400 microg, or, if sedation is needed, hyoscine hydrobromide (scopolamine) 400 microg SC. Repeat after 30 min. Or, use the scopolamine patch. If no improvement, reposition the patient on one side and with upper body elevated. Consider suction with a soft catheter. If the secretions are infected consider a single dose of 1 g ceftriaxone SC (mix with 2 mL lidocaine 1% to reduce local pain). Repeat only if symptoms recur.

Adapted from Ahmedzai and Regnard[34]
cd = clinical decision

Loose airway secretions at the end of life can be a problem in up to 92% of patients in the last hours, or occasionally days, of a patient's life.[35,36] Most comatose patients seem unaware of its presence but it is distressing for partners, relatives, and staff,[37–40] and the family will need reassurance. Current evidence has failed to show that any treatment is better than placebo.[41] However, most clinicians continue to use antimuscarinic drugs to help secretions due to accumulation of saliva, but they are probably less helpful for secretions due to lung pathology.[42] No one drug is better than any other,[43] but each has different characteristics which may be useful in different situations.[44–47] An alternative is nebulized terbutaline.[48]

Hyoscine butylbromide: cheap, widely available, non-sedating, slow onset, 1–2 hr action.
Usual starting dose 20 mg
Glycopyrronium: expensive, moderately sedating, 1 hr onset, 4–6 hr action.
Usual starting dose 200 microg
Hyoscine hydrobromide (scopolamine): cheap, widely available, most sedating, 30 min onset, 4–6 hr action.
Usual starting dose 400 microg

Antimuscarinics compared

Parenteral antibiotics can ease distressing sputum due to a chest infection at the end of life,[49] and infected secretions will respond to a single injection of a long-acting, broad-spectrum cephalosporin.[50–52] In secretions due to alveolar cell carcinoma, inhaled corticosteroids or indomethacin have been suggested, and oral erythromycin may also help.[53–55]

OTHER CONDITIONS AND TREATMENT DECISIONS

Pleural effusions: drainage should be considered if the patient is distressed and the patient agrees. If an effusion recurs in less than 2 weeks, pleurodesis should be considered. Talc remains the most commonly used agent,[56] but many other agents have been used including tetracycline, erythromycin, and bleomycin.[57,58] Pleurodesis may be performed medically or surgically.[59] A pleuroperitoneal shunt is an alternative in a patient who is deteriorating slowly (month by month).[60,61] For recurrent effusions another alternative is a permanent pleural catheter, which has been shown to be safe and effective,[62,63] although complications may occur.[64]

Radiotherapy and chemotherapy: these can help in responsive tumors but are less successful at treating breathlessness due to other tumors.[65]

Acupuncture and TENS: these may have a role in persistent breathlessness.[66–68]

Respiratory infections: whether to treat a chest infection in very advanced disease often causes concern. In most cases the disease will progress regardless of antibiotics.[69] If symptoms such as fever, purulent sputum, or pleuritic chest pain are present, and the patient is willing and able to take oral medication, oral antibiotics should be used.[70–73] Some patients respond poorly or briefly to repeated antibiotic courses, but further control is possible for some weeks or months with nebulized antibiotics such as colistin or gentamicin.[74–77] In very ill patients, symptoms can be palliated in other ways (*see* cd-5 opposite and cd-9 on p. 197).

Clinical decision	If YES carry out the action below
5 Is infection present?	• **If the patient is deteriorating day by day due to underlying disease:** *No symptoms due to the infection:* no action is required. *Symptoms due to the infection:* treat fever with cooling and acetaminophen 1 g PO or PR, reduce secretions with hyoscine, glycopyrrolate or hyoscyamine, ease pain with analgesics. *Persistent symptoms of infection* (e.g. profuse sputum): give single dose of 1 g ceftriaxone SC (mix with 2 mL lidocaine 1% to reduce local pain). Repeat only if symptoms recur. • **For all other patients:** start amoxicillin or erythromycin PO (if immunocompromised or this is a persistent infection, send sputum for microbiology). *If the infection responds poorly or briefly* to repeated courses, try colistin 0.5–1 million units nebulized q12h, or gentamicin 80–120 mg nebulized q12h. • **For *Pneumocystis carinii*** (PCP) in AIDS start high-dose co-trimoxazole (20/100 mg/kg q6–8h) for 2 weeks (can cause rash, gastritis and neutropenia), or nebulized pentamidine (600 mg daily) for 3 weeks. *If hypoxia is present* add prednisolone 40 mg q12h for 5 days. *For maintenance* use co-trimoxazole 160/800 mg daily.
6 Are hiccups present?	• **If gastric stasis or a "squashed stomach syndrome" is present:** start metoclopramide or domperidone (from compounding pharmacy in US) (*see* cd-2a in *Nausea and vomiting*, p. 169). • **Treat ascites if present:** *see Ascites*, p. 87. • **Try simple measures**, e.g. re-breathing from paper bag (but not if hypercapnia is suspected). • **If hiccups are persisting:** start baclofen 5 mg q8h, and titrate if necessary. Alternatives are gabapentin 100 mg q8h, *or* nifedipine 10 mg q12h, *or* sodium valproate 200–400 mg q12h, *or* amantadine 100 mg once daily. Doses then need to be titrated. • **If hiccups are severe:** try midazolam 2–10 mg titrated IV.
7 Has the breathlessness developed slowly? (days to weeks)	• **Exclude** ventricular failure, pleural effusion or diaphragmatic splinting (tumor, ascites). • **If anemic:** transfuse if the Hb<100 g/L.[78–80] Full benefit takes 72 hours. • **If pulmonary tumor is present:** try dexamethasone PO 6 mg daily, readjusting to lowest dose that will control symptoms. Consider chemotherapy or hormone therapy if the tumor is likely to respond. • **If respiratory muscle weakness is present** (e.g. motor neurone disease/ALS, muscular dystrophy): refer to respiratory physician for consideration of non-invasive ventilation (NIV). *See* p. 196.

Adapted from Ahmedzai and Regnard[34]
cd = clinical decision

Hiccups: gastric stasis can cause hiccups and should be treated. For persistent hiccup most treatments are based on case studies, hence the wide range of drugs reported.[81,82] Baclofen can often be helpful,[83–85] backed by parenteral midazolam if the hiccups persist.[86] Evidence is gathering on the effectiveness of gabapentin.[87,88] Other drugs that have been tried include amantadine,[89] nifedipine, and sodium valproate.

Cough: no one preparation has been shown to be consistently effective.[90] Simple linctus or humidified air are soothing preparations that can be repeated as often as required. Baclofen may help.[91,92] Lidocaine given by way of a jet nebulizer through a mouthpiece is helpful to suppress cough arising anywhere down to the larger bronchi.[93–95] To prevent the lidocaine causing bronchospasm an inhaled bronchodilator should be given beforehand.[96] The lidocaine is not always tolerated and may cause numbness of the mouth and throat, temporarily preventing safe eating or drinking. High-dose dexamethasone may reduce pleural, pericardial, or diaphragmatic irritation by tumor. If the cough is due to a chest infection it will respond to antibiotics.[97]

PERSISTENT BREATHLESSNESS

Drugs used to treat breathlessness: apart from bronchodilators and antibiotics, other drugs have a limited role in breathlessness.[98] Opioids can reduce the demand for ventilation without significant respiratory depression in cancer, end-stage heart failure, and COPD.[99–105] There is no evidence that opioids decrease survival, even in high doses.[106] There is evidence for their role in easing breathlessness,[103,107–109] although there is no means of predicting this response.[110] Opioids can be prescribed in the same way as for pain control (*see Using strong opioids*, p. 63). Nebulized opioids have been used in the past but evidence for their efficacy is equivocal, and currently they are not routinely used.[111–113] Nebulized furosemide may help in the absence of heart failure,[114,115] and at least in COPD furosemide inhalation improves the dynamic ventilatory mechanics.[116] However, more evidence is needed.[113,117]

Sedation: this is not usually the aim when managing breathless, but occasionally severe breathlessness that develops suddenly at the end of life (e.g. pulmonary embolus) will need sedation.[118] Midazolam is usually preferred because its short half-life allows doses to be adjusted to each individual while minimizing respiratory effects.[119]

Breathing retraining involves helping the patient to adapt to their new respiratory capacity through relaxation, positioning, establishing a sense of control, and improving respiratory muscle strength.[120–123] It has an important role in dyspnea that persists for several months or more. This is facilitated by specialist physiotherapists and clinical nurse specialists.

Non-invasive ventilation (NIV): at first this seems inappropriate in the context of very advanced disease. But ventilation can significantly improve the quality of life for patients with chronic hypercapnic respiratory failure due to progressive neuromuscular disease (e.g. motor neurone disease/ALS, Duchenne muscular dystrophy) or chronic obstructive pulmonary disease.[124–128] Symptoms of hypercapnia include morning headaches, daytime lethargy, and poor sleep patterns. The technique is now well established and can improve sleep and daytime symptoms.[129–132] Since NIV relies on some of the patient's respiratory function, there will still be a gradual

Clinical decision	If YES carry out the action below
8 Is a cough present?	• **Consider** the following as causes of dry cough: aspiration, asthma, drugs (e.g. ACE inhibitors, β-blockers), heart failure, esophageal reflux, persistent infection (e.g. TB), recent radiotherapy to the lungs, pulmonary fibrosis. • **Treat any chest infection present.** • **Treat troublesome airway secretions:** *see* cd-4 on p. 193. • **Humidify the room air.** Start simple linctus as required. • **If the cough is persistent and troublesome** one of the following may help: — dextromethorphan 10 mg (10 mL) q8h or codeine 30–60 mg q6h if not on strong opioids. — nifedipine 5–10 mg q8h — lidocaine as a 10% spray in single spray to back of throat (a single spray is unlikely to compromise swallowing) — nebulized lidocaine 5 mL 2% solution over 20 min (precautions: give inhaled bronchodilator beforehand and note that the lidocaine may compromise swallowing and patients need to fast for one hour after use) — nebulized ipratropium — baclofen 10–20 mg q8h. • **If bronchial tumor is present:** try beclomethasone 500 microg inhaled q6h.
9 Is the breathlessness persisting?	• **If the agitation or distress is severe:** *see* cd-4 in *Emergencies*, p. 333. • **If the patient is anxious or frightened:** when relaxation is needed give lorazepam 0.5 mg sublingually or 2.5 mg midazolam buccally or SC. Sedation is not usually the aim, but may be required in severe breathlessness at the end of life. • **Start an opioid:** e.g. oral or SC morphine or hydromorphone titrated as for analgesia. • **Consider the following:** — nabilone (if there is no cardiac impairment): 100–500 microg PO q8h — acupuncture (upper sternum and L14 points in hands) — nebulized furosemide 2 mg nebulized q6h. • **Plan future support:** — refer to dyspnea clinic if this is available, and promote "breathing retraining" — help the patient to adapt to new respiratory capacity, e.g. review demands on mobility. • **Manage the consequences of dyspnea:** for dry mouth *see* cd-4 in *Oral problems*, p. 187; for anxiety *see Anxiety*, p. 239; for immobility that risks pressure damage *see* cd-1 in *Skin problems*, p. 205; and for immobility and reduced food intake causing bowel problems *see Constipation*, p. 107.

Adapted from Ahmedzai and Regnard[34]
cd = clinical decision

deterioration into respiratory failure, but this is often gentle and peaceful. Indeed, the role of NIV in terminal breathlessness is not clear[132] and it has no role in any respiratory failure accompanying the natural process of dying from non-respiratory causes. NIV should not be started without discussion with the patient and/or family as to the likely benefits of the intervention, and the patient's goals of care.[133]

Breathlessness at the end of life

For many patients who have been breathless on exertion, becoming chair- or bed-bound can reduce the problems of breathlessness. A few patients, however, become more breathless and hypoxic despite their reduced mobility. This causes distress and fear, sometimes with gasping respiration.[134,135] This uncontrolled breathlessness can cause intense distress in patients, partners, and relatives.[136] Lorazepam or midazolam can be helpful for patients.[137] The aim is not sedation, but to allow the patient to be more relaxed and comfortable. Doses should start low, but are repeated until the patient is settled and relaxed, but not necessarily sedated. Lorazepam can be given 8–12 hourly (half-life is 12–15 hours), while midazolam can be given as a continuous subcutaneous infusion. Combining midazolam and an opioid can bring further relief.[138] While such events can be distressing, helping the patient to be settled and comfortable creates an important opportunity to further discuss the reasons for the deterioration with the patient if they are able, or with their partner or relatives.

REFERENCES: RESPIRATORY PROBLEMS

B = book; C = comment; Ch = chapter; CS-n = case study-no. of cases; CT-n = controlled trial-no. of cases; E = editorial; GC = group consensus; I = interviews; LS = laboratory study; MC = multi-center; OS-n = open study-no. of cases; R = review; RCT-n = randomized controlled trial-no. of cases; RS-n = retrospective survey-no. of cases; SA = systematic or meta analysis-no. of trials.

1 Anderson H, Ward C, Eardley A, Gomm SA, *et al.* (2001) The concerns of patients under palliative care and a heart failure clinic are not being met. *Palliative Medicine.* **15**(4): 279–86. (OS-279)

2 Reuben DB, Mor V, Hiris J. (1988) Clinical symptoms and length of survival in patients with terminal cancer. *Archives of Internal Medicine.* **148**(7): 1586–91. (RS)

3 Lloyd-Williams M. (1996) An audit of palliative care in dementia. *European Journal of Cancer Care.* **5**(1): 53–5. (RS-17)

4 Neudert C, Oliver D, Wasner M, Borasio GD. (2001) The course of the terminal phase in patients with amyotrophic lateral sclerosis. *Journal of Neurology.* **248**(7): 612–16. (I-121)

5 McCarthy M, Lay M, Addington-Hall J. (1996) Dying from heart disease. *Journal of the Royal College of Physicians of London.* **30**(4): 325–8. (I-600)

6 Shee CD. (1995) Palliation in chronic respiratory disease. *Palliative Medicine.* **9**(1): 3–12. (R, 51 refs)

7 Gibbs LME, Ellershaw JE, Williams MD. (1997) Caring for patients with HIV disease: the experience of a generic hospice. *AIDS Care.* **9**(5): 601–7. (OS-24)

8 Edmonds P, Karlsen S, Khan S, Addington-Hall J. (2001) A comparison of the palliative care needs of patients dying from chronic respiratory diseases and lung cancer. *Palliative Medicine.* **15**(4): 287–95. (I-636)

9 Abernethy AP, Wheeler JL. (2008) Total dyspnoea. *Current Opinion in Supportive and Palliative Care.* **2**(2): 110–13. (R, 21 refs)

10 Heyse-Moore L, Beynon T, Ross V. (2000) Does spirometry predict dyspnoea in advanced cancer? *Palliative Medicine.* **14**(3): 189–95. (OS-155)

11 Plant H, Bredin M, Krishnasamy M, Corner J. (2000) Working with resistance, tension and objectivity: conducting a randomised controlled trial of a nursing intervention for breathlessness . . . including commentary by Bond S. *Nursing Times Research.* **5**(6): 426–36. (R)

12 Mancini I, Body JJ. (1999) Assessment of dyspnea in advanced cancer patients. *Supportive Care in Cancer.* **7**(4): 229–32. (R, 15 refs)

13 Wilcock A, Crosby V, Clarke D, Tattersfield A. (1999) Repeatability of breathlessness measurements in cancer patients. *Thorax.* **54**(4): 375. (OS-31)

14 O'Driscoll M, Corner J, Bailey C. (1999) The experience of breathlessness in lung cancer. *European Journal of Cancer Care.* **8**(1): 37–43. (I-52)

15 Wilcock A, Crosby V, Hughes A, Fielding K,

Corcoran R, Tattersfield AE. (2002) Descriptors of breathlessness in patients with cancer and other cardiorespiratory diseases. *Journal of Pain and Symptom Management*. **23**(3): 182–9. (OS-261)

16 Bausewein C, Booth S, Higginson IJ. (2008) Measurement of dyspnoea in the clinical rather than the research setting. *Current Opinion in Supportive and Palliative Care*. **2**(2): 95–9. (R, 44 refs)

17 Cox C. (2002) Non-pharmacological treatment of breathlessness. *Nursing Standard*. **16**(24): 33–6. (R, 35 refs)

18 Davis C. (1997) ABC of palliative care: breathlessness, cough, and other respiratory problems. *British Medical Journal*. **315**: 931–4. (R)

19 Bailey C. (1996) Breathe a little easier. *Nursing Times*. **92**: 55–8. (R)

20 Bredin M, Corner J, Krishnasamy M, Plant H, Bailey C, A'Hern R. (1999) Multicentre randomised controlled trial of nursing intervention for breathlessness in patients with lung cancer. *British Medical Journal*. **318**: 901–4. (RCT-119)

21 Spence DP, Graham DR, Ahmed J, Rees K, Pearson MG, Calverley PM. (1993) Does cold air affect exercise capacity and dyspnea in stable chronic obstructive pulmonary disease? *Chest*. **103**(3): 693–6. (RCT-16)

22 Kratzing CC, Cross RB. (1984) Effects of facial cooling during exercise at high temperature. *European Journal of Applied Physiology and Occupational Physiology*. **53**(2): 118–20.

23 Armour W, Clark AL, McCann GP, Hillis WS. (1998) Effects of exercise position on the ventilatory responses to exercise in chronic heart failure. *International Journal of Cardiology*. **66**(1): 59–63. (RCT-9)

24 Yap JC, Moore DM, Cleland JG, Pride NB. (2000) Effect of supine posture on respiratory mechanics in chronic left ventricular failure. *American Journal of Respiratory and Critical Care Medicine*. **162**(4 Pt. 1): 1285–91. (CT-20)

25 Collins JV, Clark TJ, Brown DJ. (1975) Airway function in healthy subjects and patients with left heart disease. *Clinical Science and Molecular Medicine*. **49**(3): 217–28. (OS-112)

26 Hanning CD, Alexander-Williams JM. (1995) Pulse oximetry: a practical review. *British Medical Journal*. **311**: 367–70.

27 Wilcock A, England R, El Khoury B, Frisby J, Howard P, Bell S, Manderson C, Keeley V, Kinnear W. (2008) The prevalence of nocturnal hypoxemia in advanced cancer. *Journal of Pain and Symptom Management*. **36**(4): 351–7. (OS-100)

28 Uronis HE, Abernethy AP. (2008) Oxygen for relief of dyspnea: what is the evidence? *Current Opinion in Supportive and Palliative Care*. **2**(2): 89–94. (R, 68 refs)

29 Philip J, Gold M, Milner A, Di Iulio J, Miller B, Spruyt O. (2006) A randomized, double-blind, crossover trial of the effect of oxygen on dyspnea in patients with advanced cancer. *Journal of Pain and Symptom Management*. **32**(6): 541–50. (RCT-51)

30 O'Driscoll BR, Howard LS, Davison AG. (2008) British Thoracic Society guideline for emergency oxygen use in adults. *Thorax*. **63**(Suppl. 6): vi, 1–68. (GS)

31 Creagh-Brown B, Shee C. (2008) Noninvasive ventilation as ceiling of therapy in end-stage chronic obstructive pulmonary disease. *Chronic Respiratory Disease*. **5**(3): 143–8. (SA, 39 refs)

32 Robinson PJ. (2002) Dornase alfa in early cystic fibrosis lung disease. *Pediatric Pulmonology*. **34**(3): 237–41. (R)

33 Rubin BK. (2007) Mucolytics, expectorants, and mucokinetic medications. *Respiratory Care*. **52**(7): 859–65. (R)

34 Ahmedzai S, Regnard C. (1995) Dyspnoea. In: *Flow Diagrams in Advanced Cancer and Other Diseases*. London: Edward Arnold. pp. 48–53.

35 Wildiers H, Menten J. (2002) Death rattle: prevalence, prevention and treatment. *Journal of Pain and Symptom Management*. **23**(4): 310–17. (RS-107).

36 Kompanje EJ. (2006) "Death rattle" after withdrawal of mechanical ventilation: practical and ethical considerations. *Intensive and Critical Care Nursing*. **22**(4): 214–9. (R, 46 refs)

37 Watts T, Jenkins K. (1999) Palliative care nurses' feelings about death rattle. *Journal of Clinical Nursing*. **8**(5): 615–16. (OS-33)

38 Wee B, Coleman P, Hillier R, Holgate S. (2008) Death rattle: its impact on staff and volunteers in palliative care. *Palliative Medicine*. **22**(2): 173–6. (I-42)

39 Wee BL, Coleman PG, Hillier R, Holgate SH. (2006) The sound of death rattle II: how do relatives interpret the sound? *Palliative Medicine*. **20**(3): 177–81. (I-25)

40 Wee BL, Coleman PG, Hillier R, Holgate SH. (2006) The sound of death rattle I: are relatives distressed by hearing this sound? *Palliative Medicine*. **20**(3): 171–5. (I-27)

41 Wee B, Hillier R. (2008) Interventions for noisy breathing in patients near to death. *Cochrane Database of Systematic Reviews*. **1**: CD005177. (SA, R–37 refs)

42 Bennett MI. (1996) Death rattle: an audit of hyoscine (scopolamine) use and review of management. *Journal of Pain and Symptom Management*. **12**(4): 229–33. (CT-100)

43 Lawrey H. (2005) Hyoscine vs glycopyrronium for drying respiratory secretions in dying patients. *British Journal of Community Nursing*. **10**(9): 421–4. (R, 17 refs)

44 Bennett M, Lucas V, Brennan M, Hughes A, O'Donnell V, Wee B. (2002) Association for Palliative Medicine's Science Committee. Using anti-muscarinic drugs in the management of death rattle: evidence-based guidelines for palliative care. *Palliative Medicine*. **16**(5): 369–74. (GC)

45 Hughes A, Wilcock A, Corcoran R, Lucas V, King A. (2000) Audit of three antimuscarinic drugs for managing retained secretions. *Palliative Medicine*. **14**(3): 221–2. (OS)

46 Back IN, Jenkins K, Blower A, Beckhelling J. (2001) A study comparing hyoscine hydrobromide and glycopyrrolate in the treatment of death rattle. *Palliative Medicine*. **15**(4): 329–36. (OS)

47 Mutagh FEM, Thorns A, Oliver DJ. (2002) Hyoscine and glycopyrrolate for death rattle. *Palliative Medicine*. **16**: 449–50.
48 Sutton PP, Gemmell HG, Innes N, *et al.* (1988) Use of nebulised saline and nebulised terbutaline as an adjunct to chest physiotherapy. *Thorax*. **43**: 57–60.
49 Clayton J, Fardell B, Hutton-Potts J, Webb D, Chye R. (2003) Parenteral antibiotics in a palliative care unit: prospective analysis of current practice. *Palliative Medicine*. **17**(1): 44–8. (OS-41)
50 Spruyt O, Kausae A. (1998) Antibiotic use for infective terminal respiratory secretions. *Journal of Pain and Symptom Management*. **15**: 263–4. (Let, CS-11)
51 Bricaire F, Castaing JL, Pocidalo JJ, Vilde JL. (1988) Pharmacokinetics and tolerance of ceftriaxone after subcutaneous administration. [French] *Pathologie et Biologie*. **36**(5 Pt. 2): 702–5. (CS-8)
52 Borner K, Lode H, Hampel B, Pfeuffer M, Koeppe P. (1985) Comparative pharmacokinetics of ceftriaxone after subcutaneous and intravenous administration. *Chemotherapy*. **31**(4): 237–45. (RCT-8)
53 Nakajima T, Terashima T, Nishida J, Onoda M, Koide O. (2002) Treatment of bronchorrhea by corticosteroids in a case of bronchioloalveolar carcinoma producing CA19-9. *Internal Medicine*. **41**(3): 225–8. (CS-1)
54 Tamaoki J, Kohri K, Isono K, Nagai A. (2000) Inhaled indomethacin in bronchorrhea in bronchioloalveolar carcinoma: role of cyclooxygenase. *Chest*. **117**(4): 1213–14. (Let)
55 Suga T, Sugiyama Y, Fujii T, Kitamura S. (1994) Bronchioloalveolar carcinoma with bronchorrhoea treated with erythromycin. *European Respiratory Journal*. **7**(12): 2249–51. (CS-1)
56 Chen H, Brahmer J. (2008) Management of malignant pleural effusion. *Current Oncology Reports*. **10**(4): 287–93. (R, 27 refs)
57 Balassoulis G, Sichletidis L, Spyratos D, Chloros D, *et al.* (2008) Efficacy and safety of erythromycin as sclerosing agent in patients with recurrent malignant pleural effusion. *American Journal of Clinical Oncology*. **31**(4): 384–9. (OS-34)
58 Tan C, Sedrakyan A, Browne J, Swift S, Treasure T. (2006) The evidence on the effectiveness of management for malignant pleural effusion: a systematic review. *European Journal of Cardio-Thoracic Surgery*. **29**(5): 829–38. (R, 73 refs)
59 Tattersall MHN, Boyer MJ. (1990) Management of malignant pleural effusions. *Thorax*. **45**: 81–2.
60 Schulze M, Boehle AS, Kurdow R, Dohrmann P, Henne-Bruns D. (2001) Effective treatment of malignant pleural effusion by minimal invasive thoracic surgery: thoracoscopic talc pleurodesis and pleuroperitoneal shunts in 101 patients. *Annals of Thoracic Surgery*. **71**(6): 1809–12. (RS-101)
61 Genc O, Petrou M, Ladas G, Goldstraw P. (2000) The long-term morbidity of pleuroperitoneal shunts in the management of recurrent malignant effusions. *European Journal of Cardio-Thoracic Surgery*. **18**(2): 143–6. (RS-160)
62 Bertolaccini L, Zamprogna C, Barberis L, *et al.* (2007) Malignant pleural effusions: review of treatment and our experience. *Reviews on Recent Clinical Trials*. **2**(1): 21–5.
63 Tremblay A, Michaud G. (2006) Single-center experience with 250 tunnelled pleural catheter insertions for malignant pleural effusion *Chest*. **129**(2): 362–8. (RS-250)
64 Janes SM, Rahman NM, Davies RJO, Lee YCG. (2007) Catheter-tract metastases associated with chronic indwelling pleural catheters. *Chest*. **131**(4): 1232–4. (CS-4)
65 Plataniotis GA, Kouvaris JR, Dardoufas C, Kouloulias V, Theofanopoulou MA, Vlahos L. (2002) A short radiotherapy course for locally advanced non-small-cell lung cancer (NSCLC): effective palliation and patients' convenience. *Lung Cancer*. **35**(2): 203–7.
66 Filshie J, Penn K, Ashley S, Davis C. (1996) Acupuncture for the relief of cancer-related breathlessness. *Palliative Medicine*. **10**: 145–50.
67 Lau KS, Jones AY. (2008) A single session of Acu-TENS increases FEV1 and reduces dyspnoea in patients with chronic obstructive pulmonary disease: a randomised, placebo-controlled trial. *Australian Journal of Physiotherapy*. **54**(3): 179–84. (RCT-46)
68 Bausewein C, Booth S, Gysels M, Higginson I. (2008) Non-pharmacological interventions for breathlessness in advanced stages of malignant and non-malignant diseases. *Cochrane Database of Systematic Reviews*. **2**: CD005623. (SA, R-166 refs)
69 Nagy-Agren S, Haley HB. (2002) Management of infections in palliative care patients with advanced cancer. *Journal of Pain and Symptom Management*. **24**: 64–70. (R, 11 refs)
70 Chen LK, Chou YC, Hsu PS, Tsai ST, Hwang SJ, Wu BY, Lin MH, Chen TW. (2002) Antibiotic prescription for fever episodes in hospice patients. *Supportive Care in Cancer*. **10**(7): 538–41. (RS-535)
71 Oneschuk D, Fainsinger R, Demoissac D. (2002) Antibiotic use in the last week of life in three different palliative care settings. *Journal of Palliative Care*. **18**(1): 25–8. (OS-150)
72 Vitetta L, Kenner D, Sali A. (2000) Bacterial infections in terminally ill hospice patients. *Journal of Pain and Symptom Management*. **20**(5): 326–34. (OS-102)
73 Chan R, Hemeryck L, O'Regan M, Clancy L, Feely J. (1995) Oral versus intravenous antibiotics for community acquired lower respiratory tract infection in a general hospital: open, randomised controlled trial. *British Medical Journal*. **310**: 1360–2. (RCT-541)
74 Beringer P. (2001) The clinical use of colistin in patients with cystic fibrosis. *Current Opinion in Pulmonary Medicine*. **7**(6): 434–40. (R, 30 refs)
75 Lin HC, Cheng HF, Wang CH, Liu CY, Yu CT, Kuo HP. (1997) Inhaled gentamicin reduces airway neutrophil activity and mucus secretion in bronchiectasis. *American Journal of Respiratory and Critical Care Medicine*. **155**(6): 2024–9. (RCT-28)
76 Falagas ME, Agrafiotis M, Athanassa Z, Siempos II. (2008) Administration of antibiotics via the

respiratory tract as monotherapy for pneumonia. *Expert Review of Antiinfective Therapy*. **6**(4): 447–52. (R, 16 refs)

77 Wood GC, Swanson JM. (2007) Aerosolised antibacterials for the prevention and treatment of hospital-acquired pneumonia. *Drugs*. **67**(6): 903–14. (R, 72 refs)

78 Gleeson C, Spencer D. (1995) Blood transfusion and its benefits in palliative care. *Palliative Medicine*. **9**: 307–13. (OS-97)

79 Monti M, Castelleni L, Berlusconi A, Cunietti E. (1996) Use of red blood cell transfusions in terminally ill cancer patients admitted to a palliative care unit. *Journal of Pain and Symptom Management*. **12**: 18–22. (OS-31)

80 Davies A, Wang S. (1997) Blood transfusions in patients with advanced cancer. *Journal of Pain and Symptom Management*. **13**: 318. (Let)

81 Friedman NL. (1996) Hiccups: a treatment review. *Pharmacotherapy*. **16**(6): 986–95. (R, 78 refs)

82 Rousseau P. (2003) Hiccups in patients with advanced cancer: a brief review. *Progress in Palliative Care*. **11**(1): 10–12. (R, 27 refs)

83 Respiratory Symptoms. In: Twycross RG, Wilcock A, Stark Toller C. (2009) *Symptom Management in Advanced Cancer*. Nottingham: palliativedrugs.com. pp. 61–144. (Ch)

84 Launois S, Bizec JL, *et al.* (1993) Hiccup in adults: an overview. *European Respiratory Journal*. **6**: 563–75.

85 Guelaud C, Similowski T, *et al.* (1995) Baclofen therapy for chronic hiccup. *European Respiratory Journal*. **8**: 235–7.

86 Wilcock A, Twycross R. (1996) Midazolam for intractable hiccup. *Journal of Pain and Symptom Management*. **12**: 59–61. (CS)

87 Moretti R, Torre P, Antonello RM, Ukmar M, Cazzato G, Bava A. (2004) Gabapentin as a drug therapy of intractable hiccup because of vascular lesion: a three-year follow up. *Neurologist*. **10**(2): 102–6. (R-52)

88 Tegeler ML, Baumrucker SJ. (2008) Gabapentin for intractable hiccups in palliative care. *American Journal of Hospice and Palliative Medicine*. **25**(1): 52–4. (R)

89 Wilcox SK, Garry A, Johnson MJ. (2009) Novel use of amantadine: to treat hiccups. *Journal of Pain and Symptom Management*. **38**(3): 460–3. (CS-1)

90 Wee B. (2008) Chronic cough. *Current Opinion in Supportive and Palliative Care*. **2**(2): 105–9. (R, 48 refs)

91 Irwin RS, Curley FJ, Bennett FM. (1993) Appropriate use of antitussives and protussives: a practical review. *Drugs*. **46**(1): 80–91. (R, 88 refs)

92 Dicpinigaitis PV, Dobkin JB. (1997) Antitussive effect of the GABA-agonist baclofen. *Chest*. **111**(4): 996–9. (RCT-12)

93 Ahmedzai S, Davis C. (1997) Nebulised drugs in palliative care. *Thorax*. **52**(Suppl. 2): S75–77.

94 Udezue E. (2001) Lidocaine inhalation for cough suppression. *American Journal of Emergency Medicine*. **19**(3): 206–7. (OS)

95 Lingerfelt BM, Swainey CW, Smith TJ, Coyne PJ. (2007) Nebulized lidocaine for intractable cough near the end of life. *The Journal of Supportive Oncology*. **5**(7): 301–2. (Let)

96 McAlpine LG, Thomson NC. (1989) Lidocaine-induced bronchoconstriction in asthmatic patients: relation to histamine airway responsiveness and effect of preservative. *Chest*. **96**: 1012–15. (OS-20)

97 Mirhosseini M, Oneschuk D, Hunter B, Hanson J, Quan H, Amigo P. (2006) The role of antibiotics in the management of infection-related symptoms in advanced cancer patients. *Journal of Palliative Care*. **22**(2): 69–74. (OS-26)

98 Davis CL. (1994) The therapeutics of dyspnoea. *Cancer Surveys*. **21**: 85–98. (R, 78 refs)

99 Walsh TD. (1984) Opiates and respiratory function in advanced cancer. *Recent Results in Cancer Research*. **89**: 115–17.

100 Boyd KJ, Kelly M. (1997) Oral morphine as symptomatic treatment of dyspnoea in patients with advanced cancer. *Palliative Medicine*. **11**(4): 277–81. (OS-15)

101 Ward C. (2002) The need for palliative care in the management of heart failure. *Heart*. **87**: 294–8. (R, 37 refs)

102 Flowers B. (2003) Palliative care for patients with end-stage heart failure. *Nursing Times*. **99**: 30–2. (R, 14 refs)

103 Abernethy AP, Currow DC, Frith P, Fazekas BS, *et al.* (2003) Randomised, double blind, placebo controlled crossover trial of sustained release morphine for the management of refractory dyspnoea. *British Medical Journal*. **327**: 523–8. (RCT-38)

104 Clemens KE, Quednau I, Klaschik E. (2008) Is there a higher risk of respiratory depression in opioid-naive palliative care patients during symptomatic therapy of dyspnea with strong opioids? *Journal of Palliative Medicine*. **11**(2): 204–16. (OS-27)

105 Clemens KE, Klaschik E. (2008) Effect of hydromorphone on ventilation in palliative care patients with dyspnea. *Supportive Care in Cancer*. **16**(1): 93–9. (OS-14)

106 Vercovitch M, Waller A, Adunsky A. (1999) High dose morphine use in the hospice setting. *Cancer*. **86**(5): 871–7. (RS-651)

107 Jennings AL, Davies AN, Higgins JP, Gibbs JS, Broadley KE. (2002) A systematic review of the use of opioids in the management of dyspnoea. *Thorax*. **57**(11): 939–44. (SA-18)

108 Clemens KE, Klaschik E. (2007) Symptomatic therapy of dyspnea with strong opioids and its effect on ventilation in palliative care patients. *Journal of Pain and Symptom Management*. **33**(4): 473–81.

109 Viola R, Kiteley C, Lloyd NS, Mackay JA, *et al.* (2008) Supportive Care Guidelines Group of the Cancer Care Ontario Program in Evidence-Based Care. The management of dyspnea in cancer patients: a systematic review. *Supportive Care in Cancer*. **16**(4): 329–37. (SA, R-47 refs)

110 Currow DC, Plummer J, Frith P, Abernethy AP. (2007) Can we predict which patients with refractory dyspnea will respond to opioids? *Journal of Palliative Medicine*. **10**(5): 1031–6. (RCT-38)

111 Brown SJ, Eichner SF, Jones JR. (2005) Nebulized morphine for relief of dyspnea due to chronic lung disease. *Annals of Pharmacotherapy*. **39**: 1088–92. (R)
112 Charles MA, Reymond L, Israel F. (2008) Relief of incident dyspnea in palliative cancer patients: a pilot, randomized, controlled trial comparing nebulized hydromorphone, systemic hydromorphone, and nebulized saline. *Journal of Pain and Symptom Management*. **36**(1): 29–38. (RCT-20)
113 Kallet RH. (2007) The role of inhaled opioids and furosemide for the treatment of dyspnea. *Respiratory Care*. **52**(7): 900–10. (R, 80 refs)
114 Shimoyama N, Shimoyama M. (2002) Nebulized furosemide as a novel treatment for dyspnea in terminal cancer patients. *Journal of Pain and Symptom Management*. **23**(1): 73–6. (CS-3)
115 Prandota J. (2002) Furosemide: progress in understanding its diuretic, anti-inflammatory, and bronchodilating mechanism of action, and use in the treatment of respiratory tract diseases. *American Journal of Therapeutics*. **9**(4): 317–28. (R, 123 refs)
116 Jensen D, Amjadi K, Harris-McAllister V, Webb KA, O'Donnell DE. (2008) Mechanisms of dyspnoea relief and improved exercise endurance after furosemide inhalation in COPD *Thorax*. **63**(7): 606–13. (RCT-20)
117 Stone P, Rix E. (2002) Nebulized furosemide for dyspnoea in terminal cancer patients. *Journal of Pain and Symptom Management*. **23**(3): 274–5. (Let)
118 Rietjens JA, van Zuylen L, van Veluw H, van der Wijk L, *et al.* (2008) Palliative sedation in a specialized unit for acute palliative care in a cancer hospital: comparing patients dying with and without palliative sedation. *Journal of Pain and Symptom Management*. **36**(3): 228–34. (RS-157)
119 Daud ML. (2007) Drug management of terminal symptoms in advanced cancer patients. *Current Opinion in Supportive and Palliative Care*. **1**(3): 202–6. (R, 51 refs)
120 Bailey C. (1995) Nursing as therapy in the management of breathlessness in lung cancer. *European Journal of Cancer Care*. **4**: 184–90. (R, 24 refs)
121 Corner J, Plant H, A'Hern R, *et al.* (1996) Non-pharmacological intervention for breathlessness in lung cancer. *Palliative Medicine*. **10**: 299–305. (RCT-20)
122 Hately J, Laurence V, Scott A, Baker R, Thomas P. (2003) Breathlessness clinics within specialist palliative care settings can improve the quality of life and functional capacity of patients with lung cancer. *Palliative Medicine*. **17**: 410–17. (OS-30)
123 Booth S, Farquhar M, Gysels M, Bausewein C, Higginson IJ. (2006) The impact of a breathlessness intervention service (BIS) on the lives of patients with intractable dyspnea: a qualitative phase 1 study. *Palliative and Supportive Care*. **4**(3): 287–93. (I)
124 Hutchinson D, Whyte K. (2008) Neuromuscular disease and respiratory failure. *Practical Neurology*. **8**(4): 229–37. (R, 12 refs)
125 Tsolaki V, Pastaka C, Karetsi E, Zygoulis P. *et al.* (2008) One-year non-invasive ventilation in chronic hypercapnic COPD: effect on quality of life. *Respiratory Medicine*. **102**(6): 904–11. (CT-49)
126 Kuhnlein P, Kubler A, Raubold S, Worrell M, *et al.* (2008) Palliative care and circumstances of dying in German ALS patients using non-invasive ventilation. *Amyotrophic Lateral Sclerosis*. **9**(2): 91–8. (I-29)
127 Dohna-Schwake C, Podlewski P, Voit T, Mellies U. (2008) Non-invasive ventilation reduces respiratory tract infections in children with neuromuscular disorders. *Pediatric Pulmonology*. **43**(1): 67–71. (OS-24)
128 Toussaint M, Chatwin M, Soudon P. (2007) Mechanical ventilation in Duchenne patients with chronic respiratory insufficiency: clinical implications of 20 years published experience. *Chronic Respiratory Disease*. **4**(3): 167–77. (R, 133 refs)
129 Branthwaite MA. (1989) Mechanical ventilation at home. *British Medical Journal*. **298**: 1409.
130 Branthwaite MA. (1991) Non-invasive and domiciliary ventilation: positive pressure techniques. *Thorax*. **46**: 208–12.
131 Polkey MI, Lyall RA, Davidson AC, Leigh PN, Moxham J. (1999) Ethical and clinical issues in the use of home non-invasive mechanical ventilation for the palliation of breathlessness in motor neurone disease. *Thorax*. **54**(4): 367–71. (R, 43 refs)
132 Shee CD, Green M. (2003) Non-invasive ventilation and palliation: experience in a district general hospital and a review. *Palliative Medicine*. **17**(1): 21–6. (CS-10)
133 Curtis JR, Cook DJ, Sinuff T, *et al.* (2007) Non-invasive positive pressure ventilation in critical and palliative care settings: understanding the goals of therapy. *Critical Care Medicine*. **35**(3): 932–9. (R, 41 refs)
134 Tarzian AJ. (2000) Caring for dying patients who have air hunger. *Journal of Nursing Scholarship*. **32**(2): 137–43. (OS-10)
135 Shumway NM, Wilson RL, Howard RS, Parker JM, Eliasson AH. (2008) Presence and treatment of air hunger in severely ill patients. *Respiratory Medicine*. **102**(1): 27–31. (OS-198)
136 Formiga F, Olmedo C, Lopez-Soto A, Navarro M, Culla A, Pujol R. (2007) Dying in hospital of terminal heart failure or severe dementia: the circumstances associated with death and the opinions of caregivers. *Palliative Medicine*. **21**(1): 35–40. (OS-102)
137 Fainsinger RL, Waller A, Bercovici M, Bengtson K, *et al.* (2000) A multicentre international study of sedation for uncontrolled symptoms in terminally ill patients. *Palliative Medicine*. **14**(4): 257–65. (OS-287)
138 Navigante AH, Cerchietti LC, Castro MA, Lutteral MA, Cabalar ME. (2006) Midazolam as adjunct therapy to morphine in the alleviation of severe dyspnea perception in patients with advanced cancer. *Journal of Pain and Symptom Management*. **31**(1): 38–47. (RCT-101)

Skin problems

CLINICAL DECISION AND ACTION CHECKLIST

1 Is the skin healthy?
2 Is the skin dry?
3 Is the skin wet?
4 Is the skin itchy?
5 Is the skin broken?

KEY POINTS

- Preventing pressure damage starts with identifying patients at risk.
- Healing of pressure damage is not realistic if the prognosis is short.
- Dry skin is common and uncomfortable.

INTRODUCTION

A number of skin problems can occur in advanced disease, particularly dry skin, sweating, pressure ulcers, and itch. Malignant ulcers are described in *Malignant ulcers and fistulae*, p. 159. Pressure ulcers are particularly common, especially in bed-bound patients in hospital and nursing homes.[1,2]

MAINTAINING A HEALTHY SKIN

A healthy skin is supple, intact, and a good color, but the skin is easily compromised in advanced disease. Assessing the risk of pressure damage is important and a number of pressure sore prediction scores are available such as the Waterlow, Norton or Braden risk scores.[3–5] However, evidence for their effectiveness is lacking.[6–9] For those at moderate or high risk of pressure damage special mattresses, seat cushions and careful handling will reduce the risk of tissue breakdown. Even using good-quality static mattresses can significantly reduce the incidence and severity of pressure sores.[10] Adequate nutrition and hydration are important and it is possible that stress plays a part by delaying healing.[11]

DIAGNOSING SKIN PROBLEMS

Diagnosing a skin problem is mainly visual:

Character	Possible cause
Dry	Dehydration, drugs, air conditioning.
Wet	Sweating (e.g. anxiety, drugs, eczema, fever, hormonal deficiency, hyperthyroidism, infection), body fluids (e.g. urine, stool, exudates, lymphorrhea).
Bluish, purple	Venous congestion, local malignancy, cyanosis, bruising.
Gray or black	Recent bruising, necrosis due to local pressure damage or arterial insufficiency.
Pale or white	Acute arterial occlusion, anemia or hypotension.
Redness	Rash (e.g. drugs, skin irritant or systemic infection), recent trauma (e.g. scratch or injury), vasodilatation (e.g. fever or local infection).
Yellow or green	Old bruising

MANAGING SKIN PROBLEMS

Dry skin

Simple measures can prevent and treat a dry skin and avoid cracking and itch (*see* cd-2 opposite).

Wet skin

Wet skin can become macerated, sore, and prone to infection such as candida. Barrier preparations can help to protect the skin from sources of moisture such as urine or feces.

Sweating: some patients suffer profuse sweating, particularly at night. It may be due to anxiety or hormone deficiency. Occasionally, malignancy will produce a fever with sweating – measures such as cooling with a fan or sponge are effective. If the cause cannot be treated, systemic drugs can be tried, but their use is based on small numbers or case studies and include amitriptyline, cimetidine, propantheline,[12] nabilone,[13] venlafaxine,[14] gabapentin[15] and thalidomide.[16,17]

Itch (pruritus)

A wide range of skin disorders and systemic conditions are known to cause itching and an equally wide range of underlying mechanisms and treatments have been suggested.[18,19] Some antidepressants are H_1 and/or H_2 antagonists and may be more effective than conventional H_1 antagonists.[20,21] Some itching may be amenable to non-drug treatments, e.g. stenting of the bile duct for cholestatic itching, local cooling,[22] UVB light phototherapy,[23,24] and acupuncture.[25] Some drugs such as ondansetron and gabapentin have shown conflicting results in controlled trials.[26–30] Most treatments are based on small numbers or case studies and include topical agents (clobetasol,[31] capsaicin,[32] and doxepin);[33] and systemic drugs

Clinical decision	If YES carry out the action below
1 Is the skin healthy? (supple, intact, good color)	• **Check the skin and calculate a pressure risk score weekly** (daily if the risk is moderate or high). • **Ensure:** — good hydration and nutrition (especially vitamin C and zinc)[34,35] — the skin is kept supple, and prevent contact with urine or feces. • **If there is a moderate to high risk of pressure damage:** distribute pressure using special surfaces or mattresses. If tolerated, keep the patient's upper body at no more than a 30-degree tilt and take care with positioning. Prevent trauma to pressure areas by ensuring careful moving and positioning. If the skin is dry *see* cd-2 below.
2 Is the skin dry?	• **When bathing:** use tepid water and hypoallergenic soaps.[36] Use an emollient cream within 5 min of washing, then pat dry (do not rub). Avoid lotions. • **Increase ambient humidity:** if necessary with a room humidifier.
3 Is the skin wet?	• **If due to exposure to body fluids:** use a barrier preparation (e.g. zinc ointments or simethicone cream) or a barrier application, e.g. Sween cream, Cavilon solution (Canada only),[37] Secura cream (US only). • **If due to sweating:** treat causes such as anxiety, drugs, eczema, hormonal deficiency, hyperthyroidism, infection. Use fans and reduce the temperature in the room. • **If due to persistent fever:** use acetaminophen PO or PR 1 g q4h or diclofenac PO 50 mg q8h.[38] • **For hormone deficiency:** — in women try megestrol acetate 20–40 mg PO daily[39] — in men after antiandrogen treatment, cyproterone acetate 50 mg PO q12h.[40] • **If sweating persists** try *one* of the following: amitriptyline 10–50 mg at bedtime, propantheline 15–30 mg at bedtime, nabilone 0.5–1 mg q12h, venlafaxine 75 mg q12h, gabapentin, or thalidomide 50–100 mg PO daily (Special Access status in North America).
4 Is the skin itchy?	• **Correct simple causes** such as stopping or changing a drug causing an itchy rash. Avoid lotions. • **Treat any dry skin:** *see* cd-2 above. • **If the itch is localized:** try local cooling with a cold compress. Alternatives are topical clobetasol 0.05% ointment daily if inflammation is present, *or* capsaicin cream (start with 0.025%), *or* doxepin 5% cream q8h (from compounding pharmacy in Canada), but all topical applications may themselves cause local sensitivity reactions. • **If the itch is generalized:** start with sertraline 50–150 mg daily. Alternatives are paroxetine 10–20 mg PO on waking, *or* mirtazapine 15–45 mg at bedtime. • **If the itch persists:** consider adding one of the following: *If H_1 mediated:* try hydroxyzine PO 25 mg at bedtime initially, increasing to 25 mg q8h. *If cholestasis:* rifampicin PO 150–300 mg q6h, *or* (if not on opioids) naltrexone PO 25–50 mg daily. Consider UVB phototherapy. *If uremia:* treat iron deficiency anemia.[41] Consider UVB phototherapy, *or* naltrexone PO 25–50 mg daily (avoid if already on opioids), *or* gabapentin. *Other options:* thalidomide (Special Access status in North America) up to 200 mg PO at bedtime; acupuncture.

Adapted from Bale and Regnard[42]
cd = clinical decision

(sertraline,[43,44] paroxetine,[45] mirtazapine,[46] rifampicin,[47–49] naltrexone,[50,51] and thalidomide[52,53]).

Broken skin

Early damage can be difficult to identify, although one suggestion is that the skin in early damage feels warmer than surrounding skin.[54] For a deep ulcer, cleansing and healing will take several months. Patients with a short prognosis (day-by-day deterioration) are unlikely to heal, and even debridement may be incomplete, but odor and pain can be controlled. Slower deterioration (week to week) may allow some healing of shallow ulcers if nutrition is adequate, but only cleansing in deeper ulcers.

Moist dressings for pressure ulcers: the ideal dressing maintains high humidity, removes exudate and toxins, provides thermal insulation, is impermeable to bacteria, free from particles and toxins, and capable of removal without further damage or pain.[55] Traditional gauzes, antiseptics and hypochlorites (e.g. Milton), do not fulfill these needs.[56] Few trials have shown any one dressing to have an advantage, and choice will depend not only on the type of wound, but also on availability, experience of the carer, the site of the wound, and patient preference or tolerance.[57] Hydrogels (e.g. Intrasite gel) are useful where slough and infection are present. Conformable polyurethane foam dressing (e.g. Tielle, Allevyn, Lyofoam) are useful for heavy exudates. Hydrocolloids (e.g. Comfeel, Duoderm) maintain a moist environment useful for debridement and healing and are increasingly the preferred dressing for pressure ulcers.[58]

Sucralfate: sucralfate suspension can be used as a hemostatic agent (*see* cd-3, *Bleeding*, p. 95) and has been shown to improve inflammation, discomfort, and healing of venous ulcers.[59]

Debridement of pressure ulcers: necrotic tissue delays healing, produces odor, and masks the extent of damage. Dressings that maintain a moist environment remove necrotic tissue without further damage.[60] A hard, dark eschar of dead skin can occasionally prevent access to the ulcer, but the eschar can be softened with moist dressings. There is no evidence to support one cleansing solution or technique.[61] Larval therapy can help (*see Malignant ulcers and fistulae*, p. 162).

Other dressings and appliances: semipermeable adhesive film dressings (e.g. OpSite, Tegaderm) are useful in maintaining humidity in shallow ulcers (<0.5 cm) or in protecting very early damage. Silicone foam dressing (e.g. Mepilex) can be useful in cavities where frequent cleansing is required. Topical negative pressure devices are being used more frequently in complex wounds, but the evidence for their efficacy is lacking.[62,63]

Pressure relieving devices

These vary in cost and complexity:

Simple devices: these vary from sheepskins to pressure-distributing cushions.

Complex devices: air flow mattresses are being increasingly used for high-risk patients, but there is conflicting evidence whether alternating-pressure mattresses are more effective than constant-pressure mattresses.[64]

Clinical decision	If YES carry out the action below
5 Is the skin broken?	• **Exclude these causes:** infection, arterial insufficiency, venous ulceration, or trauma due to sensory loss. • **If the area is bleeding:** apply sucralfate suspension directly to the bleeding area and apply pressure with a non-adherent dressing. • **If the prognosis is too short to allow healing** (e.g. day-by-day deterioration): choose dressings for comfort such as non-adherent, soft silicone net dressings (e.g. Mepitel).[65,66] • **If odor is present:** *see* cd-4 in *Malignant ulcers and fistulae*, p. 163. • **If pain is present:** *see* cd-6 in *Malignant ulcers and fistulae*, p. 163. • **If this is a malignant ulcer:** *see Malignant ulcers and fistulae*, p. 162. • **If the skin surface is intact but damaged:** *Superficial damage:* if pressure care is fully implemented, a dressing is not usually required for discoloration of skin. A blister or abrasion may need a light dressing for protection. *Deep damage:* this is likely to develop into an ulcer. If a hard eschar is present this needs moistening with hydrocolloid or hydrogel dressing for one week followed by debridement (*see Malignant ulcers and fistulae*, p. 162). • **If this is an ulcer due to pressure damage:** *Avoid harmful chemicals:* e.g. chlorinated solutions (e.g. Dakin's) or hydrogen peroxide. *Superficial ulcer:* provide an environment for re-epithelialization: moisture-retaining dressings (e.g. Tielle, Allevyn, Lyofoam, hydrocolloid dressings, OpSite). Reassess as needed. *Deep ulcer:* provide an environment for granulation using moist cavity dressing (e.g. cavity foam dressing, calcium alginate, or hydrogel). For heavy exudate *see* cd-4 in *Malignant ulcers and fistulae*, p. 161. If debris is present use 0.9% saline for irrigation.[67] Antiseptics such as iodine-based derivatives (e.g. povidone iodine fabric dressing) can reduce infection.[68] Consider larval therapy (*see* p. 162 in *Malignant ulcers and fistulae*). Surgical debridement in the OR may be appropriate in some patients.[69] Reassess the ulcer at each dressing change using wound assessment sheets or charts.

Adapted from Bale and Regnard[42]
cd = clinical decision

Pain

This is common in several skin conditions. It is particularly common in pressure ulcers,[70] and is more severe in deeper ulcers.[71] Topical opioids have been suggested as a treatment,[72–75] but are not effective in acute skin injury.[76,77] Any benefit appears due to a local action as very little is absorbed systemically.[78]

REFERENCES: SKIN PROBLEMS

B = book; C = comment; Ch = chapter; CS-n = case study-no. of cases; CT-n = controlled trial-no. of cases; E = editorial; GC = group consensus; I = interviews; Let = letter; LS = laboratory study; MC = multi-center; OS-n = open study-no. of cases; R = review; RCT-n = randomized controlled trial-no. of cases; RS-n = retrospective survey-no. of cases; SA = systematic or meta analysis.

1 Wann-Hansson C, Hagell P, Willman A. (2008) Risk factors and prevention among patients with hospital-acquired and pre-existing pressure ulcers in an acute care hospital. *Journal of Clinical Nursing*. **17**(13): 1718–27. (OS-535)

2 Bergstrom N, Smout R, Horn S, Spector W, Hartz A, Limcangco MR. (2008) Stage 2 pressure ulcer healing in nursing homes. *Journal of the American Geriatrics Society*. **56**(7): 1252–8. (OS-774)

3 Birchall L. (1993) Making sense of pressure sore calculators. *Nursing Times*. **89**: 34–7.

4 Galvin J. (2002) An audit of pressure ulcer incidence in a palliative care setting. *International Journal of Palliative Nursing*. **8**(5): 214, 216, 218–21. (OS-542)

5 Comfort EH. (2008) Reducing pressure ulcer incidence through Braden Scale risk assessment and support surface use. *Advances in Skin and Wound Care*. **21**(7): 330–4. (SA)

6 Moore ZE, Cowman S. (2008) Risk assessment tools for the prevention of pressure ulcers. *Cochrane Database of Systematic Reviews*. **3**: CD006471 (SA, 59 refs)

7 Mortenson WB, Miller WC, SCIRE Research Team. (2008) A review of scales for assessing the risk of developing a pressure ulcer in individuals with SCI. *Spinal Cord*. **46**(3): 168–75. (R, 36 refs)

8 Brown SJ. (2004) The Braden scale: a review of the research evidence. *Orthopaedic Nursing*. **23**: 30–8. (R, 15 refs)

9 Gould D, Goldstone L, Gammon J, Kelly D, Maidwell A. (2002) Establishing the validity of pressure ulcer risk assessment scales: a novel approach using illustrated patient scenarios. *International Journal of Nursing Studies*. **39**: 215–18.

10 Hofman A, Geelkerken RH, Wille J, Hamming JJ, Hermans J, Breslau PJ. (1994) Pressure sores and pressure-decreasing mattresses: controlled clinical trial. *The Lancet*. **343**: 568–71. (RCT-44)

11 Kiecolt-Glaser JK, Marucha PT, Malarkey WB, Mercado AM, Glaser R. (1995) Slowing of healing by psychological stress. *The Lancet*. **346**: 1194–6. (CT-26)

12 Canaday BR, Stanford RH. (1995) Propantheline bromide in the management of hyperhidrosis associated with spinal cord injury. *Annals of Pharmacotherapy*. **29**(5): 489–92. (CS-2)

13 Maida V. (2008) Nabilone for the treatment of paraneoplastic night sweats: a report of four cases. *Journal of Palliative Medicine*. **11**(6): 929–34. (CS-4)

14 Loprinzi CL, Pisansky TM, Fonseca R, Sloan JA, *et al.* (1998) Pilot evaluation of venlafaxine hydrochloride for the therapy of hot flashes in cancer survivors. *Journal of Clinical Oncology*. **16**(7): 2377–81. (CT-28)

15 Porzio G, Aielli F, Verna L, Porto C, *et al.* (2006) Gabapentin in the treatment of severe sweating experienced by advanced cancer patients. *Supportive Care in Cancer*. **14**(4): 389–91. (CS-9)

16 Peuckmann V, Fisch M, Bruera E. (2000) Potential novel uses of thalidomide: focus on palliative care. *Drugs*: **60**(2): 273–92. (R, 120 refs)

17 Deaner PB. (2000) The use of thalidomide in the management of severe sweating in patients with advanced malignancy: trial report. *Palliative Medicine*. **14**: 429–31. (OS-10).

18 Bueller HA, Bernhard JD. (1998) Review of pruritus therapy. *Dermatology Nursing*. **10**(2): 101–7. (R, 66 refs)

19 Twycross R, Greaves MW, Handwerker H, Jones EA, *et al.* (2003) Itch: scratching more than the surface. *Quarterly Journal of Medicine*. **96**: 7–26. (R, 211 refs)

20 Figueiredo A, Ribeiro CA, Goncalo M, Almeida L, *et al.* (1990) Mechanism of action of doxepin in the treatment of chronic urticaria. *Fundamental and Clinical Pharmacology*. **4**: 147–58. (OS-15)

21 Preskorn SH. (2000) Imipramine, mirtazapine, and nefazodone: multiple targets. *Journal of Practical Psychiatry and Behavioral Health*. March: 97–102.

22 Fruhstorfer H, Hermanns M, Latzke L. (1986) The effects of thermal stimulation on clinical and experimental itch. *Pain*. **24**: 259–69. (OS-18)

23 Ada S, Seckin D, Budakoglu I, Ozdemir FN. (2005) Treatment of uremic pruritus with narrowband ultraviolet B phototherapy: an open pilot study. *Journal of the American Academy of Dermatology*. **53**(1): 149–51. (OS-20)

24 Hanid MA, Levi AJ. (1980) Phototherapy for pruritus in primary biliary cirrhosis. *Lancet*. **2**: 530. (Let)

25 Che-Yi C, Wen CY, Min-Tsung K, Chiu-Ching H. (2005) Acupuncture in haemodialysis patients at the Quchi (LI11) acupoint for refractory uraemic pruritus. *Nephrology Dialysis Transplantation*. **20**(9): 1912–5. (RCT-40)

26 Muller C, Pongratz S, Pidlich J, Penner E, *et al.* (1998) Treatment of pruritus in chronic liver disease with the 5-hydroxytryptamine receptor type 3 antagonist ondansetron: a randomized, placebo-controlled, double-blind cross-over trial. *European Journal of Gastroenterology and Hepatology*. **10**(10): 865–70. (RCT)

27 Jones EA, Molenaar HA, Oosting J. (2007) Ondansetron and pruritus in chronic liver disease: a controlled study. *Hepato-Gastroenterology*. **54**(76): 1196–9. (RCT-17)

28 O'Donohue JW, Pereira SP, Ashdown AC, Haigh CG, Wilkinson JR, Williams R. (2005) A controlled trial of ondansetron in the pruritus of cholestasis. *Alimentary Pharmacology and Therapeutics*. **21**(8): 1041–5. (RCT-19)

29 Vila T, Gommer J, Scates AC. (2008) Role of gabapentin in the treatment of uremic pruritus. *Annals of Pharmacotherapy*. **42**(7): 1080–4. (SA)

30 Bergasa NV, McGee M, Ginsburg IH, Engler D. (2006) Gabapentin in patients with the pruritus of cholestasis: a double-blind, randomized, placebo-controlled trial. *Hepatology*. **44**(5): 1317–23. (RCT-16)
31 Lorenz B, Kaufman RH, Kutzner SK. (1998) Lichen sclerosus: therapy with clobetasol propionate. *Journal of Reproductive Medicine*. **43**(9): 790–4. (RS-81)
32 Weisshaar E, Heyer G, Forster C, Handwerker HO. (1998) Effect of topical capsaicin on the cutaneous reactions and itching to histamine in atopic eczema compared to healthy skin. *Archives of Dermatological Research*. **290**(6): 306–11. (RCT)
33 Richelson E. (1979) Tricyclic antidepressants and histamine H1 receptors. *Mayo Clinic Proceedings*. **54**: 669–74. (R)
34 Goode HF, Burns E, Walker BE. (1992) Vitamin C depletion and pressure sores in elderly patients with femoral neck fracture. *British Medical Journal*. **305**: 925–7. (OS-21)
35 Dickerson JWT. (1993) Ascorbic acid, zinc and wound healing. *Journal of Wound Care*. **2**: 350–3.
36 Bernhard JD. (1994) General principles, overview, and miscellaneous treatments of itching. In: Bernhard JD, ed., *Itch: mechanisms and management of pruritus*. New York: McGraw-Hill, Inc. pp. 367–81. (Ch)
37 Grocott P. (1999) The management of fungating wounds. *Journal of Wound Care*. **8**(5): 232–4. (R, 24 refs)
38 Obořilová A, Jiří M, Pospíšil Z, Kořístek Z. (2002) Symptomatic intravenous antipyretic therapy: efficacy of metamizol, diclofenac and propacetamol. *Journal of Pain and Symptom Management*. **24**(6): 608–15. (OS-254).
39 Wymenga AN, Sleijfer DT. (2002) Management of hot flushes in breast cancer patients. *Acta Oncologica*. **41**(3): 269–75. (R, 56 refs)
40 Cervenakov I, Kopecny M, Jancar M, Chovan D, Mal'a M. (2000) "Hot flush," an unpleasant symptom accompanying antiandrogen therapy of prostatic cancer and its treatment by cyproterone acetate. *International Urology and Nephrology*. **32**(1): 77–9. (OS-31)
41 Polat M, Oztas P, Ilhan MN, Yalcin B, Alli N. (2008) Generalized pruritus: a prospective study concerning etiology. *American Journal of Clinical Dermatology*. **9**(1): 39–44. (CT-55)
42 Bale S, Regnard C. (1995) Pressure sores. In: *Flow Diagrams in Advanced Cancer and Other Diseases*. London: Edward Arnold. pp. 54–6. (Ch)
43 Mayo MJ, Handem I, Saldana S, Jacobe H, Getachew Y, Rush AJ. (2007) Sertraline as a first-line treatment for cholestatic pruritus. *Hepatology*. **45**(3): 666–74. (OS-21, RCT-12)
44 Browning J, Combes B, Mayo MJ. (2003) Long-term efficacy of sertraline as a treatment for cholestatic pruritus in patients with primary biliary cirrhosis. *American Journal of Gastroenterology*. **98**(12): 2736–41. (RCT-40)
45 Zylicz Z, Krajnik M, Sorge AA, Costantini M. (2003) Paroxetine in the treatment of severe non-dermatological pruritus: a randomized, controlled trial. *Journal of Pain and Symptom Management*. **26**(6): 1105–12. (RCT-26)
46 Davis MP, Frandsen JL, Walsh D, Andresen S, Taylor S. (2003) Mirtazapine for pruritus. *Journal of Pain and Symptom Management*. **25**(3): 288–91. (CS-4)
47 Tandon P, Rowe BH, Vandermeer B, Bain VG. (2007) The efficacy and safety of bile acid binding agents, opioid antagonists, or rifampin in the treatment of cholestasis-associated pruritus. *American Journal of Gastroenterology*. **102**(7): 1528–36. (R, 72 refs)
48 El-Karaksy H, Mansour S, El-Sayed R, El-Raziky M, El-Koofy N, Taha G. (2007) Safety and efficacy of rifampicin in children with cholestatic pruritus. *Indian Journal of Pediatrics*. **74**(3): 279–81. (OS-23)
49 Khurana S, Singh P. (2006) Rifampin is safe for treatment of pruritus due to chronic cholestasis: a meta-analysis of prospective randomized-controlled trials. *Liver International*. **26**(8): 943–8. (SA)
50 Peer G, Kivity S, Agami O, Fireman E, *et al.* (1996) Randomised crossover trial of naltrexone in uraemic patients. *Lancet*. **348**: 1552–4. (RCT-15)
51 Legroux-Crespel E, Cledes J, Misery L. (2004) A comparative study on the effects of naltrexone and loratadine on uremic pruritus. *Dermatology*. **208**(4): 326–30. (RCT-52)
52 Daly BM, Shuster S. (2000) Antipruritic action of thalidomide. *Acta Dermato-Veneroligica*. **80**(1): 24–5. (OS-11)
53 Silva SR, Viana PC, Lugon NV, Hoette M, Ruzany F, Lugon JR. (1994) Thalidomide for the treatment of uremic pruritus: a crossover randomized double-blind trial. *Nephron*. **67**(3): 270–3. (RCT-29)
54 Lowthian P. (1994) Pressure sores: a search for definition. *Nursing Standard*. **9**: 30–2.
55 Turner TD. (1985) Semiocclusive and occlusive dressings. In: Ryan T, ed. An environment for healing: the role of occlusion. *Royal Society of Medicine Congress and Symposium Series*. **88**: 5–14. (Ch)
56 Bale S. (1987) Dressing leg ulcers. *Journal of District Nursing*. **5**: 9–13.
57 Anonymous. (2002) Wound management products and elastic hosiery. In: *British National Formulary No 45 (March 2003)*. London: British Medical Association and the Royal Pharmaceutical Society of Great Britain.
58 Heyneman A, Beele H, Vanderwee K, Defloor T. (2008) A systematic review of the use of hydrocolloids in the treatment of pressure ulcers. *Journal of Clinical Nursing*. **17**(9): 1164–73. (SA-29, 65 refs)
59 Tumino G, Masuelli L, Bei R, Simonelli L, Santoro A, Francipane S. (2008) Topical treatment of chronic venous ulcers with sucralfate: a placebo controlled randomized study. *International Journal of Molecular Medicine*. **22**(1): 17–23. (RCT-50)
60 Miller M. (1994) The ideal healing environment. *Nursing Times*. **90**: 62–8. (Ch)
61 Moore Z, Cowman S. (2008) A systematic review of wound cleansing for pressure ulcers. *Journal of Clinical Nursing*. **17**(15): 1963–72. (SA)
62 Ubbink DT, Westerbos SJ, Nelson EA, Vermeulen

H. (2008) A systematic review of topical negative pressure therapy for acute and chronic wounds. *British Journal of Surgery*. **95**(6): 685–92. (SA-13, 12 refs)

63 Vikatmaa P, Juutilainen V, Kuukasjarvi P, Malmivaara A. (2008) Negative pressure wound therapy: a systematic review on effectiveness and safety. *European Journal of Vascular and Endovascular Surgery*. **36**(4): 438–48. (R, 34 refs, SA-14)

64 Vanderwee K, Grypdonck M, Defloor T. (2008) Alternating pressure air mattresses as prevention for pressure ulcers: a literature review. *International Journal of Nursing Studies*. **45**(5): 784–801. (SA-15, 62 refs)

65 Gotschall CS, Morrison MI, Eichelberger MR. (1998) Prospective randomized study of the efficacy of Mepitel on partial thickness scalds in children. *Journal of Burn Care Rehabilitation*. **19**: 279–283. (RCT)

66 Taylor R. (1999) Use of a silicone net dressing in severe mycosis fungoides. *Journal of Wound Care*. **8**(9): 429–30. (CS-1)

67 Glide S. (1997) Cleaning choices. *Nursing Times*. **88**: 74–8.

68 Gilchrist B on behalf of the European Tissue Repair Society. (1997) Should iodine be recognised in wound management? *Journal of Wound Care*. **6**: 148–50.

69 Bale S. (1997) A guide to wound debridement. *Journal of Wound Care*. **6**: 179–82. (R)

70 Gunes UY. (2008) A descriptive study of pressure ulcer pain. *Ostomy Wound Management*. **54**(2): 56–61. (OS-47)

71 Girouard K, Harrison MB, VanDenKerkof E. (2008) The symptom of pain with pressure ulcers: a review of the literature. *Ostomy Wound Management*. **54**(5): 30–42. (R, 52 refs)

72 Zeppetella G, Paul J, Ribeiro MD. (2003) Analgesic efficacy of morphine applied topically to painful ulcers. *Journal of Pain and Symptom Management*. **25**(6): 555–8. (RCT-5)

73 Cerchietti LC, Navigante AH, Bonomi MR, Zaderajko MA, *et al.* (2002) Effect of topical morphine for mucositis-associated pain following concomitant chemoradiotherapy for head and neck carcinoma. *Cancer*. **95**(10): 2230–6. (RCT-26)

74 Twillman RK, Long TD, Cathers TA, Mueller DW. (1999) Treatment of painful skin ulcers with topical opioids. *Journal of Pain and Symptom Management*. **17**(4): 288–92. (CS-9)

75 Krajnik M, Zylicz Z, Finlay I, Luczak J, van Sorge AA. (1999) Potential uses of topical opioids in palliative care: report of 6 cases. *Pain*. **80**(1–2): 121–5. (CS-6)

76 Welling A. (2007) A randomised controlled trial to test the analgesic efficacy of topical morphine on minor superficial and partial thickness burns in accident and emergency departments. *Emergency Medicine Journal*. **24**(6): 408–12. (RCT-59)

77 Skiveren J, Haedersdal M, Philipsen PA, Wiegell SR, Wulf HC. (2006) Morphine gel 0.3% does not relieve pain during topical photodynamic therapy: a randomized, double-blind, placebo-controlled study. *Acta Dermato-Venereologica*. **86**(5): 409–11. (RCT-26)

78 Paice JA, Von Roenn JH, Hudgins JC, Luong L, *et al.* (2008) Morphine bioavailability from a topical gel formulation in volunteers. *Journal of Pain and Symptom Management*. **35**(3): 314–20. (RCT-5)

Terminal phase and bereavement

CLINICAL DECISION AND ACTION CHECKLIST

1 Is communication difficult?
2 Are religious and spiritual needs uncertain?
3 Do the medications and interventions need reviewing?
4 Is there uncertainty that the plan of care has been discussed?
5 Are symptoms present or anticipated?
6 Is there doubt that the patient is dying?
7 Is there any uncertainty about caring for the body after death?
8 Is there uncertainty about giving further information?

KEY POINTS

- The last hours and days are a time of adjustments for the patient and carers.
- Most patients die peacefully without distress.
- If distress does occur, sedation is not first-line treatment.

INTRODUCTION

This advice refers to patients who are dying. Some patients show a steady, inexorable deterioration so that a day-by-day or hour-by-hour deterioration is likely to indicate the terminal phase. In other patients, several life-threatening episodes may precede the terminal phase, making it more difficult to predict the terminal phase.[1] However, patients in the terminal phase have several common features:

- deterioration day-by-day or faster because of their underlying condition
- brief or absent response to repeated treatments
- presence of an irreversible complication of their disease
- a realization that they are dying
- reduced cognition, drowsiness, or a comatose state
- bed bound (low or very low performance status)
- limited food or fluid intake and difficulty with oral medication
- altered breathing pattern
- peripherally cyanosed and cold – may cause skin to have a mottled appearance.

The signs and symptoms of a dying patient

Any of these features on their own can occur in a patient who is not dying, but taken together they can help a team to be as certain as it can be that a patient has reached the terminal phase. Exacerbations of pain or breathlessness are unusual in patients whose symptoms have been well controlled until this point.[2] This final phase starts a median of 23 hours before death, varying from a few hours to several days.[3] Many patients are awake and rational until this terminal phase.

A TIME OF ADJUSTMENTS

The terminal phase is a crucial time of adjustments for all:

- **Stopping unnecessary drugs:** it is often possible to simplify drug regimes as a patient deteriorates.
- **Continuing with other drugs by an appropriate route:** the subcutaneous and buccal routes are useful and kind alternatives.
- **Ensure "as required" (PRN) medication is available or prescribed:** an antiemetic, analgesic, antisecretory and sedative, e.g. metoclopramide, hydromorphone or morphine, hyoscine/scopolamine or glycopyrrolate, and midazolam should be available in the patient's home or ward.
- **Controlling physical symptoms:** adjustments (psychological or social) are impossible if there is troublesome pain, nausea, or breathlessness.
- **Giving explanations:** lack of information is a common cause of problems. Like drugs, information must be titrated to the individual. *See Breaking difficult news*, p. 23 and *Helping the person with the effects of difficult news*, p. 27.
- **Anticipating changes:** although it is not possible to anticipate every crisis, planning ahead is essential. For example, many patients suffer from bronchial secretions at the end of life and having drugs such as hyoscine/ scopolamine or glycopyrrolate available is sensible.
- **Giving and accepting adequate support:** duty demands we provide support, but clinical governance insists we also seek and accept help, advice, and support when we are unsure of the situation.
- **Setting realistic goals:** goals change as a patient deteriorates but can still foster hope even if that is now about comfort. Resuscitation issues will need to be considered – *see Issues around cardiopulmonary resuscitation*, p. 273.
- **Ensuring that religious and spiritual care is offered if wanted:** ask the patient, partner or family if they would like to talk to a chaplain or other professional.
- **Explaining changes to the partner, family, and carers:** they also need as much (or as little) information as they need (if the patient agrees).
- **Helping the patient, partner, relatives and carers understand the changes:** although changes are frightening, it can be comforting for some patients, partners, or relatives to have the natural and gentle course of a death explained.
- **Informing other team members:** the family physician, hospital physician, community nurse, and clinical nurse specialist will need to know what is happening.
- **Ensuring the environment is appropriate:** comfortable and as quiet (or noisy) as they want.
- **Anticipating the death:** for some patients, partners, families, and carers this can be a valuable time to consider issues such as funeral arrangements and organ donation. Making such decisions in advance can make the time of death, and later, less distressing. A common question is, "How long?", but even in the last hours exact predictions are impossible. However, partners, relatives, and friends can usually see the rate of deterioration and realize that hour-by-hour deterioration means only hours are left. Often all they want is for this rate of deterioration to be confirmed.

Reviewing drugs in the last hours and days

Drug	Suggested action	Alternative action
Analgesics		
acetaminophen	stop	acetaminophen 500 mg PR
weak opioids	hydromorphone SC 0.5–1.0 mg q1h PRN	hydromorphone SC infusion
strong opioids	give SC at equivalent doses	transdermal fentanyl (will need at least 12 hours to effect, and a strong opioid for breakthrough)
ketamine	continue by SC infusion or intermittent SC	–
NSAIDs	stop	diclofenac 100 mg PR once daily or ketorolac 30 mg SC
Antiemetics		
dimenhydrinate or diphenhydramine	continue by SC injection or infusion	dimenhydrinate or diphenhydramine PR q8h
haloperidol	continue by SC injection once at night	methotrimeprazine SC once at night (Canada only)
hyoscine/scopolamine	continue by SC injection or infusion	transdermal hyoscine hydrobromide/ scopolamine
methotrimeprazine (Canada only)	continue by SC injection once at night	chlorpromazine PR once at night
metoclopramide	continue by SC injection or infusion	domperidone PR q8h (from compounding pharmacy in US)
Antiepileptics		
— for neuropathic pain — for seizures	carbamazepine PR once daily carbamazepine PR once daily or clonazepam 1 mg SC twice daily	SC ketamine midazolam or phenobarbital SC bolus or infusion for prevention; buccal, IM or IV midazolam to treat seizure
Antimicrobial agents		
chest infections	hyoscine/scopolamine or glycopyrrolate SC for excess upper bronchial secretions	ceftriaxone SC as needed (*see* cd-5, p. 195)
fungal infections	stop systemic antifungal	topical miconazole
gram-negative infections	stop	metronidazole 400 mg PR q8h
Cardiovascular		
antiarrhythmics	stop	–
antihypertensives	stop	–
ACE inhibitor	stop	furosemide SC as needed
furosemide	stop	furosemide SC as needed
Corticosteroids		
e.g. dexamethasone	If used as co-analgesic give as single SC od injection, otherwise stop	

Drug	Suggested action	Alternative action
Endocrine and metabolic drugs		
bisphosphonates	stop	–
hypoglycemics	stop	–
octreotide	stop	octreotide SC injection or infusion
Gastrointestinal drugs		
antacids	stop	–
laxatives	stop	bisacodyl suppository
PPI, H_2 antagonists	stop	ranitidine SC infusion
Hematological drugs		
erythropoietin	stop	–
iron, B_{12}	stop	–
Psychotropic drugs		
antidepressants — for depression — for neuropathic pain	stop (but beware of agitation on stopping SSRI and SNRI drugs) carbamazepine PR once daily	
benzodiazepines	midazolam as SC infusion	diazepam PR once at night
haloperidol	continue by SC injection once at night	methotrimeprazine SC hs (Canada only)
methotrimeprazine	continue by SC injection once at night	chlorpromazine PR once at night
Miscellaneous		
baclofen	diazepam PR once at night	midazolam SC infusion
dantrolene	diazepam PR once at night	midazolam SC infusion
bronchodilators	stop	nebulized salbutamol as needed
enteral nutrition	stop	only SC fluids (review need daily)
wound management	minimize dressing changes	–

MANAGING SYMPTOMS

These are discussed in detail elsewhere in this book. A key issue is that when helping a distressed patient **sedation is *not* first-line treatment**. Other approaches are tried first, and even if drugs with sedative actions are used, low doses are chosen and then titrated to the individual. Opioids are never used to "settle" a patient.

Noisy or moist breathing: positional change may be enough to reduce the airway secretions, otherwise hyoscine/ scopolamine, hyoscyamine, or glycopyrrolate help at least half of such patients.

Urinary incontinence: this will probably subside as the patient's renal function reduces. Consider the use of pads or catheter (indwelling or intermittent), or use sheaths for male patients.

Clinical decision	If YES carry out the action below
Patient is deteriorating day by day: the clinical team is as certain as it can be that this is because of their underlying condition, or because of an irreversible complication of their disease. **The following is based on the Liverpool Care Pathway for the Dying Patient (LCP) v12.**[4–8]	
1 Is communication difficult?	**LCP Goal 1: The patient, partner, relatives, and carers are able to take a full and active part in communication and are aware of the current situation.** **LCP Goal 2: The relatives and carer have had a full explanation of the facilities and services available to them.** • For patients who are unconscious or have severe communication problems *see Identifying distress in the person with a severe communication difficulty*, p. 31. If a patient is conscious but an impairment of mind or brain is suspected, check their capacity for treatment decisions (*see Decisions around capacity*, pp. 267–71). • Check language, hearing, vision, speech. • Explore what the patient knows and check if they want to know more. If the patient agrees, do the same with the family (*see Breaking difficult news*, p. 23). NB. The patient, partner, and relatives may be aware, but may not feel able to discuss this openly (*see Helping the person with the effects of difficult news*, p. 27). • Ensure the health care team has up-to-date contact information.
2 Are religious and spiritual needs uncertain?	**LCP Goal 3: The patient, partner, and relatives are given the opportunity to discuss their wishes, feelings, faith, beliefs, and values.** • Assess the religious and spiritual needs with the patient, partner, and relatives. Ask if the patient, partner, or relatives wish to see a spiritual advisor, priest, cleric, or chaplain.
3 Do the medications and interventions need reviewing?	**LCP Goal 4: The patient has medication prescribed on *PRN* basis for any pain, agitation, respiratory tract secretions, nausea/vomiting, or dyspnea that may develop in the last hours or days of life, and has equipment available for CSCI if needed.** • *See* cd-6 on p. 217. • *See* table on pp. 213–14 for review of medication. Stop all non-essential medication. If unable to swallow, convert to SC route either as once daily drugs or as continuous SC infusion. **LCP Goal 5: The patient is only receiving interventions that the multi-professional team agree is in the patient's best interests and has a Do Not (Attempt) Resuscitation (DN(A)R) order in place.** • *See Issues around cardiopulmonary resuscitation*, p. 273. Ensure that an implanted defibrillator has been switched off. **LCP Goals 6 and 7: The need for clinically assisted (artificial) nutrition and hydration has been reviewed and discussed.** • *See Nutrition and hydration problems*, p. 175. **LCP Goal 8: The patient's skin integrity has been reviewed.** • *See Skin problems*, p. 203.

Based on the 2010 Liverpool Care Pathway for the Dying Patient[8]
cd = clinical decision

Pain: consider causes such as urinary retention, constipation, uncomfortable position, infection, and pressure sore pain in addition to known disease-related pain.

Restlessness/agitation/confusion: exclude pain or a full bowel or bladder. If other measures are inappropriate, consider a benzodiazepine.

Breathlessness: consider changing the patient's position, increasing air movement (fan, open windows), oxygen, relaxation, and explanation. Consider an opioid,[9,10] with or without a benzodiazepine to reduce any fear and the feeling of breathlessness.

Nausea/vomiting: continue antiemetics by the most appropriate route.

Sweating: keep the patient cool, regularly change the bed linen, and use cotton nightwear. Involve the family in sponging the patient if they wish.

Jerking/twitching/plucking: this can be myoclonic jerks due to excessive opioid, in which case reduce the dose or change opioid. Other causes are uremia or an altered neurological state. Low-dose midazolam may help.

WHEN SEDATION IS NEEDED

There are occasions when sedation may be needed at the end of life for intractable symptoms causing intolerable suffering. Sedation can be brief (e.g. for a procedure or short period of distress), intermittent (e.g. overnight only) or continuous. The aim is to titrate doses to each individual, and use the lowest doses that will reduce the distress. When used in this way there is no evidence that sedation shortens life or hastens death.[11,12] Sedation is distinct from euthanasia even in countries where euthanasia is legal.[13]

Opioids are not used for sedation because the sedative effects wear off rapidly, and there is a risk of accumulation of neuroexcitatory metabolites which would cause distress. A benzodiazepine is usually used, and because of the ability to individually titrate doses to each individual, midazolam is frequently the first-line choice.[14]

ORGAN DONATION

Organs for donation are universally in short supply. There are patients, partners, and relatives willing to consider donation, feeling that this is at least one positive outcome of the tragedy that has befallen them. Organs that can be donated depend on the circumstances, but advice should always be sought from the local transplant coordinator:

Non-heart-beating donation

Corneas

- up to 24 hours after death (ideally within 8 hours)
- any age above 1 year
- contraindications: hepatitis B or C, HIV, CMV, syphilis, Alzheimer's, MS, RA, leukemia, lymphoma, local tumor (NB. Other cancers are not a contraindication), long-term steroids, recent chemotherapy.

Bone

- up to 48 hours after death in those aged 16–70 years
- contraindications: hepatitis B or C, HIV, CMV, syphilis, Alzheimer's, MS, RA, any malignancy, recent chemotherapy.

Skin

- up to 48 hours after death in those aged 16–70 years
- contraindications: hepatitis B or C, HIV, CMV, syphilis, Alzheimer's, MS, RA, any malignancy, chronic skin disease, long-term steroids, recent chemotherapy.

Heart-beating donation (usually ITU/ICU patients)

- heart, liver, kidneys, lungs, small bowel, pancreas, bone, tissue, skin, tendons
- each organ and tissue has different limits and the transplant coordinator will advise.

Organ donation

Clinical decision	If YES carry out the action below
4 Is there uncertainty that the plan of care has been discussed?	**LCP Goal 9: The patient, partner, relatives, and family physician have had the plan explained.** If available, an explanatory leaflet is given to the relative or carer. The primary health care or hospital team should be made aware that the patient is dying. Explain the plan with the patient (if their conscious level allows) and with the partner and relative. Make sure the patient (if their conscious level allows), partner, relatives, and others express an understanding of the plan of care. Consider the option of organ donation: (corneas after death, or solid organs if patient is in ITU/ICU – *see* opposite).
5 Are symptoms present or anticipated?	• **Pain** (*see also Diagnosing and treating pain*, p. 43): *If not on a strong opioid:* If the patient is in pain: give usual breakthrough dose of oral analgesic or if unable to swallow give 2.5 mg morphine or 0.5 mg hydromorphone SC. If the pain is controlled: prescribe morphine 2.5 mg or hydromorphone 0.5 mg SC q4h as required. *If already on a strong opioid:* If the patient is in pain: give one-tenth of the 24 hr dose. If the pain is controlled: continue oral strong opioid if able to swallow, otherwise convert to hydromorphone SC infusion (conversion: 24 hr dose oral morphine ÷ 10 = 24 hr dose of hydromorphone SC infusion). Prescribe PRN dose of hydromorphone as one-tenth of 24 hr dose of SC infusion to be given q1h as required. *If any renal impairment is present:* consider using an alternative strong opioid such as a fentanyl infusion. *If on a different opioid:* contact the palliative care team for advice. • **Nausea and vomiting** (*see also Nausea and vomiting*, p. 167): *If present:* give metoclopramide 10 mg SC q6h. *If absent:* prescribe metoclopramide 10 mg SC q6h PRN. • **Respiratory tract secretions** (also *see* cd-4 in *Respiratory problems*, p. 193): *If present:* give hyoscine hydrobromide (scopolamine) 400 microg SC. *If absent:* prescribe hyoscine hydrobromide (scopolamine) 400 microg SC q4h PRN. • **Terminal restlessness and agitation** (*see* cd-4 in *Emergencies*, p. 333): *If present:* give midazolam 2.5–5 mg SC q1h. *If absent:* prescribe midazolam 2.5 mg SC q1h PRN. *If persistent:* add haloperidol 1–2.5 mg SC (*see* cd-6 in *Confusional states*, p. 247). • **Check:** the patient is free from other symptoms (dyspnea, itch, edema, skin damage, oral problems, bladder, or bowel problems). See the relevant sections for management. • **Ensure:** personal hygiene needs are met, the physical environment is adjusted to their needs, and the psychological well-being of the patient and carers (and the physical well-being of the carers) is maintained. • **After 24 hours:** review the medication and if two or more PRN doses have been needed, either consider a SC infusion with a syringe driver for 24 hours, or increase the dose of an existing infusion. *If problems are still present after 24 hours:* contact the palliative care team for advice.

Based on the 2010 Liverpool Care Pathway for the Dying Patient[8]
cd = clinical decision

THE DEATH

How it seems for the patient: what is observed for most patients with advanced illness is a gentle "winding down" of the body's systems. Even in cardiac and respiratory failure, sudden, dramatic deaths are uncommon. At the end it is more a gentle absence of life than a sudden presence of death. Peaceful silence is the most obvious feature.

How it seems for the partner and relatives:[15] some find it easy to cry, others feel as though they have dried up. Some feel the urge to speak, often to express relief. Others feel it is an anticlimax because, in a sense, the patient left hours or days before. Many are so numbed with grief that they feel helpless and useless, but they may not admit to this. Others cannot remember names, addresses, and telephone numbers. This needs to be understood when it comes to giving information about what to do now, and this information may have to be given to another member of the family.

Occasionally, a relative or partner has been unable to adjust to the deterioration of the patient and reacts with shock or anger to what is obvious to everyone else. It is rare for such people to be truly ignorant of the facts; it is just that they have not been able to face the terrible reality. Experienced help and support from a palliative care specialist (doctor, nurse, chaplain, or social worker) may be needed.

How it is for the professional carer: it often feels awkward. There is an overwhelming feeling to do something such as checking the pulse or breathing, moving a pillow, making tea. There are no rules, but there are some principles:

- Take your cue from the family or partner – enable them to do it their way.
- Silence is awkward, but it is right in the right place (there's nothing you can say that will make it better).
- If those present want to talk then talk; if they're silent then let them be silent.
- Someone (usually a qualified health care professional) *will* need to confirm that the patient has died. Don't pronounce death until at least several minutes have elapsed from the last breath. Some patients take an occasional breath for several minutes.
- After the death, ask those present if they want to stay, and if so, whether they want to be alone.
- If there are children in the family, offer the parent help in offering the children the opportunity to see the patient after death if they wish, and to answer their questions appropriately.

THE ARRANGEMENTS AFTER DEATH

The carer now has a number of responsibilities:

- helping the family contact friends and relatives
- asking them whether it is to be a burial or a cremation
- helping them choose an undertaker if the decision has not already been made
- if a post mortem (autopsy) is needed, obtaining consent and explaining the arrangements
- explaining how to register a death
- explaining what is on the death certificate.

The death certificate: the death certificate should be filled out by the doctor who saw the patient within the last few days. The cause of death is, for example, "Carcinoma of stomach," not the mode of death such as "respiratory arrest" or "coma." Because the next of kin do not receive a copy of the death certificate, or any notification of the

Clinical decision	If YES carry out the action below
6 Is there doubt that the patient is dying?	*Undertake a full multi-professional team assessment if:* — the patient has clinically improved — it is more than 3 days since the last assessment — the need for clinically assisted nutrition or hydration have not been reviewed.
7 Is there any uncertainty about caring for the body after death?	**LCP Goal 10: The patient is treated with respect and dignity and the last offices undertaken** Ensure that local policy is followed and that religious and cultural needs are addressed. Ensure there are arrangements for removal of pacemaker or defibrillator.
8 Is there any uncertainty about giving further information?	**LCP Goal 11: The relative and carer can express an understanding of what they will need to do next** Discuss the next steps. Provide information such as what to do after the death, explanation about the cause of death, collection of belongings, etc. Give information about bereavement such as a leaflet of contact numbers for adult or child bereavement services. **LCP Goal 12: The primary health care or hospital team is notified of the patient's death, and the patient's death is communicated to any other appropriate services.**

Based on the 2010 Liverpool Care Pathway for the Dying Patient[8]
cd = clinical decision

cause of death, they may wish to question the attending physician about the cause of death. Such questions should be answered honestly but considerately.

Post mortems: in many provinces in Canada and most states in the US, when death is due to industrial disease (e.g. asbestosis), injury, neglect, suspicious circumstances, or within the normal recovery time of an operation referral to the Medical Examiner (ME) is mandated. The ME may demand a post mortem, so the relative's permission is not needed, but they should be informed. For all other deaths a post mortem can be a valuable way of finding out why a disease behaved the way it did. In this case, a relative's permission is essential and usually it is not difficult to ask if this is done sensitively (e.g. "It would help us to examine Michael to find out why he had so much pain"), and it is made clear that the relative or partner can refuse. For some families, it can be helpful to discuss this ahead of the death. The funeral may be delayed by a day or two by a post mortem.

BEREAVEMENT

(adapted from CLiP)[16–18]

Grief is a common reaction to loss and can be understood more effectively when it is viewed within the emotional, cultural, social, and psychological aspects of a person's life. Bereavement is one of life's most challenging periods.

The effect on the partner, relatives, and friends

People experience grief differently:

Shock at the news is inevitable.

Anxiety about this new situation can result in fear with feelings of vulnerability and loss of security. Separation anxieties are common, and children need reassurance that diseases such as cancer and death are not "catching."

Relief and guilt. The feeling of relief seems odd at first, but relief can result from the ending of any suffering and the release from the burden of caring. Although this relief is understandable, people often feel guilty that they feel such relief. Any family member may feel guilt. Children often blame themselves and need reassurance that illness and death are not their fault.

Sadness is a normal feeling in the grieving process and is part of learning to adapt to life without the person who has died. Sometimes the sadness can be intensely overwhelming and feel more painful and profound than previous emotional encounters.

Loneliness. Grief can be a very isolating experience even if the loss is shared among family members. This isolation is increased when people avoid talking about their thoughts and feelings. Consequently, the isolation can be reduced by offering opportunities to talk about the illness and death, and to reminisce about the person who died.

Hyperactivity can occur as a means of avoiding the pain of the loss. This may be by "keeping busy," but irritability and exhaustion can develop.

Controlled v. overwhelmed: The emotions caused by the reality of their loss can overwhelm people. A common reaction is to regain control by focusing on thinking and action, e.g. "keeping busy." The extent of the oscillation between these two states defines the severity of the effect of bereavement. In the early stages these oscillations are rapid and intense. Some may even hear, smell, or see the person who has died – while some find this comforting, others find this experience disturbing. However, the oscillations gradually reduce over time as the loss and grief begin to resolve.

The effect on staff

Staff may be so involved in responding to the grief reactions of the remaining clients or patients that their own feelings go unrecognized. Sheer workload in some teams prevents staff exploring what they feel about the death of a patient. And, yet, staff need "permission to cry." Some health teams understand this and allow staff to show their feelings, but other teams cannot cope with such emotion, viewing it as "unprofessional," "letting the team down," or even seeing it as a weakness. This may lead to feelings being hidden and possible problems not being addressed. Staff most commonly take their unresolved feelings home. Although they may share the reasons with their partners or relatives, it is more common for them to "dump the feelings" on the unsuspecting partner or relative without being able to explain the reason. It will be harder if the staff member has recently had their own bereavement.

Reassurance: Care staff usually perceive themselves as being able to make things better so they may feel that they have failed in this situation. Guilt may be the result. This in-built desire to "fix things" can prevent staff from realizing that, in reality, they made a difference by being with the patient, partner, and relatives, and that this was therapeutic and helpful.

Assessing risk

The extent of the grief reaction will depend on many different past experiences, on personality, and on current issues.[19] Not surprisingly, it is not possible to talk about "normal" or "abnormal" grief. The one clear feature, however, is that most people find they begin to cope and function more effectively as time passes.

For many, this journey started at the time of diagnosis when they were first faced with the possibility of such profound losses. Some will have used that time (and been supported) to work through some of the issues they are having to face. The distressing "oscillations" of loss–restoration will have lessened and they will be better prepared for the death. Others will not have been able to use this time for the reasons below.

Factors which help resolution include close relationships, the perception of a good network of support, strong spiritual beliefs of any sort, a good relationship with the person who died, a feeling of "closure" about the life and death of the person (i.e. no "unfinished business"), a peaceful and expected death, being present at the death, and a healthy status of the bereaved.

Factors which can hinder resolution include poor relationships, little or no social support, a difficult or poor relationship with the person who died, unfinished business, difficulty in shedding tears, a sudden or unexpected death, a distressing death, being unable to fulfill a wish to be present at the death or funeral, illness in the bereaved, bad experiences of previous deaths, the presence of other sources of stress (e.g. recent divorce or death), lack of planning in financial or business affairs, and absent or inadequate care arrangements for children.

High-risk factors: in reality, *any* factor could indicate a high risk in certain circumstances, and indicate that bereavement may resolve slowly. Particular risk factors include persisting anger or guilt, extreme or obsessive crying after the first few months, previous psychiatric history or suicidal tendencies, and drug or alcohol dependence. Being absent at the time of the death is less of a risk if the bereaved person felt they had already said all that needed to be said. On the other hand, missing the opportunity to say goodbye or express their love could seriously hinder resolution of their bereavement.

Finding help

This can be difficult in some organizations and areas, but sources are:

- Caring staff – opportunities to discuss feelings/concerns with staff who have cared for the patient can be very helpful for the bereaved person.[20]
- The clergy – support for the family could be provided both in the short- and long-term.
- Medical staff – general support for the partner and relatives and discussion of unresolved issues. The family physician is often the first line of help and should be meeting the bereaved within a few weeks, and again after a few months.
- Specialist help – persistent or complicated grief will need specialist help from a bereavement service, counselor or psychiatrist.

REFERENCES: TERMINAL PHASE AND BEREAVEMENT

B = book; C = comment; Ch = chapter; CS-n = case study-no. of cases; CT-n = controlled trial-no. of cases; E = editorial; GC = group consensus; I = interviews; LS = laboratory study; MC = multi-center; OS-n = open study-no. of cases; PC = personal communication; R = review; RCT-n = randomized controlled trial-no. of cases; RS-n = retrospective survey-no. of cases; SA = systematic or meta analysis.

1 Gibbins J, McCourbrie R, Alexander N, Kinzel C, Forbesk K. (2009) Diagnosing dying in the acute hospital setting: are we too late? *Clinical Medicine*. **9**: 116–19. (RS-100)

2 Henriksen H, Riis J, Christophersen B, Moe C. (1997) Distress symptoms in hospice patients. *Ugeskrift for Laeger*. **159**(47): 6992–6. (OS-117)

3 Morita T, Ichiki T, Tsunoda J, Inoue S, Chihara S. (1998) A prospective study on the dying process in terminally ill cancer patients. *American Journal of Hospice and Palliative Care*. **15**(4): 217–22. (OS-100)

4 Ellershaw J, Gambles M, McGlinchey T. (2008) Benchmarking: a useful tool for informing and improving care of the dying? *Supportive Care in Cancer*. **16**(7): 813–9. (I-62)

5 Gambles M, Stirzaker S, Jack BA, Ellershaw JE.

(2006) The Liverpool Care Pathway in hospices: an exploratory study of doctor and nurse perceptions. *International Journal of Palliative Nursing*. **12**(9): 414–21. (I-11)

6 Matthews K, Gambles M, Ellershaw JE, Brook L, *et al*. (2006) Developing the Liverpool Care Pathway for the dying child. *Paediatric Nursing*. **18**(1): 18–21. (RS)

7 Ellershaw J, Ward C. (2003) Care of the dying patient: the last hours and days of life. *British Medical Journal*. **326**: 30–4. (R, 24 refs)

8 Liverpool Care Pathway v.12 (Jan 2010). Liverpool: Marie Curie Institute. Available on www.mcpcil.org.uk (accessed 10 January 2010).

9 Walsh TD. (1984) Opiates and respiratory function in advanced cancer. *Recent Results in Cancer Research*. **89**: 115–17.

10 Boyd KJ, Kelly M. (1997) Oral morphine as symptomatic treatment of dyspnoea in patients with advanced cancer. *Palliative Medicine*. **11**(4): 277–81. (OS-15)

11 George R, Regnard C. (2007) Lethal opioids or dangerous prescribers? *Palliative Medicine*. **21**: 77–80. (E)

12 Rietjens JA, van Zuylen L, van Veluw H, van der Wijk L, *et al*. (2008) Palliative sedation in a specialized unit for acute palliative care in a cancer hospital: comparing patients dying with and without palliative sedation. *Journal of Pain and Symptom Management*. **36**(3): 228–34. (RS-157)

13 Verkerk M, van Wijlick E, Legemaate J, de Graeff A. (2007) A national guideline for palliative sedation in the Netherlands. *Journal of Pain and Symptom Management*. **34**(6): 666–70. (R)

14 de Graeff A, Dean M. (2007) Palliative sedation therapy in the last weeks of life: a literature review and recommendations for standards. *Journal of Palliative Medicine*. **10**(1): 67–85. (GS, R-191 refs)

15 Doyle D. (1994) *Caring for a Dying Relative: a guide for families*. Oxford: Oxford University Press.

16 Regnard C, Kindlen M, Jackson J, Gibson L, Matthews D. Bereavement: the loss begins. CLiP (Current Learning in Palliative Care). Available at: www.helpthehospices.org.uk/clip (accessed 21 September 2009).

17 Regnard C, Kindlen M, Gibson L, Matthews D. Bereavement: the effect of death on staff. CLiP (Current Learning in Palliative Care). Available at: www.helpthehospices.org.uk/clip (accessed 10 January 2010).

18 Regnard C, Kindlen M, Jackson J, Nichol T, Gibson L, Matthews D. Assessing risk. CLiP (Current Learning in Palliative Care). Available at: www.helpthehospices.org.uk/clip (accessed 10 January 2010).

19 Relf M, Machin L, Archer N. (2008) Guidance for bereavement needs assessment in palliative care. London: Help the Hospices. See www.helpthehospices.org.uk/our-services/developing-practice/bereavement/assessing-bereavement-needs (accessed 10 January 2010).

20 Hebert RS, Schulz R, Copeland VC, Arnold RM. (2009) Preparing family caregivers for death and bereavement: insights from caregivers of terminally ill patients. *Journal of Pain and Symptom Management*. **37**(1): 3–12. (I-33)

Urinary problems and sexual difficulties

CLINICAL DECISION AND ACTION CHECKLIST

1. Has urinary output changed?
2. Is a UTI symptom present?
3. Has the urine changed color?
4. Is pain present?
5. Are sexual difficulties present?
6. Has urinary frequency changed?
7. Is urinary incontinence present?

KEY POINTS

- Urinary problems are common in advanced disease.
- The symptoms of a urinary tract infection may be non-specific in the elderly and neurologically impaired.
- Intermittent self-catheterization is an underused but effective technique for several urinary problems.
- Sexual problems are often not discussed or explored by professionals.

INTRODUCTION

A wide range of urinary problems can be caused by local cancer, or by any condition that impairs mobility or pelvic neurological function. Consequently, urinary problems are common in advanced disease and have a major impact on self-esteem and quality of life.[1]

Despite the many ways in which advanced disease can cause sexual dysfunction, it is uncommon for sexual problems to be discussed or explored.[2–6] In reality, many couples find it helpful that the subject has been openly discussed, whether or not it is a problem in their relationship.[7] They have often assumed it was an inevitable part of treatment or the illness and suffered in silence.[8]

URINARY OUTPUT CHANGE

Any significant change in urinary output should be investigated, since many causes are reversible. However, if it is occurring naturally at the end of life, no action is needed.

INFECTIONS

In adults, a crystal-clear straw-colored urine that is negative for nitrites and leukocyte esterase is likely to be free of infection.[9] There are four key symptoms of infection: dysuria, malodor, frequency, back pain, and sometimes hematuria.[10] Women with two of these symptoms have a 90% chance of a UTI being present.[10] In the elderly or in neurologically impaired patients, symptoms may be non-specific, e.g. delirium, myoclonic jerks, increased seizures. If bedside testing is negative, culture is unnecessary for most women,[11] but in children, a normal dipstick does not exclude infection and culture is needed.[12,13]

For women with a normal urinary tract a 3-day course of trimethoprim or trimethoprim/sulfamethoxazole (US) is sufficient.[14–17] Culture and 7-day courses are necessary for recurrent infection, in men, or if the genitourinary tract is abnormal. Patients with urethral catheters invariably have urine that contains bacteria or candida and treatment is only required in the presence of local or systemic symptoms.[18]

BLEEDING

It is unusual for blood loss to be severe, so oral iron supplements may be sufficient to prevent symptomatic anemia. Often it is the patient's anxiety that is uppermost and reassurance may be the most effective treatment. Infection should always be excluded. Palliative radiotherapy can reduce hematuria arising from a bleeding cancer in the urinary tract. Bladder irrigation with a 1% alum solution can reduce severe bleeding from the bladder.[19] Sucralfate can be used but since only a non-sterile suspension is available, this would have to be restricted to when no other options were appropriate.[20] Interventional treatments include selective embolization,[21,22] radiofrequency ablation,[23] and diathermy.[24] Aminocaproic acid (US only) or tranexamic acid may help but there are case reports of production of hard clots that can cause obstruction and are difficult to remove.[25,26]

PAIN

Trigone pain: the trigone is at the base of the bladder, surrounding the urethral opening. Irritation of this area can cause pain that radiates to the tip of the distal urethra. Catheter balloons are a common cause and reducing the balloon volume can help as well as avoiding tension on the catheter itself. Intermittent catheterization is an alternative (*see* p. 228).

Bladder pain due to tumor or persistent infection can be eased with local anesthetic instilled into the bladder. Lidocaine can be used on a once-daily basis when mixed with bicarbonate to reduce systemic absorption.[27,28] Bupivacaine may be simpler and more effective.[29] Intravesical opioid may also be effective.[30] Instillation of drugs into the bladder can be done using intermittent catheterization (*see* p. 228). Drug-induced cystitis can be caused by ketamine and some cytotoxics.[31,32]

Ureteric pain ("renal colic") can be severe. Strong opioids are as effective as NSAIDs.[33] Previous studies have shown opioids to have a higher incidence of vomiting than NSAIDs, but most used IV meperidine. There is conflicting

Clinical decision	If YES carry out the action below
1 Has urinary output changed?	• **Increased urine output:** consider these causes and treat if possible: cardiac failure with nocturia, chronic renal failure, diabetes mellitus, diabetes insipidus (pituitary or nephrogenic), diuretics, hypercalcemia. • **Decreased urine output:** *Dehydration:* may require correction (*see Nutrition and hydration problems*, p. 175). When it occurs naturally at the end of life no action is required. *Obstruction of both ureters:* start dexamethasone 8 mg in the morning. Consider referral to the urologists for insertion of a ureteric stent. *Obstruction of urethra:* distortion caused by fecal impaction (*see* cd-5 in *Constipation*, p. 109); blockage by tumor (a suprapubic catheter may be needed); or increased sphincter tone caused by antimuscarinic drugs (reduce dose or stop drugs). If due to benign prostatic hyperplasia, consider starting an alpha-blocking drug. *Obstruction of catheter:* wash out or replace. *Endocrine:* syndrome of inappropriate antidiuretic hormone (SIADH) causing fluid overload (*see* cd-7e in *Emergencies*, p. 343). *Neurological:* exclude cord compression (*see* cd-9a in *Emergencies*, p. 345).
2 Is a UTI symptom present? (dysuria, frequency, back pain, or hematuria)	• **Test the urine** for nitrites, leukocyte esterase and protein. • **If the urine test is positive for nitrites, or leukocytes:** *In women with a normal GU tract:* give trimethoprim 200 mg q12h (or trimethoprim/sulfamethoxazole (US)) for 3 days. *In all other patients:* culture the urine. Start trimethoprim 200 mg q12h (1–2 mg/kg q12h for children) (TMP/SMX 160/800 in US) for 3 days. Continue for further 3 days if symptoms persist and culture confirms sensitivity. *If the infection persists:* culture the urine and give a 7-day course of a cephalosporin or quinolone (continue for 2 weeks if pyelonephritis is present). • **If an enterovesical fistula is present** (mixed enterococci on culture): treat only if the symptoms are troublesome since eradication of infection is impossible. • **If the urine dipstick test is negative:** consider candida if local symptoms are present.
3 Has the urine changed color?	• **If the urine is positive for blood on testing:** Exclude and treat a urinary tract infection (*see* cd-2 above). *If the bleeding is severe:* exclude a clotting disorder. Insert an 18–24 Ch gauge catheter and irrigate with 0.9% saline to remove clots. Instill with 1% alum solution 50 mL for 30 minutes, continued if needed at a rate of 5 mL/hr for 24–72 hours. Alternatives are instillations of silver nitrate or formalin under anesthetic (contact urologists for advice). If no other option, use sucralfate suspension 25 mL with a 20 mL 0.9% saline flush. *If the source of bleeding is unclear:* refer to a urologist to consider a pyelogram or cystoscopy. *If a tumor is the source of bleeding:* start aminocaproic (US) or tranexamic acid 1–1.5 g PO q8–12h but there is a risk of producing hard clots that can cause obstruction. Refer to an oncologist to consider radiotherapy or to an interventional radiologist for embolization. • ***If this is not blood:*** Reassure the patient. Consider other causes of color change: orange-red (senna, bile, rifampicin, rhubarb), red-brown (Adriamycin, bile, beetroot, food dyes), green-black (mitoxantrone, bile); yellow (sulfasalazine).

Adapted from Regnard and Mannix[34]
cd = clinical decision

evidence whether NSAIDs have an opioid-sparing effect.[35] The titrated use of other opioids and the potential renal adverse effects of NSAIDs make them a second-line treatment.[36] The role for hyoscine butylbromide (Canada only; hyoscyamine, or scopolamine in the US) seems limited.[37,38] In less severe, recurrent ureteric pain, acupuncture and TENS have been used successfully.[39,40]

Persistent pain from the renal tract may require ketamine or spinal analgesia. If ketamine is used be aware that this can cause cystitis.[32,41]

SEXUAL DIFFICULTIES

Erectile dysfunction: some causes can be solved simply, such as stopping a drug that is causing erectile impotence. If erectile impotence persists, a trial of sildenafil is worthwhile as many patients with advanced disease do not have the inclination or time to wait for a full impotence assessment.

Hormonal deficiency: in women this can cause a loss of sexual interest. Painful intercourse because of dryness and vaginitis may be helped by lubrication or estrogen creams. In men hormone deficiency can cause erectile dysfunction and a loss of sexual interest.

Altered body image: this can impair a patient's perception of their sexuality. While open discussion will help, some patients will need cognitive behavioral therapy or skilled psychosexual counseling.

Urinary incontinence and discharge: incontinence has only a modest effect on sexual satisfaction,[42] but the distress of incontinence may result in reduced sexual interest. Vaginal discharge or bleeding due to tumor will often result in a cessation of intercourse.

Sex and the catheter: some patients with catheters and their partners are still able and willing to consider intercourse, but they are afraid of the catheter. Women can have intercourse with an indwelling catheter, but the catheter can reduce satisfaction.[43] Intermittent self-catheterization is a better alternative. Men who are able to achieve an erection can do so with a catheter present. Gentle intercourse is possible for men with a disconnected catheter (after draining the bladder), and placing a condom over the penis and catheter.[44] If the ejaculatory mechanism is undamaged this can still occur with a catheter, but may be painful. Alternatives are self-recatheterization or intermittent catheterization if there is no urethral obstruction, or a condom catheter if incontinence was the original reason for a catheter.

Problems preventing intercourse: local cancer, painful infection, severe incontinence, fistulae or previous surgery may prevent penetrative intercourse. Patients and their partners may wish to explore other ways of achieving sexual satisfaction. The help of a psychosexual counselor can be invaluable.

OTHER URINARY PROBLEMS

Urinary retention: constipation is a common cause of retention in the elderly, debilitated, or neurologically impaired. Morphine is an unusual cause of retention and more common causes are tricyclic antidepressants and drugs with antimuscarinic actions. Urethral obstruction is more common in older men due to an enlarged prostate. Abdominal and pelvic malignancies can cause urethral or ureteric obstruction.

Incontinence: this is a distressing symptom with effects on self-esteem, personal hygiene, and social interaction, although many patients manage to cope if the problem is mild.[45,46] A wide variety

Clinical decision	If YES carry out the action below
4 Is pain present?	• **Pain in the midline** *If the pain is in the penis or urethra:* test the urine to exclude a UTI. *If the trigone (base of bladder) is being irritated* (produces pain felt at the tip of the urethra): — by catheter: reduce the volume of balloon, try a smaller size catheter or consider intermittent catheterization. Avoid tension on the catheter. — by tumor: try a bladder instillation of bupivacaine 50 mg (e.g. 20 mL 0.25% solution) for 15 min q12h. For a once daily regimen, try instilling lidocaine 200 mg (e.g. 10 mL 2% solution) with 10 mL of 8.4% sodium bicarbonate. *If the pain is felt in the lower abdomen this may be due to:* — catheter: reduce the balloon volume. Consider intermittent catheterization — cystitis (persistent infection, NSAIDs, ketamine, some cytotoxics): treat the cause if possible, otherwise try instilling bupivacaine or lidocaine as above — unstable bladder: *see* incontinence (cd-7 on p. 229) — urinary retention: *see* decreased urine output (cd-1 on p. 225). • **Unilateral pain** *If the pain is in the groin:* this may be ureteric colic due to irritation or obstruction. — treat the cause — consider starting a strong opioid (or giving a breakthrough dose of an existing opioid). An NSAID can be tried if the renal function is normal. For ureteric obstruction due to tumor, try dexamethasone 16 mg daily. *If the pain is felt in the loin:* this may be renal capsule distension or irritation. — infection: exclude TB or pyelonephritis — hemorrhage: hydromorphone 1 mg or morphine 5 mg SC if not on an opioid, otherwise use equivalent of current analgesia. Consider ketamine (but be aware that ketamine can cause pain due to cystitis) — tumor: start opioid or increase existing opioid by up to 50% if needed. If renal function is poor, avoid NSAIDs and morphine — bilateral ureteric obstruction: *see* cd-6 on p. 229.
5 Are sexual difficulties present?	**Enable open discussion of sexuality and body image.** • **Has the couple's usual physical intimacy changed?** • **Is this a problem for them?** • **Do they want to discuss these difficulties?** If the answer is yes to all three questions consider the following: *Erectile impotence:* exclude reversible causes such as anxiety, depression, and drugs (antihypertensives, antidepressants, β-blockers, lipid-lowering drugs, thiazides, spironolactone): consider a trial of sildenafil 25–50 mg 1 hour before sexual activity (contraindicated if hypotensive, on nitrates, recent CVA, or recent myocardial infarction). *Vaginal pain on intercourse:* exclude hormonal deficiency causing dryness or vaginitis. *Intercourse physically impossible* (e.g. local tumor): explore other ways to stimulate the partner or express physical closeness.

Adapted from Regnard and Mannix[34]
cd = clinical decision

of approaches can help many patients to cope, such as regular voiding, exercises, and drugs. The advice of a continence nurse is essential.

Treatment is more difficult in older, disabled adults. Up to 60% of adults receiving care at home or in institutions have urinary incontinence.[47,48] Incontinence is more common in elderly patients, especially in the presence of cognitive impairment such as dementia or stroke in nursing or long-term care. In these patients regular prompting to void is the most helpful strategy.[49,50] Antimuscarinics can help and are well tolerated,[51] but may worsen the symptoms of Alzheimer's dementia.[52]

Permanent catheterization should be a last resort since there are many causes which can be treated (*see* clinical decision table). In intractable nocturnal incontinence, desmopressin, a synthetic analogue of vasopressin (antidiuretic hormone) which reduces urinary output overnight, is occasionally helpful in both children and adults of any age.[53–55] A fluid intake/output chart is started, and no fluids given after 6pm to ensure the patient produces a daytime output of at least 500 mL, otherwise water intoxication can occur. An intranasal or oral dose is given at bedtime. For some patients incontinence cannot be avoided and they can be helped with pads.[56]

Catheter problems: blockage is the commonest problem and is usually related to infection.[57] There is no evidence that regular bladder washouts reduce the risk of catheter blockage.[58,59] Bypassing of urine around a catheter may be due to a) a large balloon causing bladder irritability; b) a large catheter that is stretching and reducing the seal provided by the bladder sphincter; or c) obstruction of the catheter.

Choosing the correct catheter gauge is important: size 12–16 Ch catheters will drain clear and dilute urine, 16–18 Ch will drain urine containing debris, and 18 Ch or larger are needed to drain clots. Catheter balloons can deflate spontaneously (the likelihood is the same whether normal saline or water are used to fill the balloon),[60] they can stimulate bladder contractions, or they can fail to deflate when the catheter needs to be removed.

INTERMITTENT SELF-CATHETERIZATION

This is an underused procedure that is safe, effective, and is suitable for children and adult men and women.[61,62] It can be a viable alternative to indwelling catheters, even in older men.[63] It is the treatment of choice in hypotonic and unstable bladder,[64,65] but can be used in many other situations. Because the bladder is emptied completely, the risk of infection should be reduced, but the evidence for this is lacking. The following technique should be used at least four times a day by patients or carers – sterility is *not* necessary during the procedure:

1. Wash the hands.
2. Wash the skin around urethra with warm water.
3. Cover a 10 Ch reusable catheter with KY lubricant jelly.
4. Insert the catheter until urine flows.
5. Once urine has stopped flowing slowly withdraw the catheter, gently rotating the catheter until no further urine flows.
6. Rinse the catheter in tap water and leave immersed in a 0.016% sodium hypochlorite solution (Milton no.1 in 300 mL water) for at least 30 minutes.
7. Allow the catheter to dry, and cover with clean paper tissue until the next time.

Procedure for intermittent catheterization

Clinical decision	If YES carry out the action below
6 Has urinary frequency changed?	• **Increased frequency** *Causes of increased urine output: see* cd-1, p. 225. *Bladder irritability:* — infection: *see* cd-2, p. 225 — unstable bladder: *see* cd-7 below — anxiety: *see Anxiety*, p. 239 — obstruction with overflow: *see* decreased urine output (cd-1, p. 225). *Small capacity bladder* (due to tumor): ensure regular voiding or try intermittent catheterization. • **Decreased frequency** *Causes of decreased urinary output: see* cd-1, p. 225. *Antimuscarinic drugs* (e.g. hyoscine, tricyclic antidepressants) causing increased sphincter tone: reduce dose or stop drug. *Neurological problems: see* cd-7 below.
7 Is urinary incontinence present?	• **Is behavior or cognition causing inappropriate micturition?** Exclude delirium, dementia, depression, anxiety state, or a psychosis. • **If a fistula is present (vesicovaginal or vesicorectal):** Plan regular voiding through the urethra, using water-absorbent pads the rest of the time. Regular intermittent catheterization may help by keeping the bladder empty. • **In the absence of a fistula** *Exclude overflow* due to urethral or catheter obstruction (urge to micturate, full bladder on examination): *see* decreased urine output (cd-1, p. 225). *Total urinary incontinence* (i.e. no control present, usually due to local tumor): catheterization with long-term indwelling catheter. *Stress incontinence* (incontinence on straining): exclude a hypotonic bladder (*see* below). Other options are external pads, estrogen replacement, support prostheses, and urethral inserts. If there is insufficient time for these treatments to work, the drugs used for unstable bladder (*see* below) can be used. *Neurological* (caused by damage to neural control of bladder): — *hypotonic (neuropathic) bladder:* symptoms are difficulty in initiating micturition, intermittent stream, incomplete emptying, recurrent infections, stress incontinence. It is caused by damage to the sacral plexus or due to spinal cord compression below T11. It is best managed with intermittent catheterization (*see* opposite). — *unstable bladder:* symptoms are frequency, nocturia, and urgency. It is caused by damage to suprasacral pathways. Start oxybutynin 3–5 mg q8h or tolterodine 1–2 mg q12h. — *neurogenic bladder:* features are the same as unstable bladder, but symptoms are worsened by oxybutynin or other antimuscarinic drugs. It is caused by spinal cord damage or multiple sclerosis and best managed with intermittent catheterization (*see* opposite). *Bypassing catheter:* change to smaller size catheter or catheter with a smaller balloon volume. *Poor mobility:* refer to physiotherapist. Consider sheath catheter or intermittent catheterization (*see* opposite). *Benign prostatic hyperplasia:* start an alpha-blocking drug. • **If nights are disturbed by incontinence** (and only if renal function is normal): give desmopressin 10–40 microg intranasally or 100–400 microg PO at night to stop overnight renal production of urine. • **Manage the consequences of incontinence:** use barrier preparations to protect skin. Personal hygiene: provide encouragement and help to wash regularly and change clothes if needed. Consider the sexual and psychological consequences.

Adapted from Regnard and Mannix[33]
cd = clinical decision

SUPRAPUBIC CATHETERS

For some patients indwelling urethral catheters and intermittent catheterization are not possible or acceptable. A suprapubic catheter can be helpful and patients learn to adapt to this approach.[66]

REFERENCES: URINARY PROBLEMS AND SEXUAL DIFFICULTIES

B = book; C = comment; Ch = chapter; CS-n = case study-no. of cases; CT-n = controlled trial-no. of cases; E = editorial; GC = group consensus; I = interviews; Let = Letter; LS = laboratory study; MC = multi-center; OS-n = open study-no. of cases; Q-n = questionnaire-no. completed; R = review; RCT-n = randomized controlled trial-no. of cases; RS-n = retrospective survey-no. of cases; SA = systematic or meta analysis.

1 Smith DB. (1999) Urinary continence issues in oncology. *Clinical Journal of Oncology Nursing*. **3**(4): 161–7. (R, 25 refs)

2 Galbraith ME, Crighton F. (2008) Alterations of sexual function in men with cancer. *Seminars in Oncology Nursing*. **24**(2): 102–14. (R, 94 refs)

3 Shell JA. (2002) Evidence-based practice for symptom management in adults with cancer: sexual dysfunction. *Oncology Nursing Forum*. **29**(1): 53–66. (SA, 104 refs)

4 Penson RT, Gallagher J, Gioiella ME, Wallace M, *et al.* (2000) Sexuality and cancer: conversation comfort zone. *Oncologist*. **5**(4): 336–44. (R)

5 Rice A. (2000) Sexuality in cancer and palliative care 1: effects of disease and treatment. *International Journal of Palliative Nursing*. **6**(8): 392–7. (R)

6 Rice AM. Sexuality in cancer and palliative care 2: exploring the issues. *International Journal of Palliative Nursing*. **6**(9): 448–53. 2000 (R, 43 refs)

7 Ananth H, Jones L, King M, Tookman A. (2003) The impact of cancer on sexual function: a controlled study. *Palliative Medicine*. **17**: 202–5. (Q-120)

8 Hughes MK. (2000) Sexuality and the cancer survivor: a silent coexistence. *Cancer Nursing*. **23**(6): 477–82. (R, 55 refs)

9 Richards D, Toop L, Chambers S, Fletcher L. (2005) Response to antibiotics of women with symptoms of urinary tract infection but negative dipstick urine test results: double blind randomised controlled trial. *British Medical Journal*. **331**: 143. (RCT-59)

10 Bent S, Nallamothu BK, Simel DL, Fihn SD, Saint S. (2002) Does this woman have an acute uncomplicated urinary tract infection? *Journal of the American Medical Association*. **287**(20): 2701–10. (SA, 52 refs)

11 Guay DR. (2008) Contemporary management of uncomplicated urinary tract infections. *Drugs*. **68**(9): 1169–205. (R, 141 refs)

12 Sedberry-Ross S, Pohl HG. (2008) Urinary tract infections in children. *Current Urology Reports*. **9**(2): 165–71. (R, 64 refs)

13 Thayyil-Sudhan S, Gupta S. (2000) Dipstick examination for urinary tract infections. *Archive of Disease in Children*. **82**: 271–2. (Let)

14 Grude N, Tveten Y, Jenkins A, Kristiansen BE. (2005) Uncomplicated urinary tract infections: bacterial findings and efficacy of empirical antibacterial treatment. *Scandinavian Journal of Primary Health Care*. **23**(2): 115–9. (OS-184)

15 van Merode T, Nys S, Raets I, Stobberingh E. (2005) Acute uncomplicated lower urinary tract infections in general practice: clinical and microbiological cure rates after three- versus five-day treatment with trimethoprim. *European Journal of General Practice*. **11**(2): 55–8. (RCT)

16 Lutters M, Vogt-Ferrier NB. (2008) Antibiotic duration for treating uncomplicated, symptomatic lower urinary tract infections in elderly women. *Cochrane Database of Systematic Reviews*. **3**: CD001535. (SA, R-231 refs)

17 Milo G, Katchman EA, Paul M, Christiaens T, *et al.* (2005) Duration of antibacterial treatment for uncomplicated urinary tract infection in women. *Cochrane Database of Systematic Reviews*. **2**: CD004682. (SA, R-72 refs)

18 Malani AN, Kauffman CA. (2007) Candida urinary tract infections: treatment options. *Expert Review of Antiinfective Therapy*. **5**(2): 277–84. (R, 29 refs)

19 Goswami AK, Mahajan RK, Nath R, Sharma SK. (1993) How safe is 1% alum irrigation in controlling intractable vesical hemorrhage? *Journal of Urology*. **149**(2): 264–7. (CS-10)

20 Twycross R, Wilcock A, Stark Toller S. (2009) Haematuria. In: *Symptom Management in Advanced Cancer, 4th ed*. Nottingham: palliativedrugs.com.

21 Rastinehad AR, Ost MC, VanderBrink BA, Siegel DN, Kavoussi LR. (2008) Persistent prostatic hematuria. *Nature Clinical Practice Urology*. **5**(3): 159–65. (R, 35 refs)

22 Maxwell NJ, Saleem Amer N, Rogers E, Kiely D, *et al.* (2007) Renal artery embolisation in the palliative treatment of renal carcinoma. *British Journal of Radiology*. **80**(95): 96–102. (OS-19)

23 Neeman Z, Sarin S, Coleman J, Fojo T, Wood BJ. (2005) Radiofrequency ablation for tumor-related massive hematuria. *Journal of Vascular and Interventional Radiology*. **16**(3): 417–21. (CS-4)

24 Cohen JM, Cuckow P, Davies EG. (2008) Bladder wall telangiectasis causing life-threatening haematuria in ataxia-telangiectasia: a new observation. *Acta Paediatrica*. **97**(5): 667–9. (CR-2)

25 Schultz M, van der Lelie H. (1995) Microscopic haematuria as a relative contraindication for tranexamic acid. *British Journal of Haematology*. **89**(3): 663–4. (CS-3)

26 Manjunath G, Fozailoff A, Mitcheson D, Sarnak MJ. (2002) Epsilon-aminocaproic acid and renal complications: case report and review of the literature. *Clinical Nephrology*. 58: 63–7. (R)

27 Henry R, Patterson L, Avery N, Tanzola R, *et al.* (2001) Absorption of alkalized intravesical lidocaine in normal and inflamed bladders: a simple method

for improving bladder anesthesia. *Journal of Urology*. **165**(6 Pt. 1): 1900–3. (OS-24)
28 Parsons CL. (2005) Successful downregulation of bladder sensory nerves with combination of heparin and alkalinized lidocaine in patients with interstitial cystitis. *Urology*. **65**(1): 45–8. (CT-82)
29 McInerney PD, Grant A, Chawla J, Stephenson TP. (1992) The effect of intravesical Marcain instillation on hyperreflexic detrusor contractions. *Paraplegia*. **30**(2): 127–30. (OS-36)
30 McCoubrie R, Jeffrey D. (2003) Intravesical diamorphine for bladder spasm. *Journal of Pain and Symptom Management*. **25**(1): 1–2. (Let, CS-1)
31 Bramble FJ, Morley R. (1997) Drug-induced cystitis: the need for vigilance. *British Journal of Urology*. **79**(1): 3–7. (R, 18 refs)
32 Shahani R, Streutker C, Dickson B, Stewart RJ. (2007) Ketamine-associated ulcerative cystitis: a new clinical entity. *Urology*. **69**(5): 810–12. (CS-9)
33 Cordell WH, Larson TA, Lingeman JE, Nelson DR, *et al.* (1994) Indomethacin suppositories versus intravenous titrated morphine for the treatment of ureteral colic. *Annals of Emergency Medicine*. **23**: 262–9. (RCT-75)
34 Regnard C, Mannix K. (1995) Urinary problems. In: *Flow Diagrams in Advanced Cancer and Other Diseases*. London: Edward Arnold. pp. 39–43. (Ch)
35 Engeler DS, Ackermann DK, Osterwalder JJ, Keel A, Schmid HP. (2005) A double-blind, placebo controlled comparison of the morphine sparing effect of oral rofecoxib and diclofenac for acute renal colic. *Journal of Urology*. **174**(3): 933–6. (RCT-220)
36 Shokeir AA. (2002) Renal colic: new concepts related to pathophysiology, diagnosis and treatment. *Current Opinion in Urology*. **12**(4): 263–9. (R, 57 refs).
37 Lloret J, Munoz J, Monmany J, Puig X, *et al.* (1987) Treatment of renal colic with dipyrone: a double-blind comparison trial with hyoscine alone or combined with dipyrone. *Current Therapeutic Research – Clinical and Experimental*. **42**(6): 1119–28. (RCT-96)
38 Holdgate A, Oh CM. (2005) Is there a role for antimuscarinics in renal colic? A randomized controlled trial. *Journal of Urology*. **174**(2): 572–5. (RCT-178)
39 Lee Y, Lee W, Chen M, Huang JK, Chung C, Chang LS. (1992) Acupuncture in the treatment of renal colic. *Journal of Urology*. **147**: 16–18. (RCT)
40 Mora B, Giorni E, Dobrovits M, Barker R, *et al.* (2006) Transcutaneous electrical nerve stimulation: an effective treatment for pain caused by renal colic in emergency care. *Journal of Urology*. **175**(5): 1737–41. (CT-73)
41 Chu PS, Ma WK, Wong SC, Chu RW, *et al.* (2008) The destruction of the lower urinary tract by ketamine abuse: a new syndrome? *BJU International*. **102**(11): 1616–22. (RS-59)
42 Lalos O, Berglund A, Lalos A. (2001) Impact of urinary and climacteric symptoms on social and sexual life after surgical treatment of stress urinary incontinence in women: a long-term outcome. *Journal of Advanced Nursing*. **33**(3): 316–27. (OS-45)
43 Watanabe T, Rivas DA, Smith R, Staas WE Jr., Chancellor MB. (1996) The effect of urinary tract reconstruction on neurologically impaired women previously treated with an indwelling urethral catheter. *Journal of Urology*. **156**(6): 1926–8. (OS-18)
44 Rigby D. (1998) Long-term catheter care. *Professional Nurse (Study Supplement)*. **13**(5S): 14–15.
45 Bogner HR, Gallo JJ, Sammel MD, Ford DE, *et al.* (2002) Urinary incontinence and psychological distress in community-dwelling older adults. *Journal of the American Geriatrics Society*. **50**(3): 489–95. (I-781)
46 Fultz NH, Herzog AR. (2001) Self-reported social and emotional impact of urinary incontinence. *Journal of the American Geriatrics Society*. **49**(7): 892–9. (I-1326)
47 Du Moulin MF, Hamers JP, Ambergen AW, Janssen MA, Halfens RJ. (2008) Prevalence of urinary incontinence among community-dwelling adults receiving home care. *Research in Nursing and Health*. **31**(6): 604–12. (RS-2866)
48 Coffey A, McCarthy G, McCormack B, Wright J, Slater P. (2007) Incontinence: assessment, diagnosis, and management in two rehabilitation units for older people. *Worldviews on Evidence-Based Nursing*. **4**(4): 179–86. (OS-220)
49 Fink HA, Taylor BC, Tacklind JW, Rutks IR, Wilt TJ. (2008) Treatment interventions in nursing home residents with urinary incontinence: a systematic review of randomized trials. *Mayo Clinic Proceedings*. **83**(12): 1332–43. (SA, R-57 refs)
50 Thomas LH, Cross S, Barrett J, French B, *et al.* (2008) Treatment of urinary incontinence after stroke in adults. *Cochrane Database of Systematic Reviews*. **1**: CD004462. (SA, R-42 refs)
51 Armstrong RB, Dmochowski RR, Sand PK, Macdiarmid S. (2007) Safety and tolerability of extended-release oxybutynin once daily in urinary incontinence: combined results from two phase 4 controlled clinical trials. *International Urology and Nephrology*. **39**(4): 1069–77. (RCT-1168)
52 Ancelin ML, Artero S, Portet F, Dupuy AM, *et al.* (2006) Non-degenerative mild cognitive impairment in elderly people and use of anticholinergic drugs: longitudinal cohort study. *British Medical Journal*. **332**: 455–9. (OS-372)
53 Johnson TM 2nd, Miller M, Tang T, Pillion DJ, Ouslander JG. (2006) Oral ddAVP for nighttime urinary incontinence in characterized nursing home residents: a pilot study. *Journal of the American Medical Directors Association*. **7**(1): 6–11. (CT, MC)
54 Miller M. (2000) Nocturnal polyuria in older people: pathophysiology and clinical implications. *Journal of the American Geriatrics Society*. **48**(10): 1321–9. (R, 104 refs)
55 Humphreys MR, Reinberg YE. (2005) Contemporary and emerging drug treatments for urinary incontinence in children. *Paediatric Drugs*. **7**(3): 151–62. (R, 48 refs)
56 Fader M, Cottenden AM, Getliffe K. (2008) Absorbent products for moderate–heavy urinary and/or faecal incontinence in women and

men. *Cochrane Database of Systematic Reviews*. **4**: CD007408. (SA-2, 35 refs)

57 Mathur S, Suller MT, Stickler DJ, Feneley RC. (2006) Factors affecting crystal precipitation from urine in individuals with long-term urinary catheters colonized with urease-positive bacterial species. *Urological Research*. **34**(3): 173–7. (OS-21)

58 Winn C. (1998) Complications with urinary catheters. *Professional Nurse (Study Supplement)*. **13**(5): S7–10. (R)

59 Williams C, Tonkin S. (2003) Blocked urinary catheters: solutions are not the only solution. *British Journal of Community Nursing*. **8**(7): 321–6. (R, 15 refs)

60 Hui J, Ng CF, Chan LW, Chan PS. (2004) Can normal saline be used to fill the balloon of a Foley catheter? The experience of a prospective randomized study in China. *International Journal of Urology*. **11**(10): 845–7. (RCT-4000)

61 Moore KN, Fader M, Getliffe K. (2007) Long-term bladder management by intermittent catheterisation in adults and children. *Cochrane Database of Systematic Reviews*. **4**: CD006008. (SA, R-38 refs)

62 Hunt GM, Oakeshott P, Whitaker RH. (1996) Intermittent catheterisation: simple, safe, and effective but underused. *British Medical Journal*. **312**(7023): 103–7. (R, 35 refs)

63 Pilloni S, Krhut J, Mair D, Madersbacher H, Kessler TM. (2005) Intermittent catheterisation in older people: a valuable alternative to an indwelling catheter? *Age and Ageing*. **34**(1): 57–60. (OS-21)

64 Wyndaele JJ, Madersbacher H, Kovindha A. (2001) Conservative treatment of the neuropathic bladder in spinal cord injured patients. *Spinal Cord*. **39**(6): 294–300. (R, 44 refs)

65 Yavuzer G, Gök H, Tuncer S, Soygür T, Arikan N, Arasil T. (2000) Compliance with bladder management in spinal cord injury patients. *Spinal Cord*. **38**(12): 762–5. (OS-50)

66 Sweeney A, Harrington A, Button D. (2007) Suprapubic catheters: a shared understanding, from the other side looking in. *Journal of Wound, Ostomy, and Continence Nursing*. **34**(4): 418–24. (CS-6)

Psychological symptoms

NOTES

Anger

CLINICAL DECISION AND ACTION CHECKLIST

1. Acknowledge what anger does to you.
2. Acknowledge the person's anger.
3. Are several people angry?
4. Is the person controlled and contained?
5. Is the anger appropriate?
6. Is the anger inappropriate?
7. Is the anger escalating?
8. Is the anger persisting?

KEY POINTS

- Many situations in advanced disease can cause anger.
- Be aware of what anger does to you.
- Apologize if you are at fault; never apologize for others.
- Anger should defuse rapidly; if it does not, be prepared to stop the interview and leave.

INTRODUCTION

Advanced illness produces many reasons to be angry such as unrealized ambitions, loss of control, feelings of hopelessness, depression, persistent symptoms, and spiritual conflicts.[1] Anger can be an accompanying feature of pain,[2] anticipatory grief,[3] or depression.[4,5] It is more common in adult children and in caregivers not living with the patient.[3] Anger can present in six different ways:

- the expression of anger can be active (outwardly obvious) or passive (suppressed)
- the level of anger can be proportionate to the situation or out of proportion
- the target of the anger can be correctly directed or misdirected.

Anger that is actively expressed, proportionate, and correctly directed is easier to help than anger that is passive, out of proportion, or misdirected. No assumptions should be made about the anger until it has been assessed.

BE AWARE OF WHAT ANGER DOES TO YOU

It is common to be emotionally affected when confronted by an angry person. Some professionals feel irritated, in which case they need to suppress this irritation to avoid escalating the anger. Other professionals become withdrawn at the anger being directed at them, and need to be more assertive in order to be believed and help the angry person effectively. The key is to be calm but clear.[6] If your reaction makes it difficult for you to help an angry person, it would be best to ask someone else to see the angry person, and to consider getting advice or teaching on helping an angry person.

ACKNOWLEDGE THE ANGER

While this may seem unnecessary, it gives the person a clear message that you have noticed their anger and that you are taking it seriously. Most people want to know that the professional is prepared to listen and help. Acknowledging the anger may simply generate a response such as, "Well of course I'm angry." However, anger often rapidly defuses with the offer of help, "I can see you're angry, how can I help?"

The setting: with an angry person it is usually impossible to choose the right setting. If the setting seems particularly awkward (e.g. a busy corridor), as the discussion progresses it is reasonable to suggest an alternative, more private venue.

ARE SEVERAL PEOPLE ANGRY?

Friends and relatives can be angry, sometimes separately from the patient. If more than one person is angry you will need help but the process of defusing the anger is the same.

THE APPROPRIATENESS OF ANGER

The cause can be elicited by asking, "What's happened to make you feel like this?" The extent of the anger can be clarified by asking, "On a scale of 0 to 10, how angry have you been?" Most anger is understandable in that a) its reasons can be recognized; and b) some people in distressing situations become angry.

Apologizing: when the anger is correctly directed at the professional, and that anger is proportionate to the situation, it is best to apologize. For example: "I'm sorry you were kept waiting for so long – it would make me angry too." However, when the anger is about the behavior of another health professional, avoid the temptation to defend that person since a) it is not your place to defend others, and b) trying to defend the other person will fail to defuse the anger and will only result in the accusation that "You lot all stick together!" You can still show your concern without being defensive, for example, "I can see why you're angry." Then suggest that they speak or write to the individual to express their concerns.

Clinical decision	If YES carry out the action below
1 Acknowledge what anger does to you: if such situations always make you very angry or very passive, ask someone else to conduct the interview.	
2 Acknowledge the person's anger and offer help, e.g. "I can see you're angry, how can I help?" If the setting is inappropriate, suggest an alternative.	
3 Are several people angry?	• Take someone with you from a different discipline, e.g. if you are a doctor ask a nurse or social worker to join you.
4 Is the person controlled and contained?	• **Exclude conditions affecting facial expression:** e.g. myasthenia gravis, Parkinson's, drug-induced akinesia. • **If the person is passively angry:** Acknowledge the anger (e.g. "Am I right that this has made you angry?"). Negotiate to discuss the cause (e.g. "Can you explain why you're feeling like this?"). Encourage the expression of anger (e.g. "Just how angry have you been?"). • **If you (the professional) are the only person who is angry:** you should withdraw and seek advice and support.
5 Is the anger appropriate?	• **If it is correctly directed and proportionate to the situation:** (e.g. appointments are running 1 hour late): Identify the level of anger. Show understanding without being defensive (e.g. "I'd be angry too."). Enable them to express their anger. Apologize if you have made an error (do not apologize for others).
6 Is the anger inappropriate?	• **If it is misdirected** (e.g. anger at a family physician that chemotherapy failed): Check this (e.g. "I can see that you're angry that the treatment didn't work, but could you tell me why your anger is directed at me?"). Explore the causes of anger that may be uncovered. • **If the setting is difficult:** suggest moving to a quiet room. • **If the level is out of proportion to the situation:** Go to cd-7 below.
7 Is the anger escalating?	• **Position yourself near the room exit** with the door open. • **Set limits** (e.g. "I can see that this has made you very angry. I want to help, but your anger is beginning to make me feel uncomfortable. If you don't feel you can control your anger I wouldn't feel comfortable continuing.") • **If the person cannot accept limits this is likely to be pathological anger. Stop the interview and leave the room immediately.** (e.g. "In that case I have to stop this discussion now.")
8 Is the anger persisting?	• **If this is normal behavior:** usually no action is needed. Most naturally angry people recognize this and acknowledge its presence. Occasionally, limits have to be set as in cd-7 above. • **If this is unusual behavior for the person:** Is the person depressed? Are there causes unconnected to the illness? Will the person accept any offer of help or support? Ask for specialist advice and help for the person (e.g. cognitive therapy). • **If the anger is causing isolation:** — acknowledge their isolation (e.g. "Your anger seems to have left you isolated.") — explore the effects of the isolation on relationships.

Adapted from Faulkner, Maguire and Regnard[7]
cd = clinical decision

ESCALATING ANGER

The steps so far should have defused most people's anger *within a few minutes*. At the very least, it should be no worse. Occasionally, however, the anger escalates. If this happens:

- Position yourself by the nearest exit.
- Acknowledge the escalating anger, e.g. "I can see you're having difficulty controlling your anger."
- Set limits. Admitting to them that their anger is making you feel uncomfortable should switch the focus from anger to the underlying emotion such as fear or sadness. If they cannot switch, they are unlikely to calm down.
- If the person cannot accept the limits, end the interview and leave immediately to avoid the risk of being assaulted.

PERSISTING ANGER

There are several reasons for persisting anger:[8–10]

1 This is a person's normal behavior.
2 There is underlying clinical depression.
3 The person has unrealized ambitions, e.g. not seeing children grow up.
4 Loss of control.
5 Spiritual anger.

As a first step with an angry person it is worth checking if they will accept your continuing support, advice, or help. Some patients will accept such support, even if it initially appears to have brought no therapeutic benefit. Over time, sufficient trust may develop to allow the patient to express their anger in a therapeutic way. For other patients complementary approaches such as music, reminiscence or art may help.[11] For the remaining patients additional or specialist help will be needed.

REFERENCES: ANGER

B = book; C = comment; Ch = chapter; CS-n = case study-no. of cases; CT-n = controlled trial-no. of cases; E = editorial; GC = group consensus; I = interviews; LS = laboratory study; MC = multi-center; OS-n = open study-no. of cases; R = review; RCT-n = randomized controlled trial-no. of cases; RS-n = retrospective survey-no. of cases; SA = systematic or meta analysis.

1 Philip J, Gold M, Schwarz M, Komesaroff P. (2007) Anger in palliative care: a clinical approach. *Internal Medicine Journal.* **37**(1): 49–55. (R, 29 refs)
2 Sela RA, Bruera E, Conner-Spady B, Cumming C, Walker C. (2000) Sensory and affective dimensions of advanced cancer pain. *Psycho-Oncology.* **11**(1): 23–34. (OS-111)
3 Chapman KJ, Pepler C. (1998) Coping, hope, and anticipatory grief in family members in palliative home care. *Cancer Nursing.* **21**(4): 226–34. (I-61)
4 Robbins PR, Tanck RH. (1997) Anger and depressed affect: interindividual and intraindividual perspectives. *Journal of Psychology.* **131**(5): 489–500. (OS-78)
5 Koh KB, Kim CH, Park JK. (2002) Predominance of anger in depressive disorders compared with anxiety disorders and somatoform disorders. *Journal of Clinical Psychiatry.* **63**(6): 486–92. (OS-402)
6 Garnham P. (2001) Understanding and dealing with anger, aggression and violence. *Nursing Standard.* **16**(6): 37–42. (R, 11 refs)
7 Faulkner A, Maguire P, Regnard C. (1995) The angry person. In: *Flow Diagrams in Advanced Cancer and Other Diseases.* London: Edward Arnold. pp. 81–5. (Ch)
8 Brittlebank A, Regnard C. (1990) Terror or depression? A case report. *Palliative Medicine.* **4**: 317–19. (CS-1)
9 Ramsay N. (1992) Referral to a liaison psychiatrist from a palliative care unit. *Palliative Medicine.* **6**: 54–60.
10 Moorey S, Greer S. (2002) Cognitive techniques II: applications of cognitive techniques to common problems. In: *Cognitive Behaviour Therapy for People with Cancer.* Oxford: Oxford University Press. pp. 126–31. (Ch)
11 Devlin B. (2006) The art of healing and knowing in cancer and palliative care. *International Journal of Palliative Nursing.* **12**(1): 16–19. (R, 19 refs)

Anxiety

CLINICAL DECISION AND ACTION CHECKLIST

1 Does the person feel apprehensive, tense or on edge?
2 Can an anxiety state be excluded?
3 Is an anxiety state present?
4 Is the person functioning poorly?
5 Are somatic symptoms distressing?
6 Do sudden panics or phobic episodes occur?
7 Is the anxiety persisting?

KEY POINTS

- Anxiety is common in advanced disease, but not inevitable or untreatable.
- Much anxiety can be eased with clear communication and simple measures.
- Anxiety and depression often coexist.
- Specialist help is needed for persistent, severe anxiety.

INTRODUCTION

Life-threatening illness creates an uncertain future that causes anxiety which may increase as the illness progresses. Anxiety in turn makes it more difficult for the patient to cope with suffering. Anxiety is common in advanced disease,[1] but is missed in more than half of patients,[2] or not recorded in medical notes.[3] It is associated with many factors such as anorexia,[4] depression,[5] breathlessness,[6] younger adults,[7] and inadequate information.[8] It occurs in both adults and children[9] and is also common in partners and relatives.[10,11]

IDENTIFYING ANXIETY

Features of anxiety are *apprehensive expectation* (e.g. fear, rumination, tendency to perceive situations in a threatening way), *vigilance and scanning* (e.g. irritability, poor concentration, difficulty getting to sleep, tendency to perceive bodily sensations in a threatening way), *motor tension* (e.g. trembling, tension, restlessness), and *autonomic hyperactivity* (e.g. sweating, dry mouth, cold hands, tachycardia, diarrhea). In advanced disease, anxiety is often associated with depression. The Hospital Anxiety and Depression (HAD) scale is a simple screening tool that is more useful for anxiety than depression,[12] but may not be sufficiently sensitive for use in palliative care.[13]

Anxiety state: this has a persistent, dominating, and intrusive quality accompanied by at least four anxiety-related symptoms for at least two weeks. If severe, it can cause disorganized functioning (*see* cd-4 opposite).

Drug-induced restlessness (akathisia): this can mimic the motor tension aspects of anxiety, and can include a psychological restlessness. However, patients describe little or no anxiety. Examples of drugs that may cause this are haloperidol, hyoscine, methotrimeprazine, metoclopramide, and the tricyclic antidepressants (e.g. amitriptyline). Combinations of these drugs are much more likely to cause akathisia.

HELPING THE ANXIOUS PERSON

Supportive measures: enabling a person to express their feelings, to discuss their needs and fears about the end of life, and giving the information they need through open discussion can do much to ease anxiety.[14,15] Helping the individual to identify the triggers for anxiety is the preparation for reframing those triggers to ones that do not precipitate anxiety. This is the basis for cognitive behavioral therapy and basic help can be provided with brief training.[16,17] Similar approaches have been used with visualization and guided imagery.[18–20] Simple anxiety-management techniques can be helpful, such as distraction or relaxation. Muscle-relaxation techniques are best avoided as they can worsen the anxiety of some people who are excessively vigilant of their bodily sensations. Autogenic relaxation (deep relaxation and self-hypnosis) is a better alternative,[21] but there is equivocal evidence for its success in anxiety.[22] The evidence for reflexology in treating anxiety is conflicting.[23,24] Other complementary approaches include hypnosis,[25] music therapy,[26,27] and aromatherapy.[28,29]

Disorganized functioning: as anxiety worsens the individual becomes increasingly distracted from daily activities. As it becomes more severe it begins to intrude on everyday decisions such as what to wear, or whether to get washed. Decisions become increasingly erratic and are made on the spur of the moment.

Moderate disorganization will ease with anxiety suppressants such as the benzodiazepines. Lorazepam is effective in low doses with little sedation. Although there is no evidence of any absorption from the oral mucosa,[30] it is often given buccally or sublingually. Severe disorganization will require antipsychotics. Although haloperidol, olanzapine, and methotrimeprazine (Canada only) are effective in severe anxiety,[31–33] risperidone is more effective.[34–36] Given long-term, both typical and atypical antipsychotics can cause lethal cardiac arrhythmias[37] and stroke.[39–41]

Clinical decision	If YES carry out the action below
1 Does the person feel apprehensive, tense or on edge?	• **Exclude:** *Drug-induced motor restlessness (akathisia):* the patient appears restless but may deny any anxiety (*see* text for list of drugs). Stop the drug causing the reaction. *Clinical depression: see* p. 253. *Confusional state: see Confusional states,* p. 245. • **Start supportive measures:** Offer information if the patient wishes this (if the information is likely to be difficult news *see Breaking difficult news,* p. 23). Explore causes of anxiety by encouraging the patient to disclose concerns (*see Helping the person to share their problems,* p. 15). Look for links between thoughts and feelings. Explore possible solutions, e.g. by helping the person to reframe more realistic interpretations or visualize more positive images. Look at how to change procedures that are causing anxiety. Consider relaxation, massage, aromatherapy, art, or music therapy.
2 Can an anxiety state be excluded?	• **If this is moderate anxiety:** teach relaxation exercises (distraction, autogenic relaxation). Enable access to aromatherapy and massage.
3 Is an anxiety state present?	**Characteristics:** persistent apprehension for more than 2 weeks and for more than 50% of the time, and that is different to their usual mood, and with four or more features of anxiety present (*see* text). • Follow the clinical decisions below.
4 Is the person functioning poorly?	• **If disorganization is moderate** (poor concentration, but able to care for themselves): start a benzodiazepine: — for minimal sedation use lorazepam 0.5–1 mg PO or sublingually — if insomnia is the problem use temazepam 10–40 mg at bedtime. • **If disorganization is severe** (tormented, unable to care for themselves or make a decision): start an antipsychotic: — for minimal sedation use risperidone 2–4 mg (0.5–1 mg in elderly) PO once daily — if sedation is needed use olanzapine 5–10 mg PO once daily or methotrimeprazine (Canada only) 25–50 mg q8h PO or SC. There is an increased risk of cerebrovascular events if used long term in the elderly. • **If the disorganization persists:** refer for specialist help and advice.
5 Are somatic symptoms distressing?	i.e. autonomic hyperactivity (e.g. tremor, tachycardia, sweating, diarrhea). • Consider a β-blocker, e.g. propranolol 10–40 mg q8h (NB. Risk of hypotension if used with lorazepam, temazepam, or methotrimeprazine).
6 Do sudden panics or phobic episodes occur?	• **Seek out triggers and explore thoughts.** • **For panic:** provide explanation and company. *Single episodes* (e.g. during MRI scan): 2–4 mg midazolam spray intranasally or midazolam solution buccally. *Repeated episodes:* clomipramine 25 mg at night (10 mg if >70 years), or an anxiety-suppressant SSRI antidepressant such as citalopram 10–20 mg PO once in the morning. • **For phobias:** consider lorazepam 0.5–1 mg sublingually 1–2 hours before exposure to precipitating event. If persistent consider clomipramine or an SSRI as above for panic. • Refer for cognitive behavioral therapy if available.
7 Is the anxiety persisting?	• **Consider:** the concurrent presence of depression (*see Withdrawal and depression,* p. 253). Refer for specialist advice and help.

Adapted from Maguire, Faulkner and Regnard[41]
cd = clinical decision

Panic: this occurs suddenly without an obvious cause, is intense, and can last 5–20 minutes. A fear of dying and loss of control are often provoked by the episodes. Although there is no obvious warning, individuals can be taught to identify triggers or specific thoughts that precede a panic. These thoughts may give some clue as to the cause, but also provide a means of instituting self-taught controls that with practice can prevent thoughts of panic developing into a full episode. Intranasal or buccal midazolam can help reduce isolated panics related to procedures.[42]

Phobias: situations or objects are interpreted as occasions when help is impossible, difficult or embarrassing. If individuals feel humiliated by these feelings they will find it hard to disclose their phobia. Treatment often needs specialist help, requiring a combination of cognitive behavioral therapy and antidepressants.[43–45]

When problems persist

Specialist help will be needed to unravel mixed disorders (e.g. mixed anxiety and depression), to diagnose unusual presentations, deal with a persistent anxiety state, or provide further therapy.[46,47] This help may be from a psychiatrist, psychologist, counselor, or social worker.[48] Cognitive behavioral therapy with a trained therapist can be particularly helpful for anxiety.[49] In reality, however, which specialist is enlisted is more likely to depend on what is available locally.

REFERENCES: ANXIETY

B = book; C = comment; Ch = chapter; CS-n = case study-no. of cases; CT-n = controlled trial-no. of cases; E = editorial; GC = group consensus; I = interviews; LS = laboratory study; MC = multi-center; Q-n = questionnaire-no. of respondents; OS-n = open study-no. of cases; R = review; RCT-n = randomized controlled trial-no. of cases; RS-n = retrospective survey-no. of cases; SA = systematic or meta analysis.

1 Wilson KG, Chochinov HM, Skirko MG, Allard P, *et al.* (2007) Depression and anxiety disorders in palliative cancer care. *Journal of Pain and Symptom Management.* **33**(2): 118–29. (Q-381)
2 Krishnasamy M, Wilkie E, Haviland J. (2001) Lung cancer health care needs assessment: patients' and informal carers' responses to a national mail questionnaire survey. *Palliative Medicine.* **15**(3): 213–27. (Q-279)
3 Strömgren AS, Groenvold M, Pedersen L, Olsen AK, Spile M, Sjøgren P. (2001) Does the medical record cover the symptoms experienced by cancer patients receiving palliative care? A comparison of the record and patient self-rating. *Journal of Pain and Symptom Management.* **21**(3): 189–96. (OS-58)
4 Hawkins C. (2000) Anorexia and anxiety in advanced malignancy: the relative problem. *Journal of Human Nutrition and Dietetics.* **13**(2): 113–7. (Q-147)
5 Devanand DP. (2002) Comorbid psychiatric disorders in late life depression. *Biological Psychiatry.* **52**(3): 236–42. (R, 51 refs)
6 Chan CW, Richardson A, Richardson J. (2005) A study to assess the existence of the symptom cluster of breathlessness, fatigue and anxiety in patients with advanced lung cancer. *European Journal of Oncology Nursing.* **9**(4): 325–33. (OS-27)
7 Walsh D, Donnelly S, Rybicki L. (2000) The symptoms of advanced cancer: relationship to age, gender, and performance status in 1,000 patients. *Supportive Care in Cancer.* **8**(3): 175–9. (OS-100)
8 Fallowfield LJ, Jenkins VA, Beveridge HA. (2002) Truth may hurt but deceit hurts more: communication in palliative care. *Palliative Medicine.* **16**(4): 297–303. (R)
9 Kersun LS, Shemesh E. (2007) Depression and anxiety in children at the end of life. *Pediatric Clinics of North America.* 54(5): 691–708. (R, 93 refs)
10 Aranda SK, Hayman-White K. (2001) Home caregivers of the person with advanced cancer: an Australian perspective. *Cancer Nursing.* **24**(4): 300–7. (I-42)
11 Grov EK, Dahl AA, Moum T, Fossa SD. (2005) Anxiety, depression, and quality of life in caregivers of patients with cancer in late palliative phase. *Annals of Oncology.* **16**(7): 1185–91. (Q-96)
12 Le Fevre P, Devereux J, Smith S, Lawrie SM, Cornbleet M. (1999) Screening for psychiatric illness in the palliative care inpatient setting: a comparison between the Hospital Anxiety and Depression Scale and the General Health Questionnaire-12. *Palliative Medicine.* **13**(5): 399–407. (OS-79)
13 Lloyd-Williams M, Friedman T, Rudd N. (2001) An analysis of the validity of the Hospital Anxiety and Depression Scale as a screening tool in patients with advanced metastatic cancer. *Journal of Pain and Symptom Management.* **22**(6): 990–6. (OS-100)
14 Steinhauser KE, Alexander SC, Byock IR, George LK, Olsen MK, Tulsky JA. (2008) Do preparation and life completion discussions improve functioning and quality of life in seriously ill patients? Pilot randomized control trial. *Journal of Palliative Medicine.* **11**(9): 1234–40. (RCT-82)
15 Pautex S, Herrmann FR, Zulian GB. (2008)

Role of advance directives in palliative care units: a prospective study. *Palliative Medicine.* **22**(7): 835–41. (OS, MC-52)

16 Anderson T, Watson M, Davidson R. (2008) The use of cognitive behavioural therapy techniques for anxiety and depression in hospice patients: a feasibility study. *Palliative Medicine.* **22**(7): 814–21. (OS-10)

17 Mannix KA, Blackburn IM, Garland A, Gracie J, *et al.* (2006) Effectiveness of brief training in cognitive behaviour therapy techniques for palliative care practitioners. *Palliative Medicine.* **20**(6): 579–84. (RCT-20)

18 Thompson MB, Coppens NM. (1994) The effects of guided imagery on anxiety levels and movement of clients undergoing magnetic resonance imaging. *Holistic Nursing Practice.* **8**(2): 59–69. (RCT-41)

19 Hattan J, King L, Griffiths P. (2002) The impact of foot massage and guided relaxation following cardiac surgery: a randomized controlled trial. *Journal of Advanced Nursing.* **37**(2): 199–207. (RCT-25)

20 Van Fleet S. (2000) Relaxation and imagery for symptom management: improving patient assessment and individualizing treatment. *Oncology Nursing Forum.* **27**(3): 501–10. (R, 77 refs)

21 Wright S, Courtney U, Crowther D. (2002) A quantitative and qualitative pilot study of the perceived benefits of autogenic training for a group of people with cancer. *European Journal of Cancer Care.* **11**(2): 122–30. (R)

22 Ernst E, Kanji N. (2000) Autogenic training for stress and anxiety: a systematic review. *Complementary Therapies in Medicine.* **8**(2): 106–10. (SA, 11 refs)

23 Williamson J, White A, Hart A, Ernst E. (2002) Randomised controlled trial of reflexology for menopausal symptoms. *BJOG: an International Journal of Obstetrics and Gynaecology.* **109**(9): 1050–5. (RCT-75)

24 Stephenson NL, Weinrich SP, Tavakoli AS. (2000) The effects of foot reflexology on anxiety and pain in patients with breast and lung cancer. *Oncology Nursing Forum.* **27**(1): 67–72. (RCT-23)

25 Liossi C, White P. (2001) Efficacy of clinical hypnosis in the enhancement of quality of life of terminally ill cancer patients. *Contemporary Hypnosis.* **18**(3): 145–60. (RCT-50)

26 Hilliard RE. (2001) The use of music therapy in meeting the multidimensional needs of hospice patients and families. *Journal of Palliative Care.* **17**(3): 161–6. (CS-4)

27 Horne-Thompson A, Grocke D. (2008) The effect of music therapy on anxiety in patients who are terminally ill. *Journal of Palliative Medicine.* **11**(4): 582–90. (RCT-25)

28 Hadfield N. (2001) The role of aromatherapy massage in reducing anxiety in patients with malignant brain tumours. *International Journal of Palliative Nursing.* **7**(6): 279–85. (CS-8)

29 Wilkinson S, Aldridge J, Salmon I, Cain E, Wilson B. (1999) An evaluation of aromatherapy massage in palliative care. *Palliative Medicine.* **13**(5): 409–17. (RCT-103)

30 Spenard J, Caille G, de Montigny C, Vezina M, *et al.* (1988) Placebo-controlled comparative study of the anxiolytic activity and of the pharmacokinetics of oral and sublingual lorazepam in generalized anxiety. *Biopharmaceutics and Drug Disposition.* **9**(5): 457–64. (RCT-12)

31 Currier GW, Trenton A. (2002) Pharmacological treatment of psychotic agitation. *CNS Drugs.* **16**(4): 219–28. (R, 63 refs)

32 Khojainova N, Santiago-Palma J, Kornick C, Breitbart W, Gonzales GR. (2002) Olanzapine in the management of cancer pain. *Journal of Pain and Symptom Management.* **23**(4): 346–50. (OS-8)

33 Mintzer J, Faison W, Street JS, Sutton VK, Breier A. (2001) Olanzapine in the treatment of anxiety symptoms due to Alzheimer's disease: a post hoc analysis. *International Journal of Geriatric Psychiatry.* **16**(Suppl. 1): S71–7. (RCT)

34 Blin O, Azorin JM, Bouhours P. (1996) Antipsychotic and anxiolytic properties of risperidone, haloperidol, and methotrimeprazine in schizophrenic patients. *Journal of Clinical Psychopharmacology.* **16**(1): 38–44. (RCT-63)

35 Chouinard G, Jones B, Remington G, Bloom D, Addington D, *et al.* (1993) A Canadian multicenter placebo-controlled study of fixed doses of risperidone and haloperidol in the treatment of chronic schizophrenic patients. *Journal of Clinical Psychopharmacology.* **13**: 25–40. (RCT-135)

36 Conley RR, Mahmoud R. (2001) A randomized double-blind study of risperidone and olanzapine in the treatment of schizophrenia or schizoaffective disorder. *American Journal of Psychiatry.* **158**(5): 765–74. (RCT-377)

37 Maguire P, Faulkner A, Regnard C. (1995) The anxious person. In: *Flow Diagrams in Advanced Cancer and Other Diseases.* London: Edward Arnold. pp. 73–6. (Ch)

38 Ray WA, Chung CP, Murray KT, Hall K, Stein CM. (2009) Atypical antipsychotic drugs and the risk of sudden cardiac death. *New England Journal of Medicine.* **360**(3): 225–35. (MC-276907)

39 Gill SS, Bronskill SE, Normand SL, Anderson GM, *et al.* (2007) Antipsychotic drug use and mortality in older adults with dementia. *Annals of Internal Medicine.* **146**(11): 775–86.

40 Douglas IJ, Smeeth L. (2008) Exposure to antipsychotics and risk of stroke: self controlled case series study. *British Medical Journal.* **337**: a1227. (RS-6790)

41 Sacchetti E, Trifiro G, Caputi A, Turrina C, *et al.* (2008) Risk of stroke with typical and atypical anti-psychotics: a retrospective cohort study including unexposed subjects. *Journal of Psychopharmacology.* **22**(1): 39–46. (RS-74162)

42 Hollenhorst J, Munte S, Friedrich L, Heine J, *et al.* (2001) Using intranasal midazolam spray to prevent claustrophobia induced by MR imaging. *American Journal of Roentgenology.* **176**(4): 865–8. (RCT-54)

43 Rogers P, Gournay K. (2001) Phobias: nature, assessment and treatment. *Nursing Standard.* **15**(30): 37–43. (R, 29 refs)

44 Blomhoff S, Haug TT, Hellstrom K, Holme I, *et al.* (2001) Randomised controlled general practice

trial of sertraline, exposure therapy and combined treatment in generalised social phobia. *British Journal of Psychiatry*. **179**: 23–30. (RCT-387)

45 Anderson T, Watson M, Davidson R. (2008) The use of cognitive behavioural therapy techniques for anxiety and depression in hospice patients: a feasibility study. *Palliative Medicine*. **22**(7): 814–21. (OS-11)

46 Brittlebank A, Regnard C. (1990) Terror or depression? A case report. *Palliative Medicine*. **4**: 317–19.

47 Ramsay N. (1992) Referral to a liaison psychiatrist from a palliative care unit. *Palliative Medicine*. **6**: 54–60.

48 Sheldon FM. (2000) Dimensions of the role of the social worker in palliative care. *Palliative Medicine*. **14**(6): 491–8. (R, 14 refs)

49 Moorey S, Greer S. (2002) Cognitive techniques II: applications of cognitive techniques to common problems. In: *Cognitive Behaviour Therapy for People with Cancer*. Oxford: Oxford University Press. pp. 121–6. (Ch)

Confusional states (delirium and dementia)[1]

CLINICAL DECISIONS

1 Is there doubt that this is delirium?
2 Pursue the cause with a delirium screen.
3 Start treating the cause if possible.
4 Is dementia also present?
5 Is severe agitation present?
6 Is hyperactivity becoming difficult to manage?
7 Is the delirium persisting?
8 Once resolved, explore if the patient and/or relatives and/or staff understand what happened.

KEY POINTS

- The early stages of delirium are often missed and yet management of the cause is much easier at this stage.
- Hypoactive delirium is the commonest presentation and is often missed.
- Delirium can develop in the presence of a dementia.
- A delirium screen should be routine if delirium is suspected.
- Adequate staffing is essential – often having someone to sit with the patient is all that is required.
- Non-drug measures are the first-line treatment and will help any type of delirium.
- For hyperactive delirium, drugs are a last resort and should only be used under specific conditions.

INTRODUCTION

Acute confusional state (delirium): four features are typical of delirium, 1) acute onset and fluctuating course; 2) inattention; 3) disorganized thinking; and 4) altered level of alertness. Over 80% have a hypoactive type which is commonly missed. Delirium is common in the terminal stages of advanced disease,[2–7] but is not always a terminal event.[8]

Chronic confusional state (dementia) can appear similar to delirium, but with a history of years or months, symptoms that fluctuate less, and the patient's alertness is unlikely to have changed. It is not a single illness, but all variants share common features with an increasingly severe disturbance of multiple higher functions, deterioration in emotional control, social behavior, and motivation. The number of people with dementia is increasing,[9] and the effects on partners and relatives are profound.[10] However, people with dementia, their partners and relatives can be helped to cope and can achieve improvements in a patient's quality of life both at home and in residential and specialist settings. This often requires the input of a wide range of services including specialist dementia care services.

1 IS THIS A DELIRIUM?

There are several conditions that might be misinterpreted as a delirium, such as dementia, intellectual disability, severe depression, severe anxiety, hypothyroidism, severe parkinsonism, or psychosis, although all of these can be present at the same time as delirium. Hypoactive delirium is commonly missed despite this type being present in over 80% of delirium cases, since patients seem settled and comfortable.[11,12] Early delirium may present with only mild anxiety, restlessness, and insomnia.

Diagnosing delirium: it is often assumed that the diagnosis is easy, but this usually is only true for patients with hyperactive delirium. It is wrong to assume that delirium is indicated by disorientation (which is a poor indicator of delirium). In addition, tests of cognitive function cannot identify delirium. Dysgraphia is a sensitive test with good specificity,[13] and a way to test this is the clock-face drawing test.[14] Ask the patient to draw a clock face with all the numbers, and the hands in the 10-to-2pm position. Some patients, especially those with paranoid thoughts, may refuse to complete this test.

2 THE DELIRIUM SCREEN

The commonest causes of delirium are drugs, organ failure, hypoxia, infection, and hypercalcemia, many of which can be treated.[15] Dehydration may contribute to acute confusion but the evidence that rehydration alone is helpful is equivocal.[16–20]

Immediate checks include standard observations as well as S_pO_2, glucose, hydration, and excluding urinary retention and fecal loading.

In the first hour several causes need to be excluded: infection (check urine, auscultate chest, exclude cellulitis, consider septicemia); drugs (check for drug interactions and any chemicals that have been recently started or stopped, taking into account 5 half-lives of each drug or chemical (e.g. alcohol)); biochemical problems; cardiovascular problems (heart failure, bradycardia, hypotension); and cerebrovascular problems (CVA, blood hyperviscosity, hypoxia, cerebral metastases).

In a patient with cancer, a CT scan of head is the *last* test to perform, not the first!

Clinical decision	If YES carry out the action below
1 Is there doubt that this is delirium?	• **Features of delirium:** 1) Acute onset and fluctuating course; 2) Inattention; 3) Disorganized thinking; 4) Altered level of alertness. Don't miss the quiet uncomplaining patient with these symptoms (= hypoactive delirium). • **Consider** dementia, intellectual disability, severe depression, severe anxiety, hypothyroidism, severe parkinsonism or psychosis.

<table>
<tr><th>Clinical decision</th><th>If YES carry out the action below</th></tr>
<tr><td colspan="2">2 Pursue the cause with a delirium screen:
• Immediately: BP, temp, RR, HR, glucose, oxygen saturation (S_pO_2), signs of trauma, focal neurological deficit, hydration status, exclude urinary retention and fecal loading.
• In the first hour: exclude infection, check for drugs or chemicals recently started or stopped, check bloodwork (CRP/ESR, FBC, U&E, corrected calcium, LFTs, TSH, glucose), exclude any cerebro- or cardio-vascular causes.</td></tr>
<tr><td colspan="2">3 Start treating the cause if possible.
Some patients may refuse treatment. Check their capacity for making this decision. If they do not have capacity for this decision, proceed in their best interests (see Decisions around capacity, p. 267).
• Ensure that there are sufficient staff (organize a sitter if necessary), unnecessary moves are avoided, sensory aids are in place, the patient is kept hydrated, and non-essential drugs are stopped (especially anticholinergics).
• Exclude depression, "frozen terror," hypothyroidism, parkinsonism, recent physical or psychological distress.
• Explain what is happening and what you are doing to help. The explanation may have to be repeated.
• Encourage visits by friends and family, daytime activity, sleep.
• Explore creating a stable environment: ensure the bed area is light and quiet (move to single room if necessary), minimize staff changes, constantly re-orientate. Avoid urinary catheters and anything that restricts freedom around the room, bed, or chair.</td></tr>
<tr><td>4 Is dementia also present?</td><td>• If available, contact the dementia care team involved.
• If this diagnosis is new consider referral to liaison psychiatry for assessment once the delirium has settled.</td></tr>
<tr><td>5 Is severe agitation present?</td><td>Is there is an immediate risk to health or safety of staff or patient?
• Ensure: you do not challenge the patient directly; one-to-one supervision of the patient is available; you seek an urgent review by a senior member of the clinical team.
• Explore advice from the liaison psychiatry teams.</td></tr>
<tr><td>6 Is the hyperactivity becoming difficult to manage?</td><td>• Ensure the safety of the patient and staff.
• If the patient has alcohol withdrawal: start a benzodiazepine, e.g. lorazepam 0.5–1 mg q8h (follow local protocol).
• If drug management of hyperactivity is necessary:
If the distress is mild – haloperidol 0.5–1 mg PO q6h PRN (peak effect 2–6 hr). The goal is a reduction in distress without sedation.
If the distress is severe – haloperidol 1–2.5 mg SC/IM q1h PRN (peak effect 10–20 min). The goal is drowsiness, especially if urgent treatment is needed.
• Senior clinical review is essential within 24 hours especially if:
— 3 doses of haloperidol have been given without benefit
— higher doses are needed (e.g. if urgent treatment cannot be given because of persisting agitation).</td></tr>
<tr><td>7 Is the delirium persisting?</td><td>• Ensure: the senior clinician responsible has reviewed the patient and the partner and relatives have received an explanation and support.
• Consider: persisting dehydration, organic causes (e.g. hypothyroidism, subdural hematoma, limbic encephalitis), psychiatric causes (dementia, psychosis, agitated depression), unknown or hidden chemical abuse (alcohol or drugs).
• If there is still no clear solution: ask for help from the liaison psychiatry team.</td></tr>
<tr><td colspan="2">8 • Explore if the patient has unpleasant memories of the delirium episode.
• Explain what happened.
• Ensure that all the patient's key carers are informed of the delirium episode so that they can be aware of the increased risk of delirium in similar circumstances in the future.</td></tr>
</table>

Adapted from delirium guideline[1]
cd= clinical decision

3 START TREATMENT

If the cause has been identified, treatment should start.

Stop non-essential drugs

Since drugs are a common cause of delirium or may worsen its effects, any that are not essential should be stopped, especially anticholinergics.

Hydration

Dehydration is common in delirium and may cause delirium or worsen its effects. It increases the risk of falls through postural hypotension, and reduces renal function (sometimes dangerously). Look out for a dry mouth, sagging skin (reduced skin turgor), or dark urine.

Oral hydration can be encouraged by keeping a record of fluid intake, using tempting drinks (the carer, partner, or relative will tell you which ones they enjoy most), encouraging frequent small drinks (e.g. at least 3 swallows every 30 min in the day), and by making sure that water is always available and in reach. Patients may need to be reassured if they are worried about urinary incontinence related to rehydration.

If additional hydration is needed subcutaneous hydration is efficient and well tolerated in *hypo*-active delirium, but may not be tolerated in patients with *hyper*-active features. The IV route is rarely tolerated in any type of delirium unless the patient is too ill to notice and rapid hydration is urgently needed. SC or IV needle insertion can be made less distressing by using local anesthetic cream (e.g. EMLA) one hour before insertion (*see* p. 178 for advice on SC sites). Then bandage or cover the cannula to ensure it stays in place.

Working together

Confusional states can be frightening for patients, family, and staff. An informed, interdisciplinary approach is essential.[21]

Non-drug measures

Most patients are frightened and distressed by their experience, but a number of measures can help to reduce the distress:

Keep them safe: sufficient staff need to be with the patient, but in many cases this may only need a sitter to be present. Ensure they do not wander off alone or near risk areas (e.g. stairs, open windows, access to other patients' rooms or drugs).

Encourage visits: encourage visits by friends and family at times that suit the patient.

Explanation: confused patients can understand explanations, although if their concentration is impaired the explanation may have to be repeated several times. Assessing their mental capacity may be necessary since if this is lacking, treatment decisions will have to be made in their best interests (*see* p. 267). It is also important to provide the partner and relatives with information.[22] Families can help to identify if a patient is distressed.

Allow them to walk if they want to do so (supervised if necessary)

Avoid restraint: physical restriction, including the use of chairs or bed tables to block a patient in one place, often causes more agitation, while a gentle but assertive request with an explanation often works.

If sensory impairment is present arrange for the patient to have visual and hearing aids.

Ensure the environment is stable and suitable: unnecessary moves should be avoided between beds, wards, or hospitals. A stable environment is important and can be created by ensuring the bed area is light and quiet (move to a single room if necessary and available), minimizing staff changes, constantly re-orienting the patient, avoiding urinary catheters.

Encourage daytime activity: explore with the patient and relative, ways of stimulating their interest such as walking, talking, music, or watching TV.

Help with the sleep protocol: avoid tea or coffee after 6pm, and use relaxation or quiet music.

Allow patients to be up at night if necessary, under supervision (this may need a night sitter). This is often preferable to forcing a change in the day–night pattern with medication.

4 IS DEMENTIA PRESENT?

Delirium can develop on the background of dementia. Once the delirium has been treated it can become clear that cognitive impairment is present. If the patient has been previously diagnosed with dementia, the local dementia care team, if there is one, can be contacted for advice. However, if dementia is newly suspected, a referral to liaison psychiatry should be considered.

Behavioral and psychological symptoms of dementia (BPSD) can include paranoia, hallucinations, depression, and agitation. Aggression is common and remains an issue at the end of life.[23,24] Such patients often need admissions for assessment or treatment by specialist dementia teams.

5 IS SEVERE AGITATION PRESENT?

There are rare occasions in hospital or hospice when a patient is so agitated that it is impossible to keep them safe, or to ensure the safety of staff. This is unlikely to occur suddenly and highlights the need for early identification and prompt treatment of delirium.

Do not challenge the patient directly since this may prompt further agitation or aggression. Ensure that a sitter is available at all times when the patient is awake (initially this may be one-to-one supervision when the patient is awake) to limit the risk of harm to the patient or to others. If the hospice or hospital policy allows, the sitter can be a volunteer, unqualified nurse or relative who has received some basic instruction in sitting with patients who have hyperactive delirium.

Ensuring the safety of the patient: there are several considerations:
- Are they a physical danger to themselves or others?
- Can they leave the unit without being noticed?
- Are they drinking and eating?
- Are they taking their usual medication?

Ensuring the safety of staff:
- Is the patient paranoid and/or aggressive?
- Are staff aware of any paranoia or aggression in the patient?
- Do they know how to help safely?

Urgent review is needed by a senior member of the clinical team who may decide that further help is needed from the local liaison psychiatry team.

6 IS THE HYPERACTIVITY BECOMING DIFFICULT TO MANAGE?

If other measures are insufficient, medication may be required, although this should always be a last resort.

Haloperidol remains the first-line choice with few adverse effects in the short term, *but with the following conditions:*[25]

- It should not be used in Parkinson's disease (because it worsens the movement disorder) or in dementia with Lewy bodies (because these patients can develop serious adverse effects to the haloperidol).
- It is important to have an understanding of its long half-life (16 hours to several days) which means it will take at least 2 to 6 days to build to peak blood levels (possibly a week or more) when increasing drowsiness will make management more difficult.[26]
- Injectable haloperidol *taken orally* is odorless, colorless, and tasteless but if it is given covertly to a patient without capacity this must be documented and the need for covert administration must be reviewed daily (*see* Drug Information, p. 312).
- It is necessary to stop concurrent drugs that might increase the risk of extrapyramidal reactions, e.g. metoclopramide, amitriptyline.

Benzodiazepines are not first-line drugs for hyperactive delirium, since it has long been known that they can worsen delirium.[27] The only exception is delirium due to alcohol withdrawal where benzodiazepines are usually first-line treatments.[28] In addition, a benzodiazepine may have to be the first-line drug if haloperidol is contraindicated such as Lewy body dementia.

Benzodiazepines can be added to haloperidol to induce drowsiness and enable treatment if this is in the patient's best interests, but with the disadvantage that this compromises attempts to interact with the patient. Lorazepam (PO or SL) or midazolam (SC or buccal) are better choices than diazepam whose very long half-life often causes problems through accumulation.

7 IS THE DELIRIUM PERSISTING?

Most cases of delirium start to improve within one week. Persisting delirium is often due to additional causes of delirium. On other occasions there is a coexistent cause of cognitive impairment such as dementia, or a problem that mimics cognitive impairment such as severe anxiety.[29] However, some causes of delirium can persist for weeks or months such as paraneoplastic limbic encephalitis associated with cancer.[30,31] Unless the primary cause can be treated, such patients may need long-term specialist care.

REFERENCES: CONFUSIONAL STATES

B = book; C = comment; Ch = chapter; CS-n = case study-no. of cases; CT-n = controlled trial-no. of cases; E = editorial; GC = group consensus; I = interviews; Let = Letter; LS = laboratory study; MC = multi-center; OS-n = open study-no. of cases; R = review; RCT-n = randomized controlled trial-no. of cases; RS-n = retrospective survey-no. of cases; SA = systematic or meta analysis.

1 St. Oswald's Hospice, and the Northumberland Tyne&Wear NHS Trust, Delirium Guidelines Group. (2009) *Managing Delirium in the Inpatient Setting, v17.* claudregnard@stoswaldsuk.org

2 Caraceni A, Nanni O, Maltoni M, Piva L, *et al.* (2000) Impact of delirium on the short term prognosis of advanced cancer patients. Italian Multicenter Study Group on Palliative Care. *Cancer.* **89**(5): 1145–9. (OS-393)

3 Fainsinger RL, De Moissac D, Mancini I, Oneschuk D. (2000) Sedation for delirium and other symptoms in terminally ill patients in Edmonton. *Journal of Palliative Care.* **16**(2): 5–10. (OS-150)

4 Morita T, Tsunoda J, Inoue S, Chihara S. (1999) Survival prediction of terminally ill cancer patients by clinical symptoms: development of a simple indicator. *Japanese Journal of Clinical Oncology.* **29**(3): 156–9. (OS-245)

5 Hall P, Schroder C, Weaver L. (2002) The last 48 hours of life in long-term care: a focused chart audit. *Journal of the American Geriatrics Society.* **50**(3): 501–6. (RS-185)

6 Lawlor PG, Gagnon B, Mancini IL, Pereira JL, *et al.* (2000) Occurrence, causes, and outcome of delirium in patients with advanced cancer: a prospective study. *Archives of Internal Medicine.* **160**(6): 786–94. (OS-113)

7 Pereira J, Hanson J, Bruera E. (1997) The frequency and clinical course of cognitive impairment in patients with terminal cancer. *Cancer*. **79**(4): 835–42. (RS-321)

8 Leonard M, Raju B, Conroy M, Donnelly S, *et al.* (2008) Reversibility of delirium in terminally ill patients and predictors of mortality. *Palliative Medicine*. **22**(7): 848–54. (OS-121)

9 LSE (London School of Economics), King's College and the Alzheimer's Society. (2007) *Dementia UK*. All-Party Parliamentary Group on Dementia. (2008) *Always a Last Resort: inquiry into the prescription of antipsychotic drugs to people with dementia living in care homes*. HMSO: London.

10 Butler R. (2008) The carers of people with dementia. *British Medical Journal*. **336**: 1260–1.

11 Spiller JA, Keen JC. (2006) Hypoactive delirium: assessing the extent of the problem for inpatient specialist palliative care. *Palliative Medicine*. **20**(1): 17–23. (OS-100)

12 Fang CK, Chen HW, Liu SI, Lin CJ, *et al.* (2008) Prevalence, detection and treatment of delirium in terminal cancer inpatients: a prospective survey. *Japanese Journal of Clinical Oncology*. **38**(1): 56–63. (OS-228)

13 Adamis D, Reich S, Treloar A, Macdonald AJ, Martin FC. (2006) Dysgraphia in elderly delirious medical inpatients. *Aging-Clinical and Experimental Research*. **18**(4): 334–9. (OS)

14 Macleod AD, Whitehead LE. (1997) Dysgraphia and terminal delirium. *Palliative Medicine*. **11**(2): 127–32. (CT-10)

15 Morita T, Tei Y, Tsunoda J, Inoue S, Chihara S. (2001) Underlying pathologies and their associations with clinical features in terminal delirium of cancer patients. *Journal of Pain and Symptom Management*. **22**(6): 997–1006. (OS-237)

16 Cerchietti L, Navigante A, Sauri A, Palazzo F. (2000) Clinical trial: hypodermoclysis for control of dehydration in terminal-stage cancer. *International Journal of Palliative Nursing*. **6**(8): 370–4. (RCT-42)

17 Soden K, Hoy A, Hoy W, Clelland S. (2002) Artificial hydration in patients dying in a district general hospital. *Palliative Medicine*. **16**(6): 542–3. (OS-111)

18 Fainsinger RL, Bruera E. (1997) When to treat dehydration in a terminally ill patient? *Supportive Care in Cancer*. **5**(3): 205–11. (R, 54 refs)

19 Bruera E, Franco JJ, Maltoni M, Watanabe S, Suarez-Almazor M. (1995) Changing pattern of agitated impaired mental status in patients with advanced cancer: association with cognitive monitoring, hydration, and opioid rotation. *Journal of Pain and Symptom Management*. **10**(4): 287–91. (RS-279)

20 Dunphy K, Finlay I, Rathbone G, Gilbert J, Hicks F. (1995) Rehydration in palliative and terminal care: if not – why not? *Palliative Medicine*. **9**(3): 221–8. (R, 32 refs)

21 McAndrew C, Vandivort M. (2001) The six principles of excellent clinical care for dementia: nurse practitioners and physicians working together. *Nurse Practitioner Forum*. **12**(1): 12–22. (R, 29 refs)

22 Gagnon P, Charbonneau C, Allard P, Soulard C, Dumont S, Fillon L. (2002) Delirium in advanced cancer: a psychoeducational intervention for family caregivers. *Journal of Palliative Care*. **18**(4): 253–61. (CT-124)

23 O'Malley KJ, Orengo CA, Kunik ME, *et al.* (2002). Measuring aggression in older adults: a latent variable modeling approach. *Aging and Mental Health*. **6**: 231–8.

24 Eustace A, Coen R, Walsh C, *et al.* (2002). A longitudinal evaluation of behavioural and psychological symptoms of probable Alzheimer's disease. *International Journal of Geriatric Psychiatry*. **17**: 968–73.

25 Michaud L, Bula C, Berney A, Camus V, *et al.* (2007) Delirium Guidelines Development Group. Delirium: guidelines for general hospitals. *Journal of Psychosomatic Research*. **62**(3): 371–83. (R, 148 refs)

26 de Leon J, Diaz FJ, Wedlund P, Josiassen RC, Cooper TB, Simpson GM. (2004) Haloperidol half-life after chronic dosing. *Journal of Clinical Psychopharmacology*. **24**(6): 656–60.

27 Breitbart W, Marotta R, Platt MM, Weisman H, *et al.* (1996) A double-blind trial of haloperidol, chlorpromazine, and lorazepam in the treatment of delirium in hospitalized AIDS patients. *American Journal of Psychiatry*. **153**(2): 231–7. (RCT-244)

28 Bayard M, McIntyre J, Hill KR, Woodside J Jr. (2004) Alcohol withdrawal syndrome. *American Family Physician*. **69**(6): 1443–50. (R, 29 refs)

29 Brittlebank A, Regnard C. (1990) Terror or depression? A case report. *Palliative Medicine*. **4**: 317–19. (CS-1)

30 Anderson NE, Barber PA. (2008) Limbic encephalitis: a review. *Journal of Clinical Neuroscience*. **15**(9): 961–71. (CS-4, R 88 refs)

31 Tuzun E, Dalmau J. (2007) Limbic encephalitis and variants: classification, diagnosis and treatment. *Neurologist*. **13**(5): 261–71. (R, 71 refs)

NOTES

Withdrawal and depression

CLINICAL DECISION AND ACTION CHECKLIST

1 Acknowledge the withdrawal
2 Is this the patient's usual behavior?
3 Is the patient unwilling to continue talking?
4 Does the patient feel everything is meaningless?
5 Is anger present?
6 Are fears, guilt, or shame present?
7 Is the patient feeling depressed?
8 Is the withdrawal persisting?

KEY POINTS

- Withdrawal can occur for many reasons, but depression is often missed.
- Depression may respond within two weeks of starting an antidepressant.

INTRODUCTION

Withdrawal has many possible causes and these should be excluded before assuming a depression is present. The proportion of patients with advanced disease who have a clinical depression varies between studies and depends partly on the assessment tools used. It has been suggested that a median of 15% of cancer patients and up to 25% of AIDS patients suffer from depression.[1,2]

GETTING STARTED

Acknowledge what is happening

Although this may seem unnecessary, it gives the person a clear message that you have noticed their withdrawal and that you are taking it seriously.

Causes of withdrawal

This may be the person's usual behavior, but other causes include depression, distraction due to pain, a delirium, drowsiness (caused by drugs, infection or a biochemical disturbance), exhaustion, severe anxiety or fear, collusion preventing the person from talking for fear of upsetting a partner or relative, reduced facial expression due to drugs (e.g. haloperidol, metoclopramide), or neurological disease (e.g. Parkinson's, motor neurone disease/ALS).

DEPRESSION

Depression can be missed since it is easily misinterpreted as sadness or can be masked by anxiety.[3–7] Recognizing depression depends on the patient's manner, identifying clues in interviews and the use of screening tools.[8] Screening tools increase the likelihood of diagnosis and treatment,[9–11] but none is ideal.[12] The Hospital Anxiety and Depression (HAD) scale needs to have a higher cut-off threshold to be useful.[2,6] The Edinburgh postnatal depression scale or Geriatric Depression Scale may be more useful screening tools.[13–15] A simple screening question may be "Have you had a depressed mood most of the day nearly every day?".[6,16,17] Adding a second question about loss of interest increases the diagnostic sensitivity to 91% and the specificity to 86%.[18]

The diagnosis of depression is made on the following characteristics:

1 A persistent feeling of a depressed mood >2 weeks for >50% of the time in the absence of a psychosis.
2 This is a change in their usual mood.
3 There is a loss of interest and enjoyment in activities (anhedonia).
4 Three or more of the following depressive-related symptoms are present: diurnal variation in mood; repeated or early morning wakening; impaired concentration; feelings of hopelessness, guilt, shame, or feeling a burden to others; thoughts of self-harm; desire for hastened death (loss of energy, appetite, and sex drive are less useful).

The diagnostic criteria of depression (adapted from DSM IV)[19,20]

Loss of energy, appetite, and sex drive are more likely to be due to the disease itself and cannot be used as diagnostic indicators. In contrast, thoughts of self-harm and a desire for a hastened death are a strong indicator of depression.[21–23] Suicidal thoughts are not always an indicator of depression since some patients will express a realistic wish that they would prefer to be dead rather than be in pain, a burden, or immobile. Other patients may have prepared for death, and be impatient "to have it over with," but will still not be depressed. Feelings of hopelessness are more likely to indicate genuine suicidal thoughts and sustained suicidal thoughts requires closer assessment and screening for depression.[24,25] Suicides are rare in palliative care patients,[26,27] but they are associated with a fear of losing autonomy and independence.[28]

HELPING THE WITHDRAWN PATIENT

Causes of withdrawal should be treated if possible, but the most helpful approach is developing trust between the carer and the withdrawn person. Continuing to show kindness, despite the person's

Clinical decision	If YES carry out the action below
1 Acknowledge the withdrawal: e.g. "You seem quiet and withdrawn today. Can I help?"	
2 Is this the patient's usual behavior?	Normally introverted or quiet personality: offer time to establish trust.
3 Is the patient unwilling to continue talking?	• **Establish a dialogue:** acknowledge the difficulties and negotiate further discussion (e.g. "Can you bear to tell me why you find it so difficult to talk to me just now?"). • **Exclude the following:** *Confusional state: see Confusional states*, p. 245. *Distraction by a persistent symptom* such as pain. *Drugs causing dyskinesia* (e.g. amitriptyline, haloperidol, hyoscine hydrobromide (scopolamine), metoclopramide, methotrimeprazine). *Neurological causes:* motor neurone disease/ALS, Parkinson's disease, parkinsonism due to brain damage (e.g. encephalitis, dementia, tumor). *Fatigue and weakness related to the illness, or causes of drowsiness: see Fatigue, drowsiness, lethargy and weakness*, p. 149. *Collusion with a partner or relative that prevents the person from talking openly: see* p. 28 and cd-7, p. 29. *Severe anxiety or fear ("frozen terror"): see Anxiety*, p. 239. • **If no cause can be found:** acknowledge the patient's refusal to continue and express a willingness to help in the future if needed.
4 Does the patient feel everything is meaningless?	• Explore what it was that previously gave their life meaning. • Ask whether they would like to contact a spiritual advisor, priest or chaplain. • Offer counseling. • Exclude a clinical depression (*see* cd-7 on p. 257).
5 Is anger present?	• *See Anger*, p. 235.
6 Are fears, guilt, or shame present?	Identify, clarify, and specify the concerns: *see Helping the person to share their problems*, p. 15. • **If the patient is apprehensive, tense, or on edge:** *see Anxiety*, p. 239. • **If guilt or shame are present:** *If this is unrealistic:* help the patient to reframe thoughts about the emotion. *If this is realistic:* check if the patient could accept self-forgiveness. Exclude a clinical depression since guilt and shame are common in depression.

Adapted from Maguire, Faulkner and Regnard[29]
cd = clinical decision

perception of hopelessness, demonstrates to the person that they are worthwhile.

Depression should be treated if present,[30] but there is little research on treating depression in advanced disease and it is necessary to use evidence from other depressed patients.[2,31] Antidepressants are still the quickest way to achieve a response in moderate or severe depression and if the depression started recently the response may occur in less than two weeks. Consequently, antidepressants should be considered even at the end of life.[32]

Tricyclic antidepressants: low-dose tricyclics (below 100 mg/day) may be as effective as higher doses.[33]

SSRI and other antidepressants: SSRI antidepressants can have as many adverse effects as tricyclic antidepressants.[34,35] Mirtazapine may have a faster onset of action but is no more effective than other SSRIs.[36] Nausea and vomiting are common on the first dose of SSRIs and SNRIs and a withdrawal reaction (headache, nausea, paresthesia, dizziness, and anxiety) can occur on abrupt withdrawal.[37] Venlafaxine can reduce neuropathic pain and may be helpful in patients with coexisting depression and pain.[38]

Psychostimulants: methylphenidate has a role if a rapid response is needed, especially in a very withdrawn patient whose prognosis suggests there is insufficient time to respond to conventional antidepressants.[39–41] Evidence suggests that its use in cancer patients is a safe and effective treatment.[42]

Herbal treatments: if adverse effects are a problem and the depression is mild or moderate, the herb St. John's wort (*Hypericum perforatum*) is effective.[43]

Non-oral routes: there are no non-oral preparations of antidepressants available in North America. Methylphenidate can be given buccally.

Length of action: antidepressants with a longer half-life can accumulate, but they will continue to be active for a week or more if a patient is unable to take oral medication. Antidepressants with short lives are less likely to accumulate but will wear off quickly when stopped, which may cause withdrawal symptoms.

Antidepressant	Half-life	Approx. time to reach steady state
venlafaxine	5 hr	25 hr
imipramine	19 hr	4 days
clomipramine	21 hr	4–5 days
sertraline	26 hr	5–6 days
paroxetine	26 hr	5–6 days
mirtazapine	30 hr	6 days
citalopram	36 hr	7 days
fluoxetine	7 days	35 days

Antidepressant withdrawal: the commonest problem is a recurrence of depression, although this is less if cognitive behavioral therapy (CBT) has been used (*see* opposite). If any short-acting antidepressant is suddenly stopped patients can develop nausea, vomiting, and anorexia, together with headache, giddiness, "chills," insomnia, and sometimes extreme motor restlessness. Withdrawal symptoms due to stopping an SSRI include paresthesia, sleep disturbances, fatigue, influenza-like symptoms, and sweating. For most dying patients, antidepressant withdrawal is not a problem since antidepressant activity will be present for 4 days or more. However, patients on venlafaxine may develop withdrawal symptoms after 24 hours, and this may require treatment (*see* cd-4 in *Emergencies*, p. 333).

Switching antidepressants: this is sometimes needed because of adverse effects or inadequate treatment. Fluoxetine should be stopped for 3–5

Clinical decision	If YES carry out the action below
7 Is the patient feeling depressed?	**A patient is likely to have a clinical depression if the following are present:** 1 Persistent low mood (>2 weeks for >50% of time) 2 A change to their usual mood 3 A loss of interest and enjoyment 4 Three other depressive-related symptoms (*see* text on p. 254). • Start citalopram 20 mg in the morning or mirtazapine 15 mg at bedtime. *If neuropathic pain is present*, consider using venlafaxine 37.5–75 mg daily. *If adverse effects are a problem*, and the depression is of mild to moderate severity, consider St. John's wort 170 mg daily.
8 Is the withdrawal persisting?	• Refer for specialist advice and help, including cognitive behavioral therapy. • If a rapid response is needed, consider methylphenidate 5 mg in the morning, titrated up to 20 mg if necessary.[44]

Adapted from Maguire, Faulkner and Regnard[29]
cd = clinical decision

days before slowly starting the new antidepressant. Other antidepressants can be gradually reduced and the new antidepressant increased slowly at the same time, but the advice of a psychiatrist should be sought when switching antidepressants, especially between different types.

Duration of treatment: treatment with antidepressants should continue for 4–9 months.[45]

PERSISTING WITHDRAWAL

Cognitive behavioral therapy is helpful in suitable patients, particularly in preventing relapse.[32,46–48] CBT is as effective as antidepressants but takes longer to be effective.[49] If the depression persists or has complicating features (e.g. agitation, paranoia) it is essential to ask for advice and help from psychiatry colleagues.[50]

REFERENCES: WITHDRAWAL AND DEPRESSION

B = book; C = comment; Ch = chapter; CS-n = case study-no. of cases; CT-n = controlled trial-no. of cases; E = editorial; GC = group consensus; I = interviews; LS = laboratory study; MC = multi-center; OS-n = open study-no. of cases; R = review; RCT-n = randomized controlled trial-no. of cases; RS-n = retrospective survey-no. of cases; SA = systematic or meta analysis-no. of trials.

1 Breibart W. (2009) Psychiatric symptoms in palliative care. In: Hanks G, Cherney NI, Christakis NA, Fallon M, Kaasa S, Portenoy RK, eds. *Oxford Textbook of Palliative Medicine, 4th ed.* Oxford: Oxford University Press. (Ch)

2 Hotopf M, Chidgey J, Addington-Hall J, Lan Ly K. (2002) Depression in advanced disease: a systematic review. Part 1. Prevalence and case finding. *Palliative Medicine*. **16**: 81–97. (SA, 77 refs)

3 Lloyd-Williams M. (2002) Is it appropriate to screen palliative care patients for depression? *American Journal of Hospice and Palliative Care.* **19**(2): 112–14. (OS)

4 Stiefel R, Die Trill M, Berney A, Olarte JM, Razavi A. (2001) Depression in palliative care: a pragmatic report from the Expert Working Group of the European Association for Palliative Care. *Supportive Care in Cancer.* **9**(7): 477–88. (R, 113 refs)

5 Lloyd-Williams M, Friedman T, Rudd N. (1999) A survey of antidepressant prescribing in the terminally ill. *Palliative Medicine.* **13**(3): 243–8. (OS-1046)

6 Lloyd-Williams M, Spiller J, Ward J. (2003) Which depression screening tools should be used in palliative care? *Palliative Medicine*. **17**(1): 40–3. (SA, 15 refs)

7 Kessler D, Bennewith O, Lewis G, Sharp D. (2002) Detection of depression and anxiety in primary care: follow up study. *British Medical Journal.* **325**: 1016–17. (OS-179)

8 Peveler R, Carson A, Rodin G. (2002) ABC of psychological medicine: depression in medical patients. *British Medical Journal*. **323**: 149–52. (R)

9 Passik SD, Kirsh KL, Theobald D, Donaghy K, *et al.* (2002) Use of a depression screening tool and a fluoxetine-based algorithm to improve the recognition and treatment of depression in cancer patients: a demonstration project. *Journal of Pain and Symptom Management.* **24**(3): 318–27. (OS-35)

10 Lloyd-Williams M. (2001) Screening for depression in palliative care patients: a review. *European Journal of Cancer Care.* **10**(1): 31–5. (R, 40 refs)

11 Lloyd-Williams M. (2002) The stability of depression scores in patients who are receiving palliative care. *Journal of Pain and Symptom Management.* **24**(6): 593–7. (OS-72)

12 Urch CE, Chamberlain J, Field G. (1998) The drawback of the hospital anxiety and depression scale in the assessment of depression in hospice inpatients. *Palliative Medicine*. **12**: 395–6. (OS-52)

13 Lloyd-Williams M, Friedman T, Rudd N. (2000) Criterion validation of the Edinburgh postnatal depression scale as a screening tool for depression in patients with advanced metastatic cancer. *Journal of Pain and Symptom Management.* **20**(4): 259–65. (OS-100)

14 Lloyd-Williams M, Shiels C, Dowrick C. (2007) The development of the Brief Edinburgh Depression Scale (BEDS) to screen for depression in patients with advanced cancer. *Journal of Affective Disorders.* **99**(1–3): 259–64. (CT-246)

15 Crawford GB, Robinson JA. (2008) The geriatric depression scale in palliative care. *Palliative and Supportive Care*. **6**(3): 213–23. (OS-84)

16 Chochinov HM, Wilson KG, Enns M, Lander S. (1994) Prevalence of depression in the terminally ill: effects of diagnostic criteria and symptom threshold judgements. *American Journal of Psychiatry*. **154**: 674–6. (I-134)

17 Whooley MA, Avins AL, Miranda J, Browner WS. (1997) Case-finding instruments for depression: two questions are as good as many. *Journal of General Internal Medicine.* **12**(7): 439–45. (OS-536)

18 Mitchell AJ. (2008) Are one or two simple questions sufficient to detect depression in cancer and palliative care? A Bayesian meta-analysis. *British Journal of Cancer*. **98**(12): 1934–43. (SA-12)

19 American Psychiatric Association. (1994) *Diagnostic and Statistical Manual of Mental Disorders – Fourth Edition (DSM-IV)*. Washington: American Psychiatric Association. (B)

20 Lloyd-Williams M. (2002) Diagnosis and treatment of depression in palliative care. *European Journal of Palliative Care.* **9**(5): 186–8. (R, 21 refs)

21 Lloyd-Williams M. (2002) How common are thoughts of self-harm in a UK palliative care population? *Supportive Care in Cancer.* **10**(5): 422–4. (OS-248)

22 Breitbart W, Rosenfeld B, Pessin H, Kaim M, *et al.* (2000) Depression, hopelessness, and desire for hastened death in terminally ill patients with cancer. *Journal of the American Medical Association.* **284**(22): 2907–11. (OS-92)

23 Chochinov HM, Wilson KG, Enns M, Mowchun N, *et al.* (1995) Desire for death in the terminally ill. *American Journal of Psychiatry.* **152**(8): 1185–91. (I-200)

24 Chochinov HM, Wilson KG, Enns M, Lander S. (1998) Depression, hopelessness, and suicidal ideation in the terminally ill. *Psychosomatics.* **39**(4): 366–70. (OS-196)

25 Block SD. (2000) ACP–ASIM End-of-Life Care Consensus Panel. American College of Physicians – American Society of Internal Medicine. Assessing and managing depression in the terminally ill patient. *Annals of Internal Medicine.* **132**(3): 209–18. (R)

26 Ripamonti C, Filiberti A, Totis A, De Conno F, Tamburini M. (1999) Suicide among patients with cancer cared for at home by palliative-care teams. *Lancet.* **354**(9193): 1877–8. (Let, CS-5)

27 Grzybowska P, Finlay I. (1997) The incidence of suicide in palliative care patients. *Palliative Medicine.* **11**(4): 313–6. (Q)

28 Filiberti A, Ripamonti C, Totis A, Ventafridda V,

De Conno F, Contiero P, Tamburini M. (2001) Characteristics of terminal cancer patients who committed suicide during a home palliative care program. *Journal of Pain and Symptom Management.* **22**(1): 544–53. (I, CS-5)

29 Maguire P, Faulkner A, Regnard C. (1995) The withdrawn patient. In: *Flow Diagrams in Advanced Cancer and Other Diseases*. London: Edward Arnold. pp. 77–80. (Ch)

30 Block SD for the ACP–ASIM End-of-Life Care Consensus Panel. (2000) Assessing and managing depression in the terminally ill patient. *Annals of Internal Medicine.* **132**(3): 209–18. (R, 95 refs)

31 Lan Ly K, Chidgey J, Addington-Hall J, Hotopf M. (2002) Depression in advanced disease: a systematic review. Part 2. Treatment. *Palliative Medicine.* **16**: 279–84. (SA, 23 refs)

32 Qaseem A, Snow V, Shekelle P, Casey DE Jr., Cross JT Jr., *et al.* Clinical Efficacy Assessment Subcommittee of the American College of Physicians. (2008) Evidence-based interventions to improve the palliative care of pain, dyspnea, and depression at the end of life: a clinical practice guideline from the American College of Physicians. *Annals of Internal Medicine.* **148**(2): 141–6. (R)

33 Furukawa TA, McGuire H, Barbui C. (2002) Meta analysis of effects and side effects of low dosage tricyclic antidepressants in depression: systematic review. *British Medical Journal.* **325**: 991–5. (SA-141)

34 Anderson IM. (2001) Meta-analytical studies on new antidepressants. *British Medical Bulletin.* **57**: 161–78. (SA, 32 refs)

35 Moon CA, Vince M. (1996) Treatment of major depression in general practice: a double-blind comparison of paroxetine and lofepramine. *British Journal of Clinical Practice.* **50**(5): 240–4. (RCT-138)

36 Watanabe N, Omori IM, Nakagawa A, Cipriani A, *et al.* (2008) Multiple Meta-Analyses of New Generation Antidepressants (MANGA) Study Group. Mirtazapine versus other antidepressants in the acute-phase treatment of adults with major depression: systematic review and meta-analysis. *Journal of Clinical Psychiatry.* **69**(9): 1404–15. (SA-25, 54 refs)

37 Edwards JG, Anderson I. (1999) Systematic review and guide to selection of selective serotonin reuptake inhibitors. *Drugs.* **57**(4): 507–33. (R, 118 refs).

38 Tasmuth T, Hartel B, Kalso E. (2002) Venlafaxine in neuropathic pain following treatment of breast cancer. *European Journal of Pain.* **6**(1): 17–24. (RCT)

39 Rozans M, Dreisbach A, Lertora JJ, Kahn MJ. (2002) Palliative uses of methylphenidate in patients with cancer: a review. *Journal of Clinical Oncology.* **20**(1): 335–9. (R, 49 refs)

40 Pereira J, Bruera E. (2001) Depression with psychomotor retardation: diagnostic challenges and the use of psychostimulants. *Journal of Palliative Medicine.* **4**(1): 15–21. (CS-1)

41 Candy M, Jones L, Williams R, Tookman A, King M. (2008) Psychostimulants for depression. *Cochrane Database of Systematic Reviews.* **2**: CD006722. (SA-24, 126 refs)

42 Sood A, Barton DL, Loprinzi CL. (2006) Use of methylphenidate in patients with cancer. *American Journal of Hospice and Palliative Medicine.* **23**(1): 35–40. (R, 47 refs)

43 Linde K, Berner MM, Kriston L. (2008) St John's wort for major depression. *Cochrane Database of Systematic Reviews.* **4**: CD000448. (SA-29, 123 refs)

44 Homsi J, Walsh D, Nelson KA, LeGrand S, Davis M. (2000) Methylphenidate for depression in hospice practice: a case series. *American Journal of Hospice and Palliative Care.* **17**(6): 393–8. (CS-10)

45 Qaseem A, Snow V, Denberg TD, Forciea MA, Owens DK. Clinical Efficacy Assessment Subcommittee of American College of Physicians. (2008) Using second-generation antidepressants to treat depressive disorders: a clinical practice guideline from the American College of Physicians. *Annals of Internal Medicine.* **149**(10): 725–33. (R)

46 Blanch J, Rousaud A, Hautzinger M, Martinez E, *et al.* (2002) Assessment of the efficacy of a cognitive-behavioural group psychotherapy programme for HIV-infected patients referred to a consultation-liaison psychiatry department. *Psychotherapy and Psychosomatics.* **71**(2): 77–84. (CT-39)

47 Anderson T, Watson M, Davidson R. (2008) The use of cognitive behavioural therapy techniques for anxiety and depression in hospice patients: a feasibility study. *Palliative Medicine.* **22**(7): 814–21. (OS-10)

48 Teasdale JD, Scott J, Moore RG, Hayhurst H, *et al.* (2001) How does cognitive therapy prevent relapse in residual depression? Evidence from a controlled trial. *Journal of Consulting and Clinical Psychology.* **69**(3): 347–57. (CT-158)

49 Thompson LW, Coon DW, Gallagher-Thompson D, Sommer BR, Koin D. (2001) Comparison of desipramine and cognitive/behavioral therapy in the treatment of elderly outpatients with mild-to-moderate depression. *American Journal of Geriatric Psychiatry.* **9**(3): 225–40. (RCT-102)

50 Ramsay N. (1992) Referral to a liaison psychiatrist from a palliative care unit. *Palliative Medicine.* **6**: 54–60. (RS)

NOTES

Difficult decisions

NOTES

Making ethical choices

CLINICAL DECISION AND ACTION CHECKLIST

1 Is an alternative course of action available?
2 Is there any chance something could color your judgment?
3 Is the decision being made in the interest of someone other than the patient?
4 What values are part of this decision?
5 What will be the consequences of your action?
6 Are there professional issues?
7 Is a decision still unclear?

KEY POINTS

- Most clinical decisions have ethical aspects, but only some decisions need extensive ethical reviews.
- Asking for advice from team members and other professionals is essential.

INTRODUCTION

Difficult decisions in clinical care may involve ethical issues.[1–3] This does not mean that every difficult clinical decision is an ethical problem, or that it needs to include an extensive review of the ethical issues involved. For example, when the benefits and burdens of a treatment appear equally balanced it can be easier to present the situation as an ethical dilemma, when in reality there are no clear answers at that time. However, it can be helpful to screen for ethical issues.

THERE IS RARELY NO CHOICE

A common situation is the belief that there is no choice. In reality it is rare that no choices exist. Invariably, there may be solutions that were rejected as undesirable, but which advice or investigation indicates are feasible. An example might be the rejection of major surgery for bowel obstruction, when surgical advice indicates that a simple loop colostomy can be easily and quickly performed. It is also possible that advice or investigation uncovers solutions that had not been considered. For example, advice from a pain specialist could indicate the possibility of regional blocking procedures for an apparently intractable pain. The key here is to ask for advice, particularly as many apparent ethical dilemmas are simply situations in which not all the clinical solutions have been explored.

WHAT IS INFLUENCING THE DECISION?

Prejudice: it is difficult to believe that discrimination exists in health care. In reality, there is good evidence that some people find it harder than others to get access to health care.[4–9] This prejudice can result in morbidity and mortality.[10]

Whose interests? If the patient has capacity for this decision, only they can decide their best interests, but ensure that they are not being coerced by one or more of their family into a decision that they (the patient) do not really want. However, if the patient does not have capacity, decisions should be made in the best interests of the patient, taking into account his/her values, wishes, etc. (*see Decisions around capacity*, p. 267).

Which values? Different solutions reflect different underlying values. It can help to identify the best option if issues are considered such as the use of resources, whether an action is caring, or if an action breaks established rules.

CONSEQUENCES OF A DECISION

It is important to consider the effects of a course of action with regards to benefit, rights, and professional issues. Additional advice can be invaluable, if only to expand the discussion.

WHEN A DECISION IS STILL UNCLEAR

Even after checking through the issues and the consequences of different solutions, a clear solution can be elusive. It is essential to ensure that all necessary advice has been sought. If time is short, waiting to see developments can make a decision clearer.[11] If the situation is less urgent, a meeting bringing together the patient, partner or relative, advisors, and the multidisciplinary team may find a solution. A local ethics committee can provide useful advice or a formal forum for discussion. Courts are a last resort but can help to find a solution in rare cases where a solution is imperative.

Clinical decision	If YES carry out the action below
1 Is an alternative course of action available?	People may claim that they had no choice, but this is rarely true. • **Consider if there are:** — courses of action that you have discounted unfairly — desirable courses of action which you have yet to imagine. • **Are you sure this is an ethical issue?** Could it be a clinical decision for which there is insufficient information to make a clear decision? • **Ask for advice** from all the team or other specialists.

Clinical decision	If YES carry out the action below
2 Is there any chance something could color your judgment?	• **Review your prejudices** on age, class, ethnicity, gender, intellectual ability, lifestyle, culture, or religion.
3 Is the decision being made in the interest of someone other than the patient?	• **If the patient has capacity to make this decision:** only the patient can decide, but ensure it really is the patient's decision. • **If the patient does not have capacity for this decision:** Any treatment decision you make must be made according to the patient's best interests. This is not simply your opinion – there is a procedure to be followed (*see Decisions around capacity*, p. 267). Ensure that the decision is not being made solely in the best interests of the partner, relatives, society, or you.
4 What values are part of this decision?	• **Consider:** — is this course of action caring? — is this an appropriate use of resources? — what values are being sacrificed? — whose values are being sacrificed? — does this involve breaking a rule you would normally follow? — what would happen if everyone made this decision?
5 Will there be consequences to your action?	• **Consider whether this course of action will:** — cause harm — result in benefit to people other than the patient — violate anyone's rights or legitimate expectations.
6 Are there professional issues?	• **Consider:** — how would you advise a colleague to act in similar circumstances? — what would your colleagues think? — does professional guidance exist on this issue? — are you acting within the law? — how would you justify your decision to others, e.g. the media?
7 Is a decision still unclear?	• **Ensure that you have:** — involved the patient if they are able to contribute (if they cannot, ask the partner or relative about the patient's previously expressed views, or if there is an Advance Health Care Directive) — shared the issues with your team and asked their views — asked other colleagues for advice. • **If the harms and benefits of action are equally balanced:** *If time is short (rapid deterioration, terminal phase):* use the "rule of 3": — if deterioration is hour by hour wait 3 hours, if day by day wait 3 days. — after the wait, if the patient is worse this suggests that no intervention is appropriate, but if the patient is stable or better further intervention may be appropriate. *If time is less urgent, consider:* — a meeting with the team, patient, partner or relative and external advisers (e.g. palliative care specialist, ethicist, chaplain) (*see* cd-5, p. 271). — the courts can be helpful in situations where agreement cannot be reached, but are a last resort.

cd= clinical decision

NOTES

Decisions around capacity

CLINICAL DECISION AND ACTION CHECKLIST

1 Does the person have the capacity to make *this* decision for themselves?
2 Assess for capacity.
3 Is there a parent, Advance Health Care Directive, or substitute decision maker/health care proxy?
4 Is the patient without anyone who could be consulted about their best interests?
5 Act in the patient's best interests.
6 Is the test or treatment likely to be distressing?
7 Is a clear decision difficult?

KEY POINTS

- Capacity depends on the decision to be made.
- "Best interests" and decisions using estimates of quality of life are prone to error.

INTRODUCTION

Preferences for care, and consent for treatment emerge best from a process of discussion and feedback.[12] In young children, it is necessary to establish early on who has parental responsibility and who will be the proxy decision makers. This discussion is best left until a trusting relationship has developed with the care team, but this is not always possible. In situations where parental responsibility is shared (e.g. separated parents or a child under a care order), it is important to establish early on how difficult decisions will be addressed. This may involve a case conference at an early stage.

CAPACITY

"Capacity" is the ability to understand the nature and consequences of a decision, and an ability to communicate this decision. The exact definition of capacity, if one exists, varies slightly between states, provinces, and territories. Some guidance on assessing capacity can be found on the website of the attorney general for Ontario.[13]

A child can have capacity: the law in most Canadian and US jurisdictions presumes persons over 16 years of age are capable of giving consent to or refusing care. It is accepted that many children can give consent to treatment.[14] Older children may be able to consent to or refuse a proposed treatment, but this is not a clear situation.

Parents must have capacity too: occasionally parents have similar problems to a child who does not have capacity. The parent's capacity must be assessed before they can make decisions on their child's behalf.

Tests of cognition do not predict capacity: even in patients with cognitive impairment, the capacity to make a decision can vary greatly and some are able to make a valid advance directive Consequently, an abnormal cognition test does not exclude the possibility that an individual has the capacity to make a valid decision. This parallels the issue in children where capacity is not determined by age, but by maturity and the ability to understand. A young child may be able to communicate feelings through stories, play or art. An older child below 16 may be able to understand and discuss abstract and difficult issues.

Information must be understandable: clear information is crucial,[15] especially for a child or in the presence of cognitive impairment, when information may have to be presented in stages and formats suitable for that individual.

DECISIONS IN THE PATIENT WITHOUT CAPACITY

Deciding on a patient's "best interests" seems a pragmatic process that is particularly useful in emergencies,[16] but it can be misinterpreted by professionals.[17] Estimates of quality of life by professionals are poor indicators of a patient's best interests.[18] A better approach is to consider two situations:

1 **Emergency treatment:** this allows treatment to prevent death or a serious deterioration in physical or mental health.
2 **Necessary treatment:** treatment must be necessary and realistic. In many cases, with open discussion the decisions are clear to the clinical team and the partner, relatives, or parents. Relatives and parents can give invaluable information as to the current or previously expressed wishes of the patient. On occasions, consensus is difficult. This may be because more discussion is needed or the available information is incomplete. There may be a "proxy (substitute) decision maker" (in children this is usually the parents). It is rare to have to fall back on the courts for a decision. *See also Making ethical choices*, p. 263.

ADVANCE HEALTH CARE DIRECTIVE (AHCD)

This can be made only by a patient who still has capacity, but it becomes active when they lose capacity. The legislation for an AHCD varies across states, provinces, and territories. There is no legal or ethical framework that allows a patient to demand treatment.

An AHCD is invalid if it was written by someone who at that time was without relevant capacity, or the person regains capacity for the decision in question.

Clinical decision	If YES carry out the action below
1 Does the person have capacity to make this decision for themselves?	• Check that the person has all the facts. • Provide any additional information they want about the options. • Ask the patient for their opinion. NB. A person with capacity and all the relevant information has the right to make a decision that others view as unwise or eccentric. Older children below 18 can have the capacity to decide on life-sustaining treatment.
2 Start by assuming that the patient has capacity If there is doubt, proceed to a test of capacity, such as the following (based on UK legislation regarding assessment of capacity): *Stage 1:* Does the person have an impairment of, or a disturbance in the functioning of, their mind or brain? *Stage 2:* Does the impairment or disturbance mean that the person is unable to make a specific decision when they need to? Their capacity for this decision can be assessed by four functional tests: 1 Can they understand the information? *NB. This must be imparted in a way the patient can understand.* 2 Can they retain the information? *NB. This only needs to be long enough to use and weigh the information* 3 Can they use or weigh up that information? *NB. They must be able to show that they are able to consider the benefits and burdens of the alternatives to the proposed treatment.* 4 Can they communicate their decision? *NB. The carers must try every method possible to enable this.* To have capacity the answer to all four questions must be "Yes." The result of each step of this assessment should be documented, ideally by quoting the patient.	
3 Is there a parent, or AHCD?	• **If the patient is a child without capacity:** ask the parents for their decision. Ideally, there should be a consensus with the clinical team. However, the clinical team must still act in the child's best interests and this may conflict with those of the parents (*see* cd-7 on p. 271). • **If there is an AHCD:** — check that it is applicable to the current situation and that the patient has lost relevant capacity. — follow the decision(s) stated in the AHCD.
4 Is the patient without anyone who could be consulted about their best interests?	• In an emergency and in the absence of an AHCD, treatment must not be delayed if the person's life is at risk. • For any other serious medical decisions, involve a substitute decision maker/health care proxy. • Act in the person's best interests (*see* cd-5, p. 271).

cd = clinical decision

An AHCD is not applicable if the situation is not covered by the directions in the AHCD, or a more recent AHCD has been made.

If the AHCD is not valid or applicable to current circumstances the health care professionals and/or substitute decision maker/health care proxy should consider the contents of the AHCD in their assessment of the person's best interests if they have reasonable grounds to think it is a true expression of the person's wishes.

COMMUNICATION

Carers have to take all practicable steps to help a patient understand the information and communicate their decision. Professionals should take all practicable steps to include the patient in the decision, and need to understand how to proceed when a patient without capacity has no appointed decision maker. This may vary between provinces, territories, and states, so professionals should be familiar with the relevant legislation.

CARRYING OUT THE TEST OR TREATMENT/PROCEDURE

Regardless of capacity, everything should be done to minimize discomfort and distress arising from tests or treatments. Examples are a pre-appointment visit or the use of topical anesthetic for venepuncture. Occasionally, it is clear that a distressing test or procedure is needed in a patient who does not have capacity for that decision. Titrated doses of sublingual midazolam,[19–21] or lorazepam, can be used to minimize or eliminate any distress.[22,23] The sublingual and buccal routes are better tolerated in children than the intranasal route.[24]

Clinical decision	If YES carry out the action below
5 Act in the patient's best interests • **In an emergency:** treat if this is likely to succeed and will benefit the patient. • **Identify one or more decision makers** (this is usually done by discussion between the interdisciplinary team and the patient and/or their partner or relatives. Appointment of substitute decision makers or health care proxies is usually governed by provincial or state legislation.) Between them, the interdisciplinary team and the decision makers should: — encourage the participation of the patient — plan future care and/or management — identify all the relevant circumstances (clinical, social, financial, psychological, spiritual) — elicit and consider the patient's views (i.e. wishes, preferences, beliefs, and values): these may have been expressed verbally previously, or exist in an AHCD made when the patient had capacity — avoid discrimination and avoid making assumptions about the person's quality of life — assess, if able, whether the person might regain capacity — if the decision concerns life-sustaining treatment, not be motivated in any way by a desire to bring about the person's death — consult others (within the limits of confidentiality) — avoid restricting the person's rights — take all of this into account, i.e. weigh up all of these factors in order to agree the person's best interests. • **Record the decisions** • **Agree review dates** and review regularly.	
6 Is the test or treatment likely to be distressing for the patient?	• **Explore simple approaches**, such as topical anesthetic for venepuncture, and ensuring the environment is comfortable and familiar. Give explanations at the patient's cognitive level (verbal, visual). • **For a hospital appointment or procedure in hospital**, consider a pre-appointment visit to assess the patient's level of acceptance and comfort with the environment. Pre-plan any visits to ensure the minimum waiting time and good access if the patient is disabled. • **If distress is still likely AND consensus has been reached to go ahead with the treatment**, continue as follows: — have available flumazenil 200 microg IV (a reversal agent for benzodiazepines) and basic resuscitation equipment (Ambu bag, oxygen, simple airway) — three hours before test/procedure: reduce anxiety with lorazepam 0.5 mg PO or sublingual, repeated hourly up to maximum of 1.5 mg — if necessary, give 2.5 mg midazolam buccally, repeated after 10 min (maximum total 10 mg or 0.5 mg/kg for a child). NB. Retain the eyelash reflex – the aim is to reduce anxiety, not to sedate — if these doses have had no effect: cancel the test/procedure for that day. Consider repeating on another day with higher starting doses, e.g. 1 mg lorazepam and 2.5–5 mg midazolam (up to 0.75 mg/kg for child).
7 Is a clear decision difficult?	• **If there is insufficient information:** obtain information. If this is unhelpful, agree an observation period (*see* cd-7 in *Making ethical choices*, p. 265). • **If a consensus is difficult:** the senior clinician will need to make the decision. It may be helpful to arrange for a formal review by a senior clinician who is experienced in the patient's condition, but is not part of the clinical team. • **Consider involving** the local ethics committee. — It is rarely necessary to ask for legal advice unless serious differences in opinions persist.

cd = clinical decision

NOTES

Issues around cardiopulmonary resuscitation

CLINICAL DECISION AND ACTION CHECKLIST

1 Is a cardiac or respiratory arrest an *unlikely* possibility in the current circumstances of the patient?
2 Is there uncertainty about the success of CPR?
3 Is there a realistic chance that CPR *could not* be successful?
4 Is there a realistic chance that CPR *could* be successful?
— does the patient or child lack capacity for this decision?
— are the potential risks and burdens of CPR greater than the likely benefits?
5 Continue to communicate progress and elicit concerns.

KEY POINTS

- A decision about CPR made in advance can only be made if the circumstances of the arrest can be anticipated.
- If CPR is not an option, obtaining consent is impossible and patients and relatives should not be burdened with this decision.

INTRODUCTION

At the natural end of a terminal illness cardiopulmonary resuscitation (CPR) is not a treatment option since it cannot succeed. In this case the decision is *Do Not (Attempt) Resuscitation (DN(A)R)*. In other situations, however, CPR can be the correct treatment.[25,26] Despite this simple approach, clinicians have found the clinical decision process confusing.

In Canada the Joint Statement on Resuscitative Interventions guides assessment and decisions on CPR.[27] In the US there are the American Medical Association Council on Ethical and Judicial Affairs recommendations.[28] In addition, several papers have commented on the application of resuscitation guidelines in clinical practice.[29–33]

PRINCIPLES OF CPR DECISIONS

These principles are based on the Canadian Joint Statement on Resuscitative Interventions[27] and the UK Joint Statement on Cardiopulmonary Resuscitation.[34] You should know your local policies and protocols. **NB. These principles do not apply at present to US pediatric patients.**

Overview of Joint Statements

They protect adults and children who should not receive CPR and those who should receive CPR.

Adults and children who are dying are protected from receiving CPR that could not work. Equally, adults and children in whom CPR could work are enabled to have CPR.

What is CPR?

CPR decisions only apply to cardiopulmonary resuscitation (i.e. cardiac massage and artificial respiration).

A patient with a DN(A)R order in place can still have any other treatment for their health and comfort.

Individualized decisions

Decisions must be based on an *individual* assessment of each patient, not on the professional's judgment of the patient's quality of life.

Three groups of patients

Three groups of patients can be identified:

1 Patients in whom an arrest is not anticipated in the current circumstances, or the success of CPR is uncertain.
In these patients, no decision can be made. In the event of an unexpected arrest CPR is attempted, unless it is clear that it cannot succeed.

2 Patients in whom an arrest is anticipated, but CPR could not be successful.
These patients are dying of their disease and a DN(A)R decision is made. Consent cannot be obtained, but communication and information are essential.

3 Patients in whom an arrect is anticipated and CPR could be successful.
Such patients should be asked to consent for CPR (if this is an adult who does not have capacity a decision must be made in their best interests; if this is a child who does not have capacity the parents can make a CPR decision).

When no decision is in place

If no CPR decision is in place, although there is an *initial* presumption in favor of CPR, there is no obligation to start or continue CPR if it is clear that CPR could not succeed.

If a patient is dying but no CPR decision has been documented, there is no obligation to start CPR when they die naturally of their disease.

Bedside assessments at the time of an arrest

These are essential whether or not a CPR decision is in place. If it is clear that the circumstances of the arrest are different to those already documented, a different CPR decision can be made by a competent doctor or nurse. For example, an adult with motor neurone disease or a child with advanced muscular dystrophy may have a DNAR decision in place in the event of respiratory failure due to their illness. However, if they choke on some food they are eating and go into respiratory arrest, it would be reasonable to clear the airway and start CPR.

Who is responsible for making a CPR decision in advance?

This is usually the clinician responsible for the patient's care, but check local policies. Although a team consensus is helpful, the final decision rests with the clinician responsible for the patient.

Clinical decision	If YES carry out the action below
1 Is a cardiac or respiratory arrest an *unlikely* possibility in the current circumstances of the patient?	**If you cannot anticipate what you would write on the death certificate if the patient arrested, or if you are uncertain about the success of CPR, it is not possible to make the CPR decision in advance.** Consent for, or refusal of, CPR cannot be obtained. *Consequences:* • The patient should be given opportunities to receive information or an explanation about any aspect of their treatment. If the individual wishes, this may include information about CPR treatment and its likely success in different circumstances (although it is unusual for patients to discuss CPR when discussing end-of-life issues). • Continue to communicate progress to the patient (and to the partner/family if the patient agrees). • Continue to elicit the concerns of the patient, partner, or family. • Review regularly to check if circumstances have changed. **In the event of an arrest:** start CPR unless there is no reasonable chance of success.
2 Is there a realistic chance that CPR *could not* be successful?	**It is likely that the patient is going to die naturally because of an irreversible condition.** Where a decision not to attempt CPR is made on these clear medical grounds, it is not possible to obtain consent for CPR (from the patient, or from those close to the patient where the patient lacks capacity), since you should not seek consent for a treatment that cannot succeed, i.e. do not unnecessarily burden the patient and/or health care proxy/substitute decision maker/family with a CPR decision, but rather provide your valued input as a health care professional as to whether or not you feel that CPR is "medically indicated" in the present circumstances. *Consequences:* • Document the fact that CPR treatment will not benefit the patient, e.g. "The clinical team is as certain as it can be that CPR treatment cannot benefit the patient in the event of a cardiac or respiratory arrest due to advanced cancer, so DN(A)R." • Continue to communicate progress to the patient (and to the partner/family if the patient agrees or if the patient lacks capacity). This explanation may include information as to why CPR treatment is not an option. • Continue to elicit the concerns of the patient, partner, and family. • Review regularly to check if circumstances have changed. • To ensure a comfortable and natural death effective supportive care should be in place, with access if necessary to specialist palliative care, and with support for the family and partner. • If a second opinion is requested, this request should be respected, whenever possible. **In the event of the expected death, AND** (Allow Natural Dying) with effective supportive or palliative care in place.

Adapted from *Advance Decisions about Resuscitation*[35]
cd = clinical decision

If CPR could succeed, the patient's views are paramount

If CPR could succeed, but the clinical team feels the harm outweighs the benefits, the patient's views are paramount. For example, a patient with bone metastases and unstable angina is at risk of a reversible arrhythmic arrest, or a child with osteogenesis imperfecta and skeletal deformities is at risk of respiratory arrest. In both situations the clinical team may feel that CPR would fracture ribs and cause harm. However, because the CPR could be successful the patient (or the parents if the child does not have capacity) must be asked for consent, which will include explaining the potential harm. Most will refuse, but if consent is given for CPR it must be done in the event of an arrest.

Deciding in advance about hospital and ICU admission

CPR decisions are separate to decisions about ICU admission.

Although most patients go to ICU after successful CPR, a CPR decision must never be based on whether a patient is suitable for ICU.

CPR must be carried out in full

If CPR is the decision made, it must be carried out in full within the skills and facilities of the organization.

Partial CPR ("slow code") is not an acceptable advance decision. If CPR is started but the patient is not responding, CPR can stop.

When a patient does not have capacity

For those patients who do not have the capacity to make a CPR decision:

- those who previously had capacity may have made an AHCD
- if there is no AHCD the clinical team must make a decision in the patient's best interests (*see* cd-5 in *Decisions around capacity*, p. 271).

Children

These principles apply equally in Canada to children.

- If a cardiac arrest is anticipated but CPR cannot be successful, consent cannot be obtained, although the parents (or older children if they have capacity) must have clear communication and information.
- If a cardiac arrest is anticipated and CPR could be successful, the parents must be consulted when the child does not have the capacity to make this decision.
- For those with capacity their consent is paramount if cardiac arrest is anticipated and CPR could be successful.

Communication

Obtaining consent for CPR and discussing end-of-life issues are two separate processes. Consent for CPR cannot be obtained for patients in whom no CPR decision has been made, or in whom CPR cannot be successful. However, effective communication about their progress is essential if they wish to discuss any aspect of their care in the future, including at the end of life. CPR is rarely mentioned by patients in such conversations.

Training

Training about CPR decisions should be included in CPR training.

In addition to the "ABC" of CPR, "D" for "Decisions" is as important.

Advance care planning

Advance care planning is a separate, ongoing dialogue with adults and children who have capacity, and their partners and family (*see* p. 35). It will often be part of an AHCD, but in two authorities in Canada (Fraser Health, BC, and Calgary, AB) there are separate ACP policies.

Clinical decision	If YES carry out the action below
3 Is there a realistic chance that CPR *could* be successful?	• **Does the patient or child lack capacity for this decision?** (*See Decisions around capacity*, p. 267.) *In children:* discuss the options with the parents who can consent for CPR treatment. *In adults:* check if there is an Advance Health Care Directive (AHCD) refusing CPR, or an appointed substitute decision maker/health care proxy. Otherwise make a decision in the patient's best interests. • **Are the potential risks and burdens of CPR greater than the likely benefits?** *When there is only a very small chance of success and there are questions whether the burdens outweigh the benefits of attempting CPR:* the involvement of the patient who has capacity in making the decision is crucial. *When the patient is a child or young person:* those with parenteral responsibility should be involved in the decision where appropriate. *When patients have the capacity for this decision:* their own view should be the primary guide to decision making. In cases of doubt or disagreement, a second opinion should be requested. *When the adult patient does not have capacity:* proceed in their best interests (*see* cd-5 in *Decisions around capacity*, p. 271). • **In the event of the expected arrest:** carry out the wishes of the patient (or the parent or clinical team if the child or patient did not have capacity for this decision).
4 Continue to communicate progress and elicit concerns Ensure that the opportunity is always available for the patient, partner, and family to discuss end-of-life issues.	

Adapted from *Advance Decisions about Resuscitation*[35]
cd = clinical decision

CPR decisions may follow from advance care planning discussions, but they are not a requirement of such discussions. A refusal of CPR can be made by an adult or child with capacity through a valid and applicable written AHCD, or in discussion with their attending health care professionals.

Survival from CPR

At best, less than 20% of patients receiving CPR survive long enough to return home.[36] However, the discharge rate reduces to 1% in non-witnessed arrests.[37] Although some patients will request CPR even if the potential for success is as low as 10%,[38] at the end of an irreversible terminal disease (e.g. cancer) CPR will not succeed and should not be offered as a choice.

REFERENCES: DIFFICULT DECISIONS

B = book; C = comment; CC = Court Case; Ch = chapter; CS-n = case study-no. of cases; CT-n = controlled trial-no. of cases; E = editorial; GC = group consensus; I = interviews; LS = laboratory study; MC = multi-center; Q-n = questionnaire-no. of respondents; OS-n = open study-no. of cases; R = review; RCT-n = randomized controlled trial-no. of cases; RS-n = retrospective survey-no. of cases; SA = systematic or meta analysis.

1 Quill TE, Lee BC, Nunn S. (2000) University of Pennsylvania Center for Bioethics Assisted Suicide Consensus Panel. Palliative treatments of last resort: choosing the least harmful alternative. *Annals of Internal Medicine.* **132**(6): 488–93. (R)

2 Quill TE, Byock IR. (2000) ACP–ASIM End-of-Life Care Consensus Panel. American College of Physicians-American Society of Internal Medicine. Responding to intractable terminal suffering: the role of terminal sedation and voluntary refusal of food and fluids. *Annals of Internal Medicine.* **132**(5): 408–14. (R, 65 refs)

3 Latimer EJ. (1998) Ethical care at the end of life. *Canadian Medical Association Journal.* **158**(13): 1741–7. (R, 30 refs)

4 Dhruev N. (2002) Not just skin-deep: how systems sustain racism. *Nursing Times.* **98**(23): 26–7. (R, 6 refs)

5 Taywaditep KJ. (2001) Marginalization among the marginalized: gay men's anti-effeminacy attitudes. *Journal of Homosexuality.* **42**(1): 1–28. (R, 100 refs)

6 Ward D. (2000) Ageism and the abuse of older people in health and social care. *British Journal of Nursing.* **9**(9): 560–3. (R, 30 refs)

7 Surlis S, Hyde A. (2001) HIV-positive patients' experiences of stigma during hospitalization. *Journal of the Association of Nurses in AIDS Care.* **12**(6): 68–77. (R, 39 refs)

8 Garofalo R, Katz E. (2001) Health care issues of gay and lesbian youth. *Current Opinion in Pediatrics.* **13**(4): 298–302. (R, 38 refs)

9 Bonham VL. (2001) Race, ethnicity, and pain treatment: striving to understand the causes and solutions to the disparities in pain treatment. *Journal of Law, Medicine and Ethics.* **29**(1): 52–68. (R, 111 refs)

10 Mencap (2007). *Death by Indifference*. London: Mencap. (www.mencap.org.uk) (RS-6)

11 Johanson GA. (2009) The defined trial period in ethical decision making. *Journal of Pain and Symptom Management.* **38**(3): 473–6. (CS-1)

12 Prendergast TJ. (2001) Advance care planning: pitfalls, progress, promise. *Critical Care Medicine.* **29**(2): N34–39. (R, 49 refs)

13 Ontario Ministry of the Attorney General/ Dealing with Mental Capacity. Available at: www.attorneygeneral.jus.gov.on.ca/english/family/pgt/incapacity/capacity_assessment.asp#assessor

14 Dickey SB, Kiefner J, Beidler SM. (2002) Consent and confidentiality issues among school-age children and adolescents. *Journal of School Nursing.* **18**(3): 179–86 (C)

15 Taylor HA. (1999) Barriers to informed consent. *Seminars in Oncology Nursing.* **15**(2): 89–95. (R, 35 refs)

16 Larkin GL, Marco CA, Abbott JT. (2001) Emergency determination of decision-making capacity: balancing autonomy and beneficence in the emergency department. *Academic Emergency Medicine.* **8**(3): 282–4. (R, 23 refs)

17 Donnelly M. (2001) Decision-making for mentally incompetent people: the empty formula of best interests? *Medicine and Law.* **20**(3): 405–16. (R, 44 refs)

18 Costantini M, Mencaglia E, *et al.* (2000) Cancer patients as "experts" in defining quality of life domains: a multicentre survey by the Italian Group for the Evaluation of Outcomes in Oncology (IGEO). *Quality of Life Research.* **9**: 151–9.

19 Khalil S, Philbrook L, Rabb M, Wagner K, *et al.* (1998) Sublingual midazolam premedication in children: a dose response study. *Paediatric Anaesthesia.* **8**(6): 461–5. (RCT-102)

20 Scott RC, Besag FM, Boyd SG, Berry D, Neville BG. (1998) Buccal absorption of midazolam: pharmacokinetics and EEG pharmacodynamics. *Epilepsia.* **39**(3): 290–4. (CT-10)

21 Lim TW, Thomas E, Choo SM. (1997) Premedication with midazolam is more effective by the sublingual than oral route. *Canadian Journal of Anaesthesia.* **44**(7): 723–6. (RCT-100)

22 Ghanchi FD, Khan MY. (1997) Sublingual lorazepam as premedication in peribulbar anesthesia. *Journal of Cataract and Refractive Surgery.* **23**(10): 1581–4. (RCT)

23 Spenard J, Caille G, de Montigny C, Vezina M, *et al.* (1988) Placebo-controlled comparative study of the anxiolytic activity and of the pharmacokinetics of oral and sublingual lorazepam in generalized anxiety. *Biopharmaceutics and Drug Disposition.* **9**(5): 457–64. (RCT-12)

24 Karl HW, Rosenberger JL, Larach MG, Ruffle JM. (1993) Transmucosal administration of midazolam for premedication of pediatric patients: comparison of the nasal and sublingual routes. *Anesthesiology.* **78**(5): 885–91. (RCT-93).

25 Zoch TW, Desbiens NA, DeStefano F, Stueland DT, Layde PM. (2000) Short- and long-term survival after cardiopulmonary resuscitation. *Archives of Internal Medicine.* **160**(13): 1969–73. (RS-948)

26 Dumot JA, Burval DJ, Sprung J, Waters JH, *et al.* (2001). Outcome of adult cardiopulmonary resuscitations at a tertiary referral center including results of "limited" resuscitations. *Archives of Internal Medicine.* **161**(14): 1751–8. (RS-445)

27 http://policybase.cma.ca/dbtw-wpd/PolicyPDF/PD95-03.pdf

28 American Medical Association Council on Ethical and Judicial Affairs (1998). Optimal use of orders not to intervene and advance directives. *Psychology, Public Policy and Law.* **4**: 668–75.

29 Randall F. (2002) Recent guidance on resuscitation: patients' choices and doctors' duties. *Palliative Medicine.* **15**: 449–50. (E)

30 Willard C. (2000) Cardiopulmonary resuscitation for palliative care patients: a discussion of ethical issues. *Palliative Medicine*. **14**(4): 308–12. (R, 16 refs)

31 Regnard C. (2006) Please do not resuscitate: solution is flawed. *British Medical Journal*. **332**: 608.

32 Regnard C, Randall F. (2005) A framework for making advance decisions on resuscitation. *Clinical Medicine*. **5**(4): 354–60.

33 Regnard C, Randall F. (2009) Should hospices be exempt from national CPR guidelines? *British Medical Journal*. **338**: 986. (C)

34 British Medical Association, Resuscitation Council, Royal College of Nursing (2007). *Joint Statement on Cardiopulmonary Resuscitation*. London: BMA, RC and RCN.

35 Regnard C, Matthews D, Gibson L. (2009) *Advance Decisions about Resuscitation: documentation*. Newcastle: St. Oswald's Hospice and Northumberland Tyne & Wear NHS Trust.

36 Peberdy MA, Ornato JP, Larkin GL, Braithwaite RS, *et al.* (2008) National Registry of Cardiopulmonary Resuscitation Investigators. Survival from in-hospital cardiac arrest during nights and weekends. *Journal of the American Medical Association*. **299**(7): 785–92. (RS-86,748)

37 Brindley PG, Markland DM, Mayers I, Kutsogiannis DJ. (2002) Predictors of survival following in-hospital adult cardiopulmonary resuscitation. *Canadian Medical Association Journal*. **167**(4): 343–8. (RS-247)

38 Murphy DJ, Burrows D, Santilli S, Kemp AW, *et al.* (1994) The influence of the probability of survival on patients' preferences regarding cardiopulmonary resuscitation. *New England Journal of Medicine*. **330**(8): 545–9. (I-287)

NOTES

Drug Information

For current drug information see

- www.palliativedrugs.com for palliative care drugs (free access after registration, and is UK oriented).
- www.e-therapeutics.ca (the eCPS) for drug prescribing in Canada (subscriber only, also available in French).
- http://webstore.lexi.com/Store/Individual-Databases/Lexi-Drugs for drug prescribing in US (subscriber only).

KEY POINTS

- Many patients with advanced disease are on multiple medications.
- Potential drug interactions are common.
- Children tolerate some drugs very differently from adults and there is considerable variability between individuals.
- Many drugs can be given by a variety of non-oral routes.
- In Canada and the US, drugs can be prescribed for off-label uses and routes, but basic rules about reducing risk apply.

NOTES

Drug interactions

INTERACTIONS OCCUR FOR THE FOLLOWING REASONS:

What the body does to the drug

Pharmacokinetic interactions:
These can cause changes in drug absorption, distribution of the drug in the body, metabolism, and elimination.

What the drug does to the body

Pharmacodynamic interactions:
These can be additive effects, alterations to receptor transport, changes in fluid or electrolyte balance, and difficulty in titration of drugs with a narrow therapeutic window.

What drugs do to each other

Pharmaceutical interactions:
These are when two drugs interact when mixed to change the absorption or activity of one or both drugs.

THE RISK OF AN ADVERSE REACTION CAN BE MINIMIZED BY

- keeping doses low (many interactions are dose-related)
- monitoring more closely for the potential interaction, e.g. more frequent serum potassium checks for furosemide-dexamethasone interaction
- taking action to prevent the adverse effect, e.g. using a proton-pump inhibitor to reduce the risk of gastrointestinal mucosal damage caused by an NSAID-steroid interaction.

It is important to report any serious interactions to MedWatch in the USA (1-800-FDA-1088), or online at www.fda.gov/medwatch; in Canada to Health Canada (tel: 1-866-234-2345; fax 1 866-678-6789); or online at www.healthcanada.gc.ca/medeffect.

INSTRUCTIONS FOR USE OF DRUG INTERACTION TABLES

1. Drugs are listed alphabetically (some drugs may be available only in one or other of the US or Canada).
2. Find the interacting drug.
3. Check the likely importance of the interaction (based on the UK eBNF):
   ▲ = **interaction potentially hazardous.** Combination should be avoided (or only undertaken with caution and appropriate monitoring)
   △ = **interaction possible, but not usually serious.** Caution is needed.
4. Read the effect of the interaction.
5. Read the necessary action.

Important note: the list that follows is not comprehensive and is restricted to drugs that may be used in palliative care. **Any drug that is new to the patient should be checked in a comprehensive list for potential interactions with existing drugs.**

Most, if not all, pharmacies have reliable computer-based drug interaction programs that alert to potential interactions. If there is any doubt in the prescriber's mind about a particular drug combination, consultation with a pharmacist is recommended. Not all drugs listed here are available in both the USA and Canada, and some that are available may not be listed.

	Interacting drug	Effect of Interaction	Action/Precaution
▲ Potentially hazardous	**△ Interaction possible, but infrequent or not serious**		
ACE Inhibitor (ACEi)			
▲	**cyclosporin, high K^+ foods, K^+ sparing diuretics, ketorolac, potassium salts, salt substitutes**	Hyperkalemia	Avoid combination
▲	**lithium**	↑ lithium levels (↓ excretion)	Monitor lithium levels
	α-blockers, alcohol, antipsychotics baclofen, β-blockers, benzodiazepines CCBs, clonidine nitrates, phenothiazines	Risk of hypotension	Monitor BP, and symptoms of hypotension
△	allopurinol	Toxicity in renal impairment	Monitor renal function
△	antacids	↓ absorption of ACEi	Take at least 2 hours apart
△	corticosteroid, rifampicin	↓ hypotensive effect	Monitor BP more frequently
△	digoxin	↑ plasma level of digoxin	Monitor digoxin level closely
△	diuretics	Risk of severe hypotension on starting	Monitor BP, and symptoms of hypotension
△	erythropoietin	↓ hypotensive effect, hyperkalemia	Monitor BP and electrolytes more frequently
△	heparins	Hyperkalemia	Monitor electrolytes more frequently
△	insulin, metformin, sulphonylureas	Risk of hypoglycemia	Monitor blood glucose more frequently
△	NSAID	Renal impairment, ↓ hypotensive effect	Monitor renal function and BP more frequently
Acetaminophen			
△	carbamazepine	↑ metabolism of acetaminophen	Monitor efficacy
△	cholestyramine	↓ acetaminophen absorption and effect	Take at least 2 hours apart
△	domperidone, metoclopramide	↑ effects of acetaminophen	Take at least 2 hours apart
△	warfarin	↑ anticoagulant effect	Monitor INR more frequently
Alfentanil			
▲	**voriconazole**	↑ plasma level of alfentanil	Consider reducing alfentanil dose and monitor for opioid side-effects
△	erythromycin, ketoconazole	↑ plasma level of alfentanil	Monitor for opioid side-effects
Amiodarone (long half-life)			
▲	**antiarrhythmics (all), antipsychotics, erythromycin**	Myocardial depression	Avoid combination
▲	**haloperidol, methotrimeprazine, moxifloxacin, tricyclic antidepressants, trimethoprim**	Ventricular arrhythmias	Avoid combination
▲	**digoxin**	Increase plasma level of digoxin	Halve dose of digoxin
▲	**lithium**	Ventricular arrhythmias, hypothyroidism	Avoid combination
▲	**phenytoin**	↑ plasma level of phenytoin (↓ metabolism)	Avoid combination
▲	**verapamil, β-blockers**	Bradycardia, AV block	Avoid combination
▲	**warfarin**	↑ risk of bleeding (↓ metabolism)	Avoid combination
△	bupivacaine (systemic absorption)	Myocardial depression	Avoid combination
△	cimetidine, grapefruit	↑ plasma level of amiodarone	Monitor for amiodarone side-effects
△	diuretics – loop, thiazide	Hyperkalemia	Monitor electrolytes closely
Amitriptyline (*see also* tricyclic antidepressants)			
△	cimetidine	↑ plasma level of amitriptyline	Observe for adverse effects

	Interacting drug	Effect of Interaction	Action/Precaution
▲ Potentially hazardous	**△ Interaction possible, but infrequent or not serious**		
△	morphine	↑ risk of myoclonus	Observe for myoclonic jerks Consider an opioid change
Amlodipine			
△	St. John's wort	↓ plasma level of amlodipine	Monitor efficacy
△	sildenafil	Risk of hypotension	Monitor BP, and symptoms of hypotension
Amoxicillin			
△	allopurinol	Rash	Observe for rash
△	warfarin	May alter effect of warfarin	Monitor INR closely
Angiotensin II receptor antagonists (A2RAs)			
▲	**cyclosporin, diuretics (potassium-sparing), K+ salts**	↑ risk of hyperkalemia	Monitor K^+ levels closely
▲	**diuretics**	Enhanced hypotensive effect	Monitor BP closely
▲	**lithium**	↑ plasma concentration of lithium	Check lithium levels
△	ACEi, heparin, tacrolimus	↑ risk of hyperkalemia	Monitor K^+ levels
△	alcohol, α-blocker, antipsychotic, anxiolytic, baclofen, β-blocker, CCB, clonidine, diazoxide, levodopa, MAOI, nitrates	Enhanced hypotensive effect	Monitor BP
△	corticosteroids, erythropoietin, NSAIDs, estrogen	Hypotensive effect of A2RA antagonized	Monitor BP
△	NSAIDs	Increased risk of renal impairment	Monitor renal function
Antacids (including sucralfate)			
△	ACEi, aspirin, azithromycin, bisphosphonates, cefaclor, ciprofloxacin, digoxin, gabapentin, iron, itraconazole, lansoprazole, methotrimeprazine, ketoconazole, moxifloxacin, norfloxacin, olanzapine, phenytoin, rifampicin, tetracycline	↓ absorption of interacting drug	Take at least 2 hours apart
△	enteral feeds	Coagulates with feeds	Dilute with 60 mL of water and flush well
Antidepressants – SSRI and SNRI			
	(NB. Fluoxetine: long half-life can delay effect for weeks. Beware of withdrawal syndrome with paroxetine.)		
▲	**antiepileptics/anticonvulsants**	↑ risk of seizures	Observe for adverse effect
▲	**haloperidol, phenytoin, TCA**	↑ plasma level of interacting drug	Observe for adverse effect
▲	**lithium, MAOIs**	↑ CNS side-effects	Do not start fluoxetine until 2 weeks after stopping MAOIs. Do not start MAOIs until 5 weeks after stopping fluoxetine
▲	**NSAIDs**	Risk of bleeding	Observe for adverse effect
▲	**St. John's wort**	↑ serotonergic side-effects	Observe for adverse effect
▲	**tramadol**	CNS toxicity	Avoid combination
▲	**warfarin**	↑ anticoagulant effect	Monitor INR closely
△	alcohol	↑ sedative effect	Observe for adverse effect
△	barbiturates	↓ anticonvulsant effects	Observe for adverse effect
△	benzodiazepines, methadone, olanzapine	↑ plasma levels of interacting drug (fluvoxamine)	Observe for adverse effect
△	cimetidine	↑ plasma levels of sertraline and escitalopram	Reduce dose of SSRI or use ranitidine

	Interacting drug	Effect of Interaction	Action/Precaution
▲ Potentially hazardous	△ Interaction possible, but infrequent or not serious		
△	clozapine, nifedipine, risperidone metoprolol, omeprazole	↑ plasma level of interacting drug	Observe for adverse effect
△	methylphenidate	↑ plasma level of SSRIs	Observe for adverse effect
Antidepressants – tricyclic (*see also* amitriptyline)			
▲	**alcohol**	↑ sedative effect	Observe for adverse effect
▲	**antiarrhythmics, antipsychotics, moxifloxacin**	Risk of ventricular arrhythmias	Observe for adverse effect
▲	**antiepileptics**	↑ risk of seizures	Observe for adverse effect
▲	**barbiturates**	↑ risk of seizures, ↓ plasma level of TCAs	Observe for adverse effect
▲	**clonidine**	Hypotensive effect antagonized by tricyclics, risk of withdrawal hypertension on ceasing clonidine	Observe for adverse effect
▲	**MAOIs**	↑ risk of hypertension and CNS excitation	TCAs/MAOIs should not be started until 2 weeks after stopping MAOIs/TCAs (3 weeks if starting clomipramine or imipramine)
▲	**phenytoin, SSRI**	↑ plasma level of TCAs	Observe for loss of therapeutic effects
▲	**tramadol**	CNS toxicity	Observe for adverse effect
▲	**warfarin**	↑ anticoagulant effect	Monitor INR closely
△	baclofen	↑ muscle relaxant effect	Observe for adverse effect
△	cimetidine, methylphenidate	↑ plasma level of TCAs	Observe for adverse effect
△	hyoscine (scopolamine), methotrimeprazine	↑ antimuscarinic side-effects	Observe for adverse effect
△	diuretics	↑ risk of postural hypotension	Observe for adverse effect
△	lithium	Lithium toxicity	Observe for adverse effect
△	opioids	↑ sedative effect	Observe for adverse effect
△	rifampicin	↓ plasma level of TCAs	Observe for adverse effect
Antiepileptics (*see also* under individual names)			
▲	**Antidepressants (SSRI and TCAs), St. John's wort**	↑ risk of seizures	Monitor closely for seizure activity, consider increasing antiepileptic dose
Antimuscarinics			
△	antihistamine, clozapine, hyoscine (scopolamine), MAOIs, oxybutynin, tricyclic antidepressants	↑ risk of antimuscarinic side-effects	Observe for dry mouth, confusion, blurred vision and hypotension. Avoid combination or reduce doses
△	domperidone, haloperidol, metoclopramide	↑ risk of movement disorder (↓ action on bowel)	Observe for tremor, Parkinsonian features or restlessness
△	ketoconazole	↓ absorption of ketoconazole	Take at least 2 hours apart
Aspirin			
▲	**SSRI, heparin, warfarin, venlafaxine**	↑ risk of bleeding	Avoid combination
▲	**methotrexate**	Methotrexate toxicity (↓ excretion)	Monitor levels
△	antacids	↓ plasma level of aspirin	Take at least 2 hours apart
△	corticosteroids	GI ulceration and bleeding	PPI to protect stomach
△	NSAIDs	↑ risk of bronchospasm in asthmatics	Avoid combination
△	oral hypoglycemic agents	Risk of hypoglycemia	Monitor blood glucose more frequently
△	phenytoin	↑ phenytoin effects	Monitor levels and side-effects

	Interacting drug	Effect of Interaction	Action/Precaution
▲ Potentially hazardous	**△ Interaction possible, but infrequent or not serious**		
△	spironolactone	↓ diuretic effect	Increase spironolactone if necessary
△	valproate	↑ valproate effect	Monitor levels and side-effects
Baclofen			
△	ACEi, A2RA, β-blockers, clonidine, α-blockers, CCBs, diuretics, methyldopa, nitrates	Risk of hypotension	Monitor BP and symptoms of hypotension
△	alcohol, anxiolytics, hypnotics	↑ sedation	Observe for excessive drowsiness
△	levodopa	Risk of agitation, hallucinations, confusion	Observe for adverse effects
△	NSAIDs, ibuprofen, tricyclic antidepressants	↑ effect of baclofen (↓ excretion) ↑ muscle relaxant effect	Observe for drowsiness or hypotonicity
β-blocker (*see also* esmolol, labetolol, metoprolol and sotalol)			
▲	**α-blockers, amiodarone, antiarrhythmics**	Bradycardia and myocardial depression	Avoid combination
▲	**clonidine**	Risk of withdrawal hypertension	Withdraw β-blocker several days before stopping clonidine
▲	**diltiazem**	AV block and bradycardia	Avoid combination
▲	**verapamil**	Asystole, hypotension, and heart failure	Avoid combination
△	ACEi, anxiolytics and hypnotics, baclofen, CCBs, diuretics, methotrimeprazine, phenothiazines	Risk of hypotension	Monitor BP and symptoms of hypotension
△	antidiabetics	Masking of hypoglycemic symptoms	Monitor blood glucose closely
△	corticosteroids	↓ hypotensive effect	Monitor BP
△	insulin	Risk of hypoglycemia	Monitor blood glucose frequently
△	pilocarpine	Risk of arrhythmias	Avoid combination
Buspirone			
△	diltiazem, erythromycin, haloperidol, grapefruit, itraconazole, rifampicin, verapamil	↑ plasma level of buspirone	Reduce dose of buspirone, observe for side-effects
△	MAOIs	Manufacturer advises against concomitant use	Avoid combination
Calcium channel blockers (CCBs) (*see also* under individual names)			
▲	**α-blockers, ACEi, β-blockers, alcohol, anxiolytics, hypnotics, antipsychotics, diuretics, baclofen, clonidine**	Risk of hypotension	Monitor BP and symptoms of hypotension
△	cimetidine, grapefruit	↑ plasma level of CCB	Monitor BP
△	corticosteroids, NSAIDs	↓ hypotensive effect	Monitor efficacy
△	itraconazole	↑ negative inotropic effect	Change to fluconazole
Carbamazepine			
▲	**antipsychotics**	↓ seizure threshold	Avoid combination if seizures a risk
▲	**cyclosporin, clozapine, corticosteroids**	↓ plasma level of interacting drug	Monitor efficacy
▲	**cimetidine**	↑ plasma level of cimetidine (↓ metabolism)	Avoid combination. Use valproate instead of carbamazepine or ranitidine instead of cimetidine
▲	**clarithromycin, diltiazem, erythromycin, fluoxetine, fluvoxamine, verapamil**	↑ plasma level of carbamazepine	Observe for adverse effect
▲	**MAOIs, SSRIs**	↓ seizure threshold, ↓ effects of carbamazepine	Avoid combination if seizures are a risk

	Interacting drug	Effect of Interaction	Action/Precaution
▲ Potentially hazardous	△ Interaction possible, but infrequent or not serious		
▲	**St. John's wort**	↓ plasma level of carbamazepine	Avoid combination
▲	**TCA antidepressants**	↓ seizure threshold, ↑ metabolism of TCA	Avoid combination if seizures are a risk
▲	**warfarin**	↓ anticoagulant effect	Monitor INR closely
△	alcohol	↑ CNS side-effects of carbamazepine	Observe for adverse effect
△	clonazepam, haloperidol, methadone, mirtazapine, olanzapine, ondansetron, paroxetine, phenytoin, phenobarbital, risperidone, tramadol, valproate	↓ plasma level of interacting drug (↑ metabolism)	Monitor efficacy of interacting drug
△	diuretics	Risk of hyponatremia	Monitor electrolytes
△	doxycycline	↓ effect of doxycycline (↑ metabolism)	Monitor efficacy
△	fluconazole, ketoconazole	↑ plasma level of carbamazepine	Observe for side-effects
△	lithium	Neurotoxicity	Seek specialist advice. May need to increase lithium dose.
Cefaclor			
▲	**antacids**	↓ absorption of cefaclor	Take at least 2 hours apart
Cefpodoxime			
△	antacids, cimetidine, ranitidine	↓ absorption of cefaclor	Take at least 2 hours apart. Avoid or increase cefpodoxime dose
Celecoxib			
▲	**warfarin**	↑ risk of bleeding	Avoid combination
△	fluconazole	↑ plasma level of celecoxib	Halve dose of celecoxib
Cephalosporins			
▲	**warfarin**	↑ anticoagulant effect	Monitor INR more frequently
△	bumetanide, furosemide	Renal impairment	Avoid combination in renal failure
Chlorpropamide			
△	ACEi, octreotide, salicylates	Risk of hypoglycemia	Monitor blood glucose
△	alcohol	Risk of hypoglycemia, flushing	Monitor blood glucose
△	corticosteroids	↓ hypoglycemic effect	Monitor blood glucose
△	diuretics	↑ risk of hyponatremia	Check electrolytes more frequently
Cimetidine			
▲	**carbamazepine, cyclosporin, lidocaine, phenytoin, valproate**	↑ plasma level of interacting drug	Avoid combination
▲	**warfarin**	↑ anticoagulant effect	Monitor INR closely
△	antiarrhythmics, antipsychotics, β-blockers, CCBs, benzodiazepines, erythromycin, clozapine, metformin, metronidazole, opioids, sildenafil, sulphonylureas, SSRI, escitalopram, mirtazapine, TCA	↑ plasma level of interacting drug	Observe for adverse effects
△	octreotide	↓ absorption of cimetidine	Take at least 2 two hours apart
Ciprofloxacin			
▲	**cyclosporin**	Renal impairment	Avoid combination, monitor renal function closely
▲	**duloxetine**	↓ metabolism of duloxetine	Avoid combination
▲	**NSAIDs**	↑ risk of seizures	Avoid combination
▲	**warfarin**	↑ anticoagulant effect	Monitor INR closely

	Interacting drug	Effect of Interaction	Action/Precaution
▲ Potentially hazardous	**△ Interaction possible, but infrequent or not serious**		
△	antacids, enteral feeds, oral iron, sucralfate	↓ absorption of ciprofloxacin	Take at least 2 hours apart
△	clozapine, olanzapine	↑ plasma level of interacting drug	Avoid combination
△	methadone	↑ plasma level of interacting drug	Observe for opioid side-effects
Clarithromycin			
▲	**carbamazepine, cyclosporin, disopyramide, phenytoin**	↑ plasma level of interacting drug	Avoid combination
▲	**colchicine**	Colchicine toxicity	Avoid combination
▲	**midazolam**	↑ sedative effect (↓ metabolism)	Observe for excessive sedation
▲	**ritonavir**	↑ plasma level of clarithromycin	Avoid combination
▲	**verapamil**	↓ metabolism of verapamil	Avoid combination
▲	**warfarin**	↑ anticoagulant effect	Avoid combination
△	digoxin, itraconazole, omeprazole, methylprednisolone, sildenafil	↑ plasma level of interacting drug	Observe for adverse effects
Clodronate			
△	antacids, oral iron	↓ absorption of clodronate	Use IV route instead of oral
Clonazepam			
▲	**lithium**	↑ plasma level of lithium	Check lithium levels
▲	**olanzapine**	Cardiac, respiratory and CNS depression	Monitor CNS and cardiorespiratory effect
△	carbamazepine, phenobarbital, phenytoin	↓ plasma level of clonazepam	Monitor efficacy
△	tramadol	CNS and respiratory depression	Monitor for drowsiness, avoid activity requiring alertness
△	valproate	Severe drowsiness and ↓ seizure threshold	Seek specialist advice
Corticosteroids			
▲	**amphotericin**	Risk of hypokalemia	Monitor electrolytes closely
▲	**barbiturates, carbamazepine, phenytoin, primidone, rifampicin**	↓ plasma level of corticosteroids	Monitor efficacy
▲	**warfarin**	Unpredictable anticoagulant effect	Monitor INR closely
△	ACEi, clonidine	↓ hypotensive effect	Monitor efficacy
△	phenobarbital	↓ plasma level of corticosteroids	Monitor efficacy
△	antidiabetic agents	↓ hypoglycemic effect	Monitor blood glucose level
△	aspirin, NSAIDs	Risk of GI bleeding and ulceration	Avoid combination or protect with PPI
△	β-blockers, CCBs	↓ hypotensive effect	Monitor efficacy
△	erythromycin, itraconazole, ketoconazole	↑ plasma level of corticosteroids	Observe for adverse effects
△	loop or thiazide diuretics	Risk of hypokalemia	Monitor electrolytes closely
Co-trimoxazole			
▲	**amiodarone**	Risk of ventricular arrhythmia	Avoid combination
▲	**phenytoin, warfarin**	↑ plasma level of interacting drugs	Avoid combination
△	diuretics – thiazide and loop	Risk of severe hyponatremia	Monitor electrolytes closely
Dantrolene (IV)			
△	diltiazem	Risk of arrhythmias	Avoid IV dantrolene
△	verapamil	Hyperkalemia, myocardial depression	Avoid IV dantrolene

	Interacting drug	Effect of Interaction	Action/Precaution
▲ Potentially hazardous	△ Interaction possible, but infrequent or not serious		
Diazepam			
△	enteral feeds	↓ absorption of diazepam	Dilute drug with 30–60 mL of water and flush well
△	esomeprazole, fluvoxamine, omeprazole, valproate, phenytoin	↑ plasma level of diazepam	Observe for adverse effects and altered efficacy
△	phenytoin	Altered plasma level of phenytoin	Observe for adverse effects and altered efficacy
Diltiazem			
▲	**amiodarone, β-blockers**	Risk of severe myocardial depression	Avoid combination
▲	**barbiturates, phenytoin, rifampicin**	↓ effects of diltiazem	Avoid combination
▲	**carbamazepine, cyclosporin, digoxin**	↑ plasma level of interacting drug	Avoid combination
▲	**phenytoin**	↓ plasma concentration of phenytoin	Use alternative CCB
△	buspirone	↑ plasma level of buspirone	Observe for adverse effects
△	dantrolene IV	Risk of arrhythmias	Avoid IV administration of dantrolene
△	imipramine, midazolam, TCA	↑ plasma level of interacting drug	Observe for adverse effects/ excessive sedation
Dimenhydrinate			
△	alcohol, anxiolytic, hypnotics	↑ sedative effect	Observe for drowsiness
△	antimuscarinics, MAOIs, tricyclic antidepressants	↑ antimuscarinic effect	Observe for drowsiness, dry mouth, confusion, blurred vision, hypotension. Avoid/Reduce dose
△	procarbazine	CNS depression	Use combination with caution
△	theophylline	False increase in theophylline levels	Discontinue dimenhydrinate before measuring theophylline level
Diphenhydramine			
△	alcohol, anxiolytic, hypnotics	↑ sedative effect	Observe for drowsiness
△	antimuscarinics, MAOIs, tricyclic antidepressants, linezolid	↑ antimuscarinic effect	Observe for drowsiness, dry mouth, confusion, blurred vision, hypotension. Avoid/Reduce dose
△	procarbazine	CNS depression	Use combination with caution
△	metoprolol	↑ metoprolol levels	Monitor for bradycardia, hypotension, bronchospasm
Disopyramide			
▲	**amiodarone, itraconazole, ketoconazole, methotrimeprazine, moxifloxacin, sotalol, TCA**	Ventricular arrhythmias (Amiodarone has a long half-life)	Avoid combination
▲	**antiarrhythmics, verapamil, β-blocker**	Myocardial depression	Avoid combination
▲	**antipsychotics**	QT prolongation	Avoid combination
▲	**clarithromycin, erythromycin**	↑ plasma level of disopyramide	Avoid combination
▲	**diuretics**	Hypokalemia – cardiac toxicity	Avoid combination
▲	**rifampicin, ritonavir**	↓ plasma level of disopyramide	Avoid combination
△	antimuscarinics	↑ antimuscarinic effect	Observe for antimuscarinic side-effects
△	bupivacaine	Myocardial depression	Observe for cardiac effects
△	phenobarbital, phenytoin	↓ plasma level of disopyramide	Monitor efficacy
Diuretics – all (*see also* loop diuretics, thiazide diuretics and potassium-sparing diuretics)			
▲	**ACEi, α-blocker, alcohol, A2RA**	Risk of hypotension	Monitor closely the BP and symptoms of hypotension

	Interacting drug	Effect of Interaction	Action/Precaution
▲ **Potentially hazardous**	△ **Interaction possible, but infrequent or not serious**		
△	anxiolytics, β-blockers, baclofen, CCB, phenothiazines, TCA	Risk of hypotension	Monitor BP
△	carbamazepine	Risk of hyponatremia	Monitor electrolytes
△	corticosteroids	↓ diuretic effect	Monitor efficacy
△	NSAIDs	Risk of renal impairment, ↓ diuretic effect	Monitor BP and renal function
Diuretics – loop			
▲	**aminoglycosides, vancomycin**	↑ risk of ototoxicity	Avoid combination
▲	**antiarrhythmics, digoxin**	Hypokalemia – cardiac toxicity	Monitor electrolytes closely
▲	**lithium**	↓ excretion of lithium (toxicity)	Monitor lithium levels
△	amphotericin	↑ risk of hypokalemia	Monitor electrolytes closely
△	antidiabetics	↑ blood glucose level	Monitor blood glucose more frequently
△	cephalosporin	Risk of renal impairment	Monitor electrolytes closely
△	cholestyramine	↓ absorption of loop diuretics	Take at least 2 hours apart
△	corticosteroids	↑ risk of hypokalemia	Monitor electrolytes closely
Diuretics – potassium sparing			
▲	**lithium**	Lithium toxicity (↓ excretion)	Monitor lithium levels
▲	**ACEi, cyclosporin, A2RAs, potassium salts, high potassium foods, NSAIDs**	Risk of hyperkalemia	Monitor electrolytes closely
△	chlorpropamide	Risk of hyponatremia	Monitor electrolytes
Diuretics – thiazide			
▲	**antiarrhythmics, digoxin**	Hypokalemia – cardiac toxicity	Monitor electrolytes closely
▲	**lithium**	Lithium toxicity (↓ excretion)	Monitor lithium levels
△	allopurinol	↑ risk of hypersensitivity	Monitor for adverse effects
△	amphotericin, corticosteroids	↑ risk of hypokalemia	Monitor electrolytes closely
△	antidiabetics	↑ glucose levels	Monitor blood glucose
△	calcium salts, vitamin D	Risk of hypercalcemia	Monitor calcium levels
△	chlorpropamide, trimethoprim	Risk of hyponatremia	Monitor electrolytes
△	cyclosporin	Renal impairment and hypermagnesemia	Monitor electrolytes
Domperidone			
▲	**antimuscarinics, opioid analgesics**	↓ effects of domperidone on GI motility	Monitor effect on upper GI motility
▲	**clarithromycin, erythromycin, haloperidol, methadone**	Prolongation of the QT interval	ECG before starting to exclude pre-existing prolonged QT interval
▲	**ketoconazole**	Risk of arrhythmias	Avoid combination or change to metoclopramide
Doxycycline (for other tetracyclines, *see* below)			
▲	**cyclosporin**	↑ plasma level of cyclosporin	Avoid combination
▲	**warfarin**	↑ anticoagulant effect	Monitor INR closely
△	carbamazepine, phenytoin	↓ plasma level of doxycycline	Use alternative tetracycline or increase dose
△	iron – oral	↓ absorption of iron and doxycycline	Use alternative teracycline
Enteral feeds			
▲	**phenytoin**	Binds to tubes	Dilute drug with 30–60 mL water and flush well
▲	**warfarin**	↓ absorption of warfarin	Monitor INR frequently, stop feed for 1 hour before, and 2 hours after, drug administration

	Interacting drug	Effect of Interaction	Action/Precaution
▲ Potentially hazardous	△ Interaction possible, but infrequent or not serious		
△	antacids	Coagulates with feed	Dilute drug with 60 mL water and flush well
△	carbamazepine	Binds to tubes	Dilute drug with 30–60 mL water and flush well
△	diazepam	Binds to tubes	Stop feed for 1 hour before to 2 hours after drug
△	ciprofloxacin, flucloxacillin, ketoconazole, penicillin V, tetracycline	↓ absorption of interacting drug	Stop feed for 1 hour before to 2 hours after drug
Erythromycin			
▲	**amiodarone, moxifloxacin**	Risk of ventricular arrhythmias	Avoid combination
▲	**carbamazepine**	↓ plasma level of carbamazepine	Observe closely for adverse effects or avoid combination
▲	**cyclosporin, verapamil**	↓ metabolism of interacting drug	
▲	**clozapine**	↑ risk of seizures	
▲	**colchicine**	Risk of colchicine toxicity	
▲	**disopyramide**	↑ plasma level of disopyramide	
▲	**midazolam**	↑ sedation (↓ metabolism)	
▲	**domperidone, clarithromycin, haloperidol, methadone**	Prolongation of QT interval	ECG before starting to exclude pre-existing prolonged QT interval
▲	**warfarin**	↑ anticoagulant effect	Monitor INR closely, avoid combination
△	alfentanil, buspirone, corticosteroids, digoxin, felodipine, omeprazole, valproate, zopiclone	↑ plasma level of interacting drug	Monitor for adverse effects (for digoxin measure blood levels)
△	cimetidine	↑ plasma level of erythromycin	Observe for erythromycin toxicity
Esmolol			
△	morphine	↑ plasma level of esmolol	Monitor BP closely
Esomeprazole (*see also* Proton pump inhibitor)			
▲	**phenytoin**	↑ plasma level of phenytoin	Observe for adverse effects
▲	**warfarin**	↑ anticoagulant effect	Monitor INR closely
△	diazepam, voriconazole	↑ plasma level of interacting drug	Observe for adverse effects
Famotidine			
△	itraconazole, ketoconazole	↓ plasma level of interacting drug	Use cimetidine
Felodipine (*see also* calcium channel blocker)			
▲	**barbiturates**	↓ effects of felodipine	Monitor efficacy
▲	**itraconazole, ketoconazole**	↓ metabolism of felodipine	Change to fluconazole
△	carbamazepine, phenytoin	↓ effects of felodipine	Use alternative anticonvulsant
△	erythromycin, grapefruit	↑ plasma level of felodipine	Monitor BP
Flecainide			
▲	**antiarrhythmics, β-blockers, bupivacaine, verapamil**	Myocardial depression	Avoid combination
▲	**clozapine**	Arrhythmias	Avoid combination
▲	**diuretics**	Hypokalemia – cardiac toxicity	Avoid combination
▲	**tricyclic antidepressants**	Ventricular arrhythmias	Avoid combination
△	cimetidine	↑ plasma level of flecainide	Change to ranitidine
△	fluoxetine	↑ plasma level of flecainide	Use alternative SSRI
Fluconazole			
▲	**cyclosporin**	↓ metabolism of cyclosporin	Observe for adverse effect

	Interacting drug	Effect of Interaction	Action/Precaution
▲ Potentially hazardous	△ Interaction possible, but infrequent or not serious		
▲	**midazolam**	↑ plasma level of midazolam	Observe for excessive sedation
▲	**phenytoin**	↑ plasma level of phenytoin	Consider reducing dose of phenytoin
▲	**rifampicin**	↑ metabolism of fluconazole	Monitor efficacy
▲	**sulphonylureas**	↑ plasma level of sulphonylureas	Monitor blood glucose more frequently
▲	**thiazide diuretics**	↑ plasma level of fluconazole	Observe for adverse effect
▲	**warfarin**	↑ anticoagulant effect	Monitor INR closely
△	carbamazepine, celecoxib	↑ plasma level of interacting drug	Observe for adverse effect
Gabapentin			
△	antacids	↓ absorption of gabapentin	Take at least 2 hours apart
Glibenclamide, Gliclazide, Glipizide			
▲	**warfarin**	Altered warfarin effect	Monitor blood glucose and INR closely
▲	**ACEi, alcohol, ciprofloxacin, fluconazole, NSAID, octreotide, salicylates**	Risk of hypoglycemia	Monitor blood glucose closely
△	corticosteroids, diuretics, methotrimeprazine	↓ hypoglycemic effect	Monitor blood glucose
Haloperidol			
▲	**amiodarone, moxifloxacin, TCA**	Risk of ventricular arrhythmias	Avoid combination
▲	**clozapine**	Risk of neutropenia	Avoid depot haloperidol
▲	**domperidone, clarithromycin, erythromycin, methadone**	Prolongation of the QT interval	ECG before starting to exclude pre-existing prolonged QT interval
▲	**fluoxetine, fluvoxamine**	↑ plasma level of haloperidol	Observe for adverse effects
▲	**phenytoin, valproate**	↓ anticonvulsive effect	Avoid combination
▲	**rifampicin**	↑ metabolism of haloperidol	Monitor efficacy
△	ACEi	Risk of hypotension	Monitor BP and symptoms of hypotension
△	alcohol, indomethacin	↑ sedative effect	Use alternative NSAID
△	antimuscarinics	↓ effects of haloperidol	Monitor efficacy
△	buspirone, venlafaxine	↑ plasma level of haloperidol	Observe for drowsiness/ extrapyramidal side-effects
△	carbamazepine, phenobarbital	↑ metabolism of haloperidol	If necessary, increase haloperidol dose
△	morphine	↑ risk of myoclonus	Observe for myoclonic jerks
△	tramadol	↑ risk of seizures	Avoid if seizures are a risk
Heparin			
▲	**aspirin, diclofenac(IV), NSAIDs**	↑ risk of bleeding	Monitor clotting. Use with PPI cover
▲	**ketorolac**	↑ risk of bleeding	Avoid combination
△	ACEi	Risk of hyperkalemia	Monitor electrolytes
Iron			
△	bisphosphonates, ciprofloxacin, levodopa, mycophenolate, norfloxacin	↓ absorption of interacting drug	Take at least 2 hours apart
△	calcium salts, magnesium salts	↓ absorption of oral iron	Take at least 2 hours apart
△	tetracyclines	↓ absorption of iron and tetracycline	Take at least 2 hours apart
Itraconazole			
▲	**atorvastatin, simvastatin**	↑ risk of myopathy	Use fluconazole

	Interacting drug	Effect of Interaction	Action/Precaution
▲ Potentially hazardous	△ Interaction possible, but infrequent or not serious		
▲	**cyclosporin, digoxin**	↑ plasma level of interacting drug	Observe for adverse effects
▲	**ritonavir**	↑ plasma level of both drugs	Observe for adverse effects
▲	**disopyramide**	Manufacturer advises against use	Avoid combination
▲	**midazolam**	↑ sedative effect	Reduce dose of midazolam
▲	**phenytoin, rifampicin**	↓ plasma level of itraconazole	Use fluconazole
▲	**warfarin**	↑ anticoagulant effect	Monitor INR closely – reduce dose
△	alfentanil	↓ metabolism of alfentanil	Observe for adverse effects.
△	alprazolam	↑ plasma level of alprazolam	Observe for adverse effects
△	antacids, phenobarbital, ranitidine, PPIs, carbamazepine	↓ plasma level of itraconazole	Increase itraconazole dose or use fluconazole
△	buspirone	↑ plasma level of buspirone	Reduce dose of buspirone
△	CCBs	Negative inotropic effect	Observe for cardiac effects
△	clarithromycin	↑ plasma level of itraconazole	Observe for adverse effects. Switch antifungals
△	corticosteroids	↓ metabolism of corticosteroid	Reduce dose of corticosteroids
Ketamine			
▲	**memantine**	CNS toxicity	Avoid combination
△	theophylline	↑ risk of seizures	Observe for any seizure activity
Ketoconazole			
▲	**cyclosporin**	↓ metabolism of interacting drugs	Avoid combination
▲	**domperidone**	Risk of arrhythmias	Avoid combination
▲	**midazolam**	↑ sedative effect	Reduce dose of midazolam
▲	**phenytoin**	↓ plasma level of ketoconazole	Avoid combination
▲	**rifampicin**	↓ plasma level of both drugs	Avoid combination
▲	**simvastatin**	Risk of myopathy	Avoid combination
△	carbamazepine	↑ plasma level of carbamazepine	Observe for carbamazepine adverse effects or use topical antifungal
△	enteral feeds	↓ absorption of ketoconazole	Stop feed for 1 hour before and 2 hours after drug administration
△	PPIs – omeprazole, lansoprazole, ranitidine, sucralfate	↓ plasma level of ketoconazole	Use fluconazole
Labetolol (*see also* β-blocker)			
△	cimetidine	↑ plasma level of labetolol	Monitor BP closely
△	imipramine	↑ plasma level of imipramine	Observe for adverse effects
Lansoprazole (*see also* proton pump inhibitor)			
△	antacids, sucralfate	↓ absorption of interacting drug	Take at least 2 hours apart
Lorazepam			
△	valproate	↑ plasma level of lorazepam	Observe for adverse effects
Metformin			
△	ACEi, cimetidine, MAOIs	Risk of hypoglycemia	Monitor blood glucose more frequently
△	alcohol	Risk of lactic acidosis	
△	octreotide	↑ effects of metformin	
Methadone			
▲	**voriconazole**	↑ plasma level of methadone	Avoid combination

	Interacting drug	Effect of Interaction	Action/Precaution
▲ Potentially hazardous	△ Interaction possible, but infrequent or not serious		
▲	**domperidone, clarithromycin, erythromycin**	Prolongation of the QT interval	ECG before starting to exclude pre-existing prolonged QT interval
△	carbamazepine	↓ plasma level of methadone	Monitor efficacy
△	ciprofloxacin	↓ effects of methadone	Monitor efficacy
△	fluvoxamine	↑ plasma level of methadone	Observe for adverse effects
△	phenytoin	↑ metabolism of methadone (↓ effect)	Monitor efficacy
Methotrimeprazine			
▲	**amiodarone, disopyramide, pimozide, procainamide, sotalol, tricyclic antidepressants**	Risk of ventricular arrhythmia	Avoid combination
▲	**barbiturates, carbamazepine**	↓ anticonvulsant effect	Avoid combination
▲	**tricyclic antidepressants**	↑ antimuscarinic side-effects	Observe for adverse effects
△	ACEi, β-blocker, CCB, clonidine, diuretics, nitrates	Risk of hypotension	Monitor BP
△	antacids	↓ absorption of methotrimeprazine	Monitor efficacy
△	antimuscarinics	↑ antimuscarinic side-effects	Monitor for side-effects
△	anxiolytics and hypnotics	↑ sedative effect	Observe for drowsiness
△	sulphonylureas	↑ blood glucose level	Monitor blood glucose
Methylphenidate			
▲	**clonidine**	Cardiac toxicity, sudden death, rebound ↑BP (unsure mechanism)	Avoid combination
▲	**MAOIs**	Risk of hypertensive crisis	Avoid methylphenidate for at least 2 weeks after stopping MAOIs
▲	**warfarin**	↑ anticoagulant effect	Monitor INR closely
△	antidepressant – tricyclic and SSRI, phenobarbital, phenytoin	↑ plasma level of interacting drugs	Observe for adverse effects
Metoclopramide			
▲	**cyclosporin**	↑ plasma level of cyclosporin	Avoid combination
△	antimuscarinics, opioids, TCA	↓ effects of metoclopramide	Increase metoclopramide dose
△	antipsychotics	↑ risk of extrapyramidal side-effects	Observe for adverse effects
Metoprolol (*see* also β-blocker)			
△	cimetidine, citalopram, paroxetine	↑ plasma level of metoprolol	Monitor BP and heart rate
△	rifampicin	↓ plasma level of metoprolol	Monitor BP closely
Metronidazole (NB. Interaction with alcohol is rare)			
▲	**phenytoin**	Antifolate effect, ↓ metabolism of phenytoin	Avoid combination
▲	**warfarin**	↑ anticoagulant effect	Monitor INR closely
△	cimetidine	↑ plasma level of metronidazole	Observe for adverse effects
△	lithium	↑ plasma level of lithium (toxicity)	Monitor lithium levels closely
△	prednisolone	↓ plasma level of metronidazole	Monitor efficacy
Mexiletine			
▲	**antiarrhythmics – all**	Myocardial depression	Avoid combination
▲	**antipsychotics**	QT prolongation – ventricular arrhythmias	Avoid combination
▲	**diuretics**	Hypokalemia – cardiac toxicity	Monitor electrolytes closely
△	fluvoxamine	↑ plasma level of mexiletine	Observe for adverse effects

	Interacting drug	Effect of Interaction	Action/Precaution
▲ Potentially hazardous	△ Interaction possible, but infrequent or not serious		
△	phenobarbital, phenytoin, rifampicin	↓ plasma level of mexiletine	May need to increase mexiletine dose
Miconazole (NB. Systemic absorption can occur from topical oral miconazole)			
▲	**cyclosporin, gliclazide, glipizide, phenytoin, sulphonylureas**	↑ plasma level of interacting drug	Observe for adverse effects
▲	**simvastatin**	Risk of myopathy	Use fluconazole
▲	**warfarin**	↑ anticoagulant effect	Monitor INR closely
△	carbamazepine	↑ plasma level of carbamazepine	Observe for adverse effects
Midazolam			
▲	**clarithromycin, erythromycin, fluconazole, itraconazole, ketoconazole**	↓ metabolism of midazolam	Avoid combination
▲	**indinavir, ritonavir**	↑ sedative effect	Reduce midazolam dose
△	diltiazem, verapamil	↑ sedative effect	Observe for excessive drowsiness
△	carbamazepine, rifampicin	↓ plasma level of interacting drug	Monitor efficacy
Mirtazapine (*see also* antidepressants)			
▲	**alcohol, sedatives**	Risk of severe sedation	Observe closely for sedation
△	cimetidine, ketoconazole	↑ plasma level of mirtazapine	Observe for adverse effects
△	carbamazepine, phenytoin	↓ plasma level of mirtazapine	Observe for loss of effect
△	tramadol, venlafaxine	↑ risk of serotonergic effects	Observe for adverse effects
△	warfarin	↑ effect of warfarin	Observe INR closely
Morphine			
△	amitriptyline, chlorpromazine, doxepin, haloperidol	↑ risk of myoclonus	Monitor for myoclonic jerks
△	esmolol	↑ plasma level of esmolol	Monitor β-blocker side-effects
Nicardipine			
▲	**cyclosporin, digoxin**	↑ plasma level of interacting drug	Observe for adverse effects
▲	**rifampicin, carbamazepine, phenytoin**	↓ plasma level of nicardipine	Monitor efficacy
△	grapefruit	↑ plasma level of nicardipine	Observe for adverse effects
Nifedipine			
▲	**β-blockers**	Severe hypotension and heart failure	Monitor BP closely
▲	**digoxin**	↑ plasma level of digoxin	Observe for adverse effects
▲	**magnesium IV**	Severe hypotension	Monitor BP closely
▲	**phenytoin**	↓ effects of nifedipine	Use alternative anticonvulsant
▲	**rifampicin, carbamazepine**	↓ plasma level of nifedipine	Monitor efficacy
△	diltiazem, fluoxetine, grapefruit	↑ plasma level of nifedipine	Monitor for side-effects
△	diltiazem	↑ plasma level of diltiazem	Monitor for side-effects
△	insulin	↓ hypoglycemic effect	Monitor blood glucose closely
NSAIDs			
▲	**cyclosporin**	Renal impairment	Monitor renal function
▲	**digoxin**	Digoxin toxicity, renal impairment	Monitor digoxin levels and renal function
▲	**corticosteroid, heparin, SSRI, venlafaxine, warfarin**	↑ risk of bleeding	Avoid combination
▲	**lithium**	↑ plasma level of lithium (toxicity)	Monitor lithium levels closely
▲	**methotrexate**	Methotrexate toxicity (↓ excretion)	Use with specialist advice

	Interacting drug	Effect of Interaction	Action/Precaution
▲ Potentially hazardous	△ Interaction possible, but infrequent or not serious		
▲	**phenytoin**	↑ effects of phenytoin	Avoid combination
▲	**sulphonylureas**	Risk of hypoglycemia	Monitor glucose levels closely
△	ACEi, loops and thiazide diuretics	Renal impairment, ↓ effects of ACEi	Monitor BP and renal function
△	baclofen	↑ plasma level of baclofen	Monitor for side-effects
△	Diuretics – K+ sparing	Hyperkalemia	Monitor electrolytes
Nystatin			
△	chlorhexidine	↓ effects of nystatin	Take at least 2 hours apart
Olanzapine			
▲	**benzodiazepine parenteral (with IM olanzapine)**	↓ BP, bradycardia, respiratory depression	Avoid combination
▲	**valproate**	Risk of neutropenia	Avoid combination
△	carbamazepine, ciprofloxacin, fluvoxamine	↓ plasma level of olanzapine (↑ metabolism)	Monitor efficacy
Omeprazole			
▲	**warfarin**	↑ anticoagulant effect	Monitor INR closely
△	clarithromycin, diazepam, escitalopram, phenytoin	↑ plasma level of interacting drug	Observe for adverse effects
△	voriconazole, clarithromycin	↑ plasma level of omeprazole	Consider reducing omeprazole dose
△	clozapine	↓ plasma level of clozapine	Monitor efficacy
Opioids (*see also* alfentanil, morphine, and methadone)			
▲	**MAOIs**	CNS excitation or depression	Avoid until 2 weeks after stopping MAOIs
△	antipsychotics, TCAs	↑ sedative effect	Observe for excessive sedation
△	cimetidine	↑ plasma level of some opioids	Use ranitidine instead
△	ciprofloxacin	↓ plasma level of ciprofloxacin	Avoid premedication with opioids
△	domperidone, metoclopramide	↓ effect on GI motility	Use higher dose of domperidone or metoclopramide
Pamidronate			
△	aminoglycosides	Risk of hypocalcemia	Avoid combination
Phenobarbital			
▲	**antipsychotics**	↓ seizure threshold, ↓ anticonvulsant effect	Observe for adverse effects
▲	**CCB, cyclosporin, corticosteroids, verapamil, voriconazole**	↓ effects of interacting drug	Monitor efficacy
▲	**St. John's wort**	↓ plasma level of phenobarbital	Monitor efficacy
▲	**TC antidepressants**	↓ anticonvulsant effect, ↑ metabolism of TCAs	Monitor efficacy
▲	**warfarin**	↓ anticoagulant effect	Monitor INR closely
△	carbamazepine, clonazepam, ethosuximide, haloperidol, lamotrigine, paroxetine, phenytoin, valproate	↓ plasma level of interacting drug	Monitor efficacy
△	methylphenidate, phenytoin, valproate	↑ plasma level of phenobarbital	Observe for adverse effect
△	SSRI	↓ seizure threshold, ↓ anticonvulsant effect	Observe for adverse effect
Phenytoin			
▲	**amiodarone, cimetidine, esomeprazole, fluconazole, fluoxetine, fluvoxamine, metronidazole, NSAID**	↑ plasma level of phenytoin (↓ metabolism)	Monitor for phenytoin toxicity
▲	**rifampicin, St. John's wort**	↓ plasma level of phenytoin (↑metabolism)	Monitor efficacy

	Interacting drug	Effect of Interaction	Action/Precaution
▲ Potentially hazardous		**△ Interaction possible, but infrequent or not serious**	
▲	**antipsychotics**	↓ anticonvulsant effect	Observe for adverse effect
▲	**corticosteroids, warfarin**	↑ metabolism of interacting drug	Monitor efficacy, monitor INR
▲	**diltiazem**	↑ level of phenytoin, ↓ effects of diltiazem	Observe for adverse effect
▲	**itraconazole, ketoconazole, TCA**	↓ plasma levels of interacting drug	Monitor efficacy
▲	**nifedipine**	↓ effect of nifedipine	Monitor efficacy
▲	**sucralfate**	↓ absorption of phenytoin	Take at least 2 hours apart
▲	**trimethoprim**	↑ antifolate effect, ↑ phenytoin level	Monitor for phenytoin toxicity
△	antacids, carbamazepine, clonazepam, digoxin, haloperidol, lamotrigine, methadone, paroxetine, phenytoin, valproate, verapamil	↓ plasma level of interacting drug	Monitor efficacy
△	aspirin, clarithromycin, omeprazole	↑ plasma level of phenytoin	Monitor for phenytoin toxicity
△	sulfonamides, tolbutamide, valproate	Altered level of phenytoin (↑or↓)	Monitor for phenytoin toxicity
△	lithium	Risk of neurotoxicity	Observe for adverse effect
△	ondansetron, quetiapine	↑ metabolism of interacting drug	Monitor efficacy
△	phenobarbital	↑ plasma level of phenobarbital, altered plasma level of phenytoin (↑or↓)	Observe for adverse effect

Primidone

	Interacting drug	Effect of Interaction	Action/Precaution
▲	**antipsychotics, SSRI, TCA**	↓ anticonvulsant effects	Monitor efficacy
▲	**CCBs**	↓ effects of dihydropyridines	Monitor efficacy
▲	**chloramphenicol, cyclosporin, corticosteroids, voriconazole, valproate**	↑ metabolism of interacting drug	Monitor efficacy
▲	**diltiazem, verapamil**	↓ effects of diltiazem	Monitor efficacy
▲	**St. John's wort**	↓ plasma level of primidone	Avoid combination
▲	**warfarin**	↓ anticoagulant effect	Monitor INR closely
▲	**valproate**	↑ plasma level of primidone	Observe for adverse effect
△	carbamazepine	↓ plasma level of carbamazepine	Monitor efficacy
△	alcohol	↑ sedative effect	Observe for adverse effect
△	clonazepam, carbamazepine	↓ plasma level of interacting drug	Monitor efficacy
△	doxycycline, haloperidol	↑ metabolism of interacting drug	Monitor efficacy
△	MAOIs	↓ anticonvulsant effects	Monitor efficacy
△	phenytoin	Altered plasma level of both drugs	Monitor closely for adverse effects

Propranolol

	Interacting drug	Effect of Interaction	Action/Precaution
▲	**α-blockers**	Risk of hypotension	Avoid combination
▲	**antiarrhythmics – all**	Myocardial depression	Avoid combination
▲	**antipsychotics**	QT prolongation – ventricular arrhythmias	Avoid combination
▲	**bupivacaine**	Bupivacaine toxicity	Avoid combination
▲	**verapamil**	Asystole, severe hypotension, heart failure	Avoid combination
▲	**chlorpromazine, lidocaine**	↑ plasma levels of both drugs	Monitor for adverse effects

	Interacting drug	Effect of Interaction	Action/Precaution
▲ Potentially hazardous	△ Interaction possible, but infrequent or not serious		
▲	**clonidine**	Withdrawal hypotension	Withdraw β-blockers several days before slowly withdrawing clonidine
△	alcohol, anxiolytics, hypnotics	Risk of hypotension	Monitor BP
△	antidiabetic	Mask signs of hypoglycemia (e.g. tremor)	Monitor blood glucose
△	cimetidine	↑ plasma levels of propranolol	Use ranitidine instead
△	corticosteroids, NSAIDs	↓ hypotensive effect	Monitor BP
△	insulin	Risk of hypoglycemia	Monitor blood glucose
△	MAOIs	Risk of hypotension	Monitor BP
△	muscle relaxants	↑ muscle relaxation	Observe mobility and tone
△	rifampicin	↑ metabolism of propranolol	Monitor BP
Ranitidine			
△	itraconazole, ketoconazole	↓ plasma level of interacting drugs	Use cimetidine
Risperidone			
▲	**clozapine**	Risk of neutropenia	Do not use with depot risperidone
△	carbamazepine	↓ plasma level of risperidone	Observe for loss of therapeutic effect
△	fluoxetine, paroxetine	↑ plasma level of risperidone	Observe for adverse effect
Sotalol (*see also* β-blocker)			
▲	antiarrhythmics, diuretics, moxifloxacin, TCA	↑ risk of ventricular arrhythmias	Avoid combination
Sucralfate			
▲	**phenytoin**	↓ absorption of phenytoin	Take at least 2 hours apart
▲	**warfarin**	↓ anticoagulant effect	Monitor INR closely
△	ciprofloxacin, digoxin, ketoconazole, lansoprazole, olanzapine, tetracyclines	↓ absorption of interacting drug	Take at least 2 hours apart
Tetracycline			
▲	**warfarin**	↑ anticoagulant effect	Monitor INR closely
△	antacids, enteral feeds	↓ absorption of tetracycline	Take at least 2 hours apart
△	iron, zinc	↓ absorption of both drugs	Take at least 2 hours apart
Tizanidine			
▲	**ciprofloxacin, fluvoxamine**	↑ plasma level of tizanidine	Monitor for adverse effects
△	ACEi, A2RA, CCB, β-blockers, α-blockers, clonidine, diuretics, methyldopa, nitrates	Risk of hypotension	Monitor BP
△	alcohol, anxiolytics, hypnotics	↑ sedative effect	Monitor for excessive drowsiness
Tramadol			
▲	**antidepressants – TCA and SSRI**	CNS toxicity	Avoid combination
▲	**warfarin**	↑ risk of bleeding	Monitor INR closely
△	antipsychotics	↑ risk of seizures	Change to alternative weak opioid
△	carbamazepine	↓ effect of tramadol	Monitor for increased pain
△	digoxin	Digoxin toxicity	Monitor digoxin levels
Trimethoprim			
▲	**amiodarone**	Risk of ventricular arrhythmia	Avoid combination
▲	**cyclosporin**	Renal impairment, ↓ plasma level of cyclosporin with IV trimethoprim	Monitor renal function
▲	**phenytoin**	Antifolate effect, ↓ metabolism of phenytoin	Observe for adverse effect

	Interacting drug	Effect of Interaction	Action/Precaution
▲ Potentially hazardous	△ Interaction possible, but infrequent or not serious		
△	digoxin, sulphonylureas	↑ plasma level of interacting drug	Monitor digoxin levels
△	rifampicin	↓ plasma level of trimethoprim	Monitor efficacy
△	warfarin	↑ anticoagulant effect	Monitor INR closely
Valproate			
▲	**antipsychotics, SSRI, St. John's wort, TCA**	↓ anticonvulsant effect, ↓ seizure threshold	Avoid if risk of seizure
▲	**cimetidine**	↑ plasma level of valproate ↑ risk of neutropenia	Observe for adverse effect
▲	**primidone**	↑ level of primidone, ↓ level of valproate	Observe for adverse effect
▲	**olanzapine**	↑ risk of side-effects	Monitor bloods
△	amitriptyline	Altered level of amitriptyline	Observe for adverse effect
△	aspirin, lorazepam, diazepam	↑ plasma level of interacting drug	Observe for adverse effect
△	carbamazepine, phenytoin	↓ plasma level of valproate	Observe for efficacy
△	clonazepam	↑ risk of side-effects	Observe for adverse effect
△	erythromycin	↓ plasma level of valproate	Observe for adverse effect
△	MAOIs	↓ anticonvulsant effect	Observe for efficacy
△	phenytoin	Altered plasma level of both drugs	Observe for efficacy
△	cholestyramine	↓ absorption of valproate	Take at least 2 hours apart
△	warfarin	↑ anticoagulant effect enhanced	Monitor INR closely
Verapamil			
▲	**amiodarone, β-blockers**	Myocardial depression	Avoid combination
▲	**barbiturates**	↓ effects of verapamil	Avoid combination
▲	**carbamazepine, digoxin, cyclosporin**	↑ plasma level of interacting drug	Avoid combination
▲	**clarithromycin, erythromycin**	↓ metabolism of verapamil	Observe for adverse effect
▲	**rifampicin**	↑ metabolism of verapamil	Avoid combination
△	buspirone	↑ plasma level of buspirone	Observe for adverse effect
△	dantrolene IV	Risk of arrhythmias	Avoid IV administration of dantrolene
△	grapefruit	↑ plasma level of verapamil	Observe for adverse effect
△	imipramine, midazolam, TCA	↑ plasma level of interacting drug	Observe for adverse effect
△	phenytoin	↓ plasma level of phenytoin	Use alternative CCB
Warfarin			
▲	**alcohol, phenytoin**	Altered coagulation	Avoid combination
▲	**barbiturates, carbamazepine, St. John's wort, sucralfate, vitamin K**	↓ anticoagulant effect	Avoid combination
▲	**acetaminophen, amiodarone, azithromycin, celecoxib, cephalosporin, cimetidine, clopidogrel, ciprofloxacin, clarithromycin, corticosteroids, co-trimoxazole, cranberry juice, dextropropoxyphene, erythromycin, fluconazole, flurbiprofen, ketoconazole, methylphenidate, metronidazole, NSAIDs, omeprazole, SSRI, TCA, tetracycline, venlafaxine, voriconazole**	↑ anticoagulant effect and bleeding risk	Avoid combination if possible, otherwise monitor INR closely
▲	**enteral feeds**	↓ absorption of warfarin	Monitor INR closely

	Interacting drug	Effect of Interaction	Action/Precaution
▲ Potentially hazardous	△ Interaction possible, but infrequent or not serious		
▲	**sulphonylurea**	Risk of hypoglycemia, altered coagulation	Monitor blood glucose and INR more closely
△	allopurinol	Unpredictable risk of hypothrombinemia	Monitor INR and platelets more frequently
△	ampicillin, lactulose, trimethoprim, valproate	↑ anticoagulant effect and bleeding risk	Monitor INR closely

Zoledronic acid

	Interacting drug	Effect of Interaction	Action/Precaution
△	aminoglycosides	Risk of hypocalcemia	Monitor serum calcium level closely

Zopiclone

	Interacting drug	Effect of Interaction	Action/Precaution
△	erythromycin	↑ plasma level of zopiclone ↓ plasma level of zopiclone	Observe for adverse effects
△	rifampicin	↓ plasma level of zopiclone	Monitor efficacy

Effects of renal or hepatic impairment on common palliative care drugs

NB. Check with current drug formularies and ask for advice from the local liver or renal team.

HEPATIC IMPAIRMENT

Drug	Action
ACEi	Monitor closely for adverse effects
Amitriptyline, A2RA, anticoagulants-parenteral, antidepressants – SSRI, antidepressants – TCA, antiepileptics, antipsychotics, benzodiazepines, buprenorphine, buspirone, CCB, ceftriaxone, clonazepam, fentanyl, hyoscine hydrobromide, methadone, metoclopramide, olanzapine, oxybutynin, oxycontin	Reduce dose, avoid in severe liver disease
Antacids	In patients with fluid retention avoid antacids with high sodium content
Anticoagulants – oral, antidiabetics, co-trimoxazole, demeclocycline, domperidone, NSAIDs	Avoid
Antidepressants – MAOI, antifungals, clarithromycin, amoxicillin/clavulanic acid, erythromycin, acetaminophen, sodium valproate	Can cause hepatotoxicity
Antihistamines (incl. dimenhydrinate and diphenhydramine)	Can cause sedation – avoid in severe liver disease
Morphine, haloperidol, phenobarbital	May cause encephalopathy in severe liver disease
Diuretics – loop and thiazide	Hypokalemia may precipitate coma
Lansoprazole, LMW heparin, metronidazole, ondansetron	Reduce dose in severe liver disease
Prednisolone	Adverse effects more common

RENAL IMPAIRMENT

Drug	Action
Acetaminophen	Reduce dose
ACEi, carbamazepine, oxybutynin, hyoscine hydrobromide (scopolamine), haloperidol	Monitor closely for adverse effects
A2RA, benzodiazepines, baclofen, buprenorphine, cephalosporins, cimetidine, amoxicillin/clavulanic acid, co-trimoxazole, domperidone, erythromycin, insulin, midazolam, mirtazapine, olanzapine, pregabalin, sodium valproate, tinzaparin, tranexamic acid, zoledronic acid	Reduce dose
Antacids – aluminum salts, chlorpropamide, demeclocycline, tolbutamide, spironolactone	Avoid
Anticoagulants – oral or parenteral, glibenclamide, gliclazide, metoclopramide	Avoid if eGFR <10 mL/min
Antidepressants – SSRI, CCB	Caution if eGFR <30 mL/min
Bisphosphonates	Avoid if eGFR <30 mL/min. Can be used in patients on hemodialysis if renal team agrees
Codeine, dihydrocodeine, morphine, oxycodone	Reduce dose if renal impairment is stable, otherwise switch to hydromorphone or fentanyl
Gabapentin, fluconazole, itraconazole, methotrimeprazine	Reduce dose if eGFR <80 mL/min
Magnesium salts and antacids	Avoid or reduce dose
Metformin	Avoid if eGFR <60 mL/min
NSAIDs	Avoid if some renal function is still present.
Ranitidine	Reduce dose if eGFR <50 mL/min

Drugs in palliative care for children: starting doses

NB. All information on the use of drugs in children should be checked with local pediatric formularies and practice.

DRUG PHARMACOKINETICS

Children absorb, distribute, metabolize, and eliminate drugs differently from adults:

Neonates (under 1 month) have a low renal and hepatic clearance with a higher volume of distribution. This prolongs the half-life of many drugs so that they require smaller doses relative to their size, but they may need a loading dose to avoid a delay in effect. Drug and drug dose selection should be monitored by a pediatrician experienced in neonatology.

Infants (1 month to 2 years) and children (2–12 years): these children have relatively high drug clearances with a normal volume of distribution. This leads to shorter half-lives compared with adults so that they may need comparatively higher doses at shorter intervals.

Older children: children older than 12 years have similar pharmacokinetic profiles to adults.

DRUG PRESENTATION AND ROUTES

Choice of route: care and imagination are needed when selecting appropriate routes and preparations. The oral route is first line, unless a gastrostomy is present. Contrary to popular belief, children often prefer tablets rather than sickly sweet syrups or suspensions. Tablets can be halved or dissolved in liquid. Some tablets can be crushed, but not coated or controlled-release tablets. Some capsule contents can be dispersed in water, but can block feeding tubes (e.g. hydromorphone). If liquids are used their taste can be improved with fizzy drinks or fruit juice. Masking drugs in food is not recommended since the amount of drug taken is unpredictable.

Gastrostomy: many children with neurodegenerative diseases have a gastrostomy, allowing easy access for drugs that are difficult to administer through other routes, such as anticonvulsants.

Subcutaneous infusions using portable, battery-driven pumps are a valuable method of administering many drugs with minimum trouble to the child.

Other routes: in situations where oral dosing is difficult (e.g. reluctance, dysphagia, vomiting) rectal dosing is often acceptable. This route provides effective and rapid absorption and some children are willing to self-administer drugs this way. The sublingual or buccal routes are alternatives.[1] Some children already have central venous access catheters in place, often with several months' experience of their use.

Excipients: many drugs contain other chemicals necessary for their formulation – these are called excipients. Some of these can cause problems in children:

- sweeteners (mannitol, maltitol, sorbitol, or xylitol) can cause diarrhea
- propylene glycol can cause adverse effects in renal impairment and in children who metabolize it slowly.

OPIOIDS

Dosing

Infants in the first year of life are particularly sensitive to opiates. Hence a smaller recommended starting dose per kg compared with those in older children (*see* table). Children also metabolize morphine faster, so some may need short-acting preparations q2–3h rather than q4h and long-acting preparations q8h rather than q12h. As in adults, dose requirements can vary greatly between individuals.[2]

Opioid choice

This is the same as in adults (*see Using strong opioids*, p. 63).

Morphine: this remains the first-line opioid and comes in a wide range of doses and preparations.

Fentanyl has a place in the management of stable pain, but it should be used with caution. Fentanyl is a potent opioid and the smallest transdermal patch (12.5 microg/hour) is approximately equivalent to 37 mg/24 hours of oral morphine. The pharmacokinetics of transdermal fentanyl are complex, resulting in delays of up to 14 hours in steady state blood levels and up to 30 hours in reducing to low levels.[3,4] The alternative of using a subcutaneous infusion of fentanyl is less suitable in mobile children. Buccal/sublingual fentanyl can be used for brief breakthrough pain.[5,6] Fentanyl lollipops are available in the US, but it is not possible to know exactly how much fentanyl has been given or absorbed. Buccal fentanyl tablets (US only) are only available in doses that are too high for younger children at present (100 microg, equivalent to a 200 microg lollipop). Giving the injection solution sublingually, or buccally is an alternative. There is limited experience of using intranasal fentanyl in children.

USE OF DRUGS OFF-LABEL

This is common in palliative care, but especially so in pediatric care. For more information *see* p. 312.

STARTING DOSES

Doses for children can be complex since

- calculations based on weight are often needed
- doses can vary greatly between different children
- dose/kg requirements may be higher than adults, but maximum adult doses should not be exceeded
- information sources can be presented in many different ways:

micrograms	microg/m²
milligrams	mg/m²
microg/kg body weight	dose per hour
mg/kg body weight	single dose
total daily dose	24 hour infusion

Different ways of expressing doses in children

The tables that follow contain suggested starting doses and suggested frequency of dosing. Doses are in microg/kg or mg/kg as appropriate. To convert microg to mg divide by 1000. Information on different routes (including through gastrostomies) are on pp. 313–20.

Suggested starting doses				
Drug (route)	**Neonates (under 1 month)**	**Infants (1 month to 2 years)**	**Children (2–18 years)**	**Comments**
Non-opioid primary analgesics				
acetaminophen[7] (oral, PEG, rectal)	10 mg/kg q12h	1–3 m = 30 mg q8h 3–12 m = 60 mg q8h 1–2 yrs = 120 mg q6h	2–5 yrs = 120 mg q6h 6–12 yrs = 250 mg q8h >12 yrs = 500 mg q6h	Halve doses if jaundiced. In Canada licensed for use from 6 months.
ibuprofen (PEG, oral)	Not recommended	<5 kg: not recommended 1–3 m = 5 mg/kg q8h 3–12 m = 50 mg q8h 1–2 yrs = 100 mg q8h	2–4 yrs = 100 mg q8h 4–7 yrs = 150 mg q8h 7–10 yrs = 200 mg q8h >10 yrs = 300 mg q8h	Not for use in children under 5 kg weight.
diclofenac (PEG, oral)	Not recommended	1–6 m: not recommended 6–24 m = 1.5 mg/kg q12h Max = 75 mg q12h	>2 yrs = 1.5 mg/kg q12h Max = 75 mg q12h	Not licensed for use in children under 12 yrs.
Weak oral opioid primary analgesics				
codeine (PEG, oral)	500 microg/kg q6h	500 microg/kg q6h	2–12 yrs = 0.5 mg/kg q6h >12 yrs = 15 mg q6h Max = 240 mg daily	Reduce doses by 50% in renal impairment. Do not use in renal failure.
First-line strong opioid primary analgesics				
Please note: These are starting doses for children NOT previously on weak opioids – for dose conversions *see* pp. 66–7.				
morphine oral or PEG (instant release)	50 microg/kg q6h (under advice of specialist)	100 microg/kg q6h	2–12 yrs = 200 microg/kg q4h >12 yrs = 2.5 mg q4h	Can be made up in suppository form.
morphine oral or PEG (controlled release)	Not recommended	500 microg/kg (q8–12h)	2–12 yrs = 500 microg/kg >12 yrs = 5 mg (q8–12h)	–
morphine (SC injection)	25 microg/kg q6h (under advice of specialist)	50 microg/kg q6h	2–12 yrs = 100 microg/kg q4h >12 yrs = 1 mg q4h	If needed more than 3 times/24 hr, consider SC infusion.
morphine (24 hr SC infusion)	100 microg/kg over 24 hr (under advice of specialist)	200 microg/kg over 24 hr	>2 yrs = 500 microg/kg over 24 hr	–
Second-line strong opioid primary analgesics				
fentanyl hydromorphone methadone oxycodone	• *For children already on strong opioids:* convert to equivalent dose and then re-titrate if necessary (*see Using strong opioids*, p. 67). • *For children on weak opioids or no opioids:* ask for specialist advice from palliative care specialist with experience of using these opioids in children.			

Suggested starting doses				
Drug (route)	**Neonates (under 1 month)**	**Infants (1 month to 2 years)**	**Children (2–18 years)**	**Comments**
Other drugs				
amitriptyline (PEG, oral)	Not recommended	Not recommended	2–12 yrs = 200 microg/kg once at bedtime Max = 25 mg >12 yrs = 10 mg once at bedtime	Use with caution in children with cardiac dysfunction. Not for depression.
alginate (Gaviscon) (PEG, oral)	<4.5 kg = half dual sachet q6–8h >4.5 kg = one dual sachet q6–8h	<4.5 kg = half dual sachet q6–8h >4.5 kg = one dual sachet q6–8h	2–12 yrs = 2.5 mL of susp. >12 yrs = 5 mL of susp. Give after meals and bedtime	
baclofen (PEG, oral)	Not recommended	1–2 yrs = 2.5 mg q6h Max. 24 hr dose 20 mg	2–10 yrs = 2.5 mg q6h >10 yrs = 5 mg q8h Max. 24 hr doses: 2–6 yrs = 30 mg 6–10 yrs = 60 mg >10 yrs = 100 mg	Divided doses reduce adverse effects. Start with low dose and titrate at 3-day intervals until effective or adverse effects are a problem.
bisacodyl (PEG, oral, PR)	Not recommended	Not recommended	2–4 yrs = 5 mg suppository at bedtime 4–10 yrs = 5 mg tablet once in the morning >10 yrs = 10 mg tablet once in the morning	If colic is a problem try splitting the dose into two daily doses.
carbamazepine (PEG, oral or rectal)	Not recommended	5 mg/kg at night	2–12 yrs = 5 mg/kg at night >12 yrs = 100 mg once daily Max = 20 mg/kg	For rectal route, use approximately 25% more than oral dose. Start once daily, then move to q8–12h divided doses.
chloral hydrate (PEG, oral or rectal)	20 mg/kg at night	30 mg/kg at night	2–12 yrs = 30 mg/kg at night >12 yrs = 500 mg at night	–
dantrolene (PEG, oral)	Not recommended	Not recommended	2–5 yrs = not recommended 5–12 yrs = 500 microg/kg >12 yrs = 25 mg Once daily dosing initially	Not recommended for use in children <5 yrs.
desmopressin (PEG, oral)	*Diabetes insipidus* 1 microg q12h	*Diabetes insipidus* 10 microg q12h	*Diabetes insipidus* 2–12 yrs = 50 microg q12h >12 yrs = 100 microg q12h *Enuresis* >5 yrs = 200 microg at night	Not all oral preparations licensed for *Diabetes insipidus*.
(intranasal)	*Diabetes insipidus* 100 nanograms once daily	*Diabetes insipidus* 2.5 microg once daily	*Diabetes insipidus* 2–12 yrs = 5 microg daily >12 yrs = 10 microg daily	

Suggested starting doses				
Drug (route)	**Neonates (under 1 month)**	**Infants (1 month to 2 years)**	**Children (2–18 years)**	**Comments**
dexamethasone (oral, PEG, SC)	10 microg/kg once daily In emergency 4 mg daily or more (under specialist advice)	100 microg/kg once daily In emergency 4 mg daily or more	500 microg once daily In emergency 4 mg daily or more	Higher starting doses often needed for urgent treatment (e.g. raised ICP) – 0.25 mg/kg.
diazepam (PEG or oral for spasm)	Not recommended	1–12 m = 250 microg/kg q12h 1–2 yrs = 2.5 mg q12h	2–5 yrs = 2.5 mg q12h 5–12 yrs = 5 mg q12h >12 yrs = 10 mg q12h (max dose 40 mg daily)	
(IV for seizures)	300 microg/kg repeated after 10 min if needed	300 microg/kg repeated after 10 min if needed	2–12 yrs = 300 microg/kg >12 yrs = 10 mg Repeated after 10 min if needed	Maximum 10 mg as a single dose.
(rectal for seizures)	1.25–2.5 mg repeated after 10 min if necessary	5 mg repeated after 10 min if necessary	2–12 yrs = 5–10 mg >12 yrs = 10 mg Repeated after 10 min if necessary	
docusate (PEG, oral)	Not recommended	1–6 m = not recommended 6–24 m = 12.5 mg q8h	3–6 yrs = 20–60 mg/24 hr 6–12 yrs = 40–120 mg/24 hr	May give in divided doses. Takes 24–48 hours to act.
(rectal)	Not recommended	Not recommended	>12 yrs = 120 mg as single dose	Acts within 1 hour.
domperidone (PEG, oral)	100 microg/kg q6h	200 microg/kg q8h	2–12 yrs = 200 microg/kg q8h >12 yrs = 10 mg q8h	Reduce dose in renal impairment.
(rectal) (From compounding pharmacy in US)	Not recommended	<15 kg = not recommended 15–35 kg = 30 mg q12h >35 kg = 60 mg q12h	15–35 kg = 30 mg q12h >35 kg = 60 mg q12h	Reduce dose in renal repair.
fluconazole (PEG, oral)	<2 w = 3 mg/kg every 72 hrs 2–4 w = 3 mg/kg every 48 hrs	3 mg/kg daily	2–12 yrs = 3 mg/kg daily >12 yrs = 50 mg daily	Reduce dose or frequency in renal impairment.
furosemide (PEG, oral, IV)	500 microg/kg daily	500 microg/kg q12h	2–12 yrs = 500 microg/kg q12h >12 yrs = 20 mg q8h	
gabapentin (PEG, oral)	Not recommended	Not recommended	2–12 yrs = 5 mg/kg q12h >12 yrs = 100 mg q8h	Reduce dose in renal impairment. Not licensed for children <18 yrs
glycopyrrolate (SC)	5 microg/kg q8h	4 microg/kg q6h or 12 microg/kg as a 24 hr SC infusion	2–12 yrs = 40 microg/kg q6h or 12 microg/kg as a 24 hr SC infusion >12 yrs = 600 microg/24 hrs	Alternative to hyoscine hydrobromide (scopolamine).
haloperidol (PEG, oral, SC)	Not recommended	25 microg/kg q12h	2–12 yrs = 25 microg/kg q12h >12 yrs = 1.5 mg as single dose at night	Avoid high doses or prolonged courses if possible. Use lowest doses for nausea.

Suggested starting doses				
Drug (route)	**Neonates (under 1 month)**	**Infants (1 month to 2 years)**	**Children (2–18 years)**	**Comments**
hyoscine butylbromide (SC TD)	Not recommended	250 microg/kg q8h or 1 mg/kg as a 24 hr SC infusion	2–5 yrs = 5 mg q8h 5–12 yrs = 10 mg q8h >12 yrs = 10 mg q8h	Less sedating alternative to glycopyrrolate. Ineffective orally.
hyoscine hydrobromide (TD)	Not recommended	250 microg q72h as ¼ TD patch	2–3 yrs = 250 microg q72h with ¼ TD patch 3–10 yrs = 500 microg q72h with ½ TD patch >10 yrs = 1 mg q72h with whole patch	More sedating than glycopyrrolate.
(buccal, SC)		10 microg/kg q6h or 50 microg/kg as 24 hr SC infusion	2–12 yrs = 10 microg/kg q6h or 50 microg/kg as 24 hr SC infusion >12 yrs = 150 microg q6h	
imipramine (PEG, oral)	Not recommended	Not recommended	2–5 yrs = not recommended >6 yrs = 25 mg at bedtime (Off-label use)	Alternative to amitriptyline for neuropathic pain. Increase by 50% every 2–3 days.
itraconazole (PEG, oral)	Not recommended	3 mg/kg as single daily dose	2–12 yrs = 3 mg/kg as single daily dose >12 yrs = 100 mg once daily	Not licensed for children <18 yrs.
ketamine (SC, PEG, oral) (as analgesic)	50 microg/kg as single dose 1 mg/kg as 24 hr SC infusion	50 microg/kg as single dose 1 mg/kg as 24 hr SC infusion	1 mg as single dose 2.5 mg/kg as 24 hr SC infusion	Analgesic doses are approximately 10% of anesthetic doses. Only for use in specialist units
lactulose (PEG, oral)	Not recommended	1–12 m = 2.5 mL q12h 1–2 yrs = 5 mL q12h	2–5 yrs = 5 mL q12h 5–10 yrs = 10 mL q12h >10 yrs = 15 mL q12h	Takes 36–48 hr to act. High doses can cause abdominal bloating and dehydration.
lansoprazole (PEG, oral)	Not recommended	500 microg/kg (max 15 mg/24 hr)	<30 kg = 500 microg/kg >30 kg = 15 mg once daily	Not licensed for use in children Available as dissolvable tablet.
loperamide (PEG, oral)	Not recommended	Acute diarrhea – not recommended Chronic diarrhea = 100 microg/kg q12h	Acute diarrhea: 2–4 yrs = not recommended 4–8 yrs = 1 mg q8h (3 days only) 8–12 yrs = 2 mg q6h (5 days only) >12 yrs = 2 mg after each loose stool Chronic diarrhea: 2–12 yrs = 100 microg/kg q8h >12 yrs = 2 mg after each loose stool	Maximum 16 mg daily. In chronic diarrhea regular q6–8h dosing may be necessary.

Suggested starting doses				
Drug (route)	**Neonates (under 1 month)**	**Infants (1 month to 2 years)**	**Children (2–18 years)**	**Comments**
lorazepam (PEG, oral for anxiety)	25 microg/kg as single dose	50 microg/kg as single dose	2–12 yrs = 50 microg/kg q12h >12 yrs = 500 microg q8h	Sedating at higher doses.
(IV or rectal for seizure)	100 microg/kg repeated after 10 min if necessary	100 microg/kg repeated after 10 min if necessary	2–12 yrs = 100 microg/kg repeated after 10 min if necessary >12 yrs = 4 mg repeated after 10 min if necessary	IV should be a slow injection.
methotrimeprazine (PEG, oral, SC)	Not recommended	1–12 m = not recommended 1–2 yrs = 350 microg/kg as 24 hr SC infusion	2–12 yrs = 350 microg/kg as 24 hr SC infusion >12 yrs = 5 mg once at night	Found to be useful in pediatric palliative care.
metoclopramide (PEG, oral)	100 microg/kg q8h	100 microg/kg q12h (max 2 mg/24 hr)	<10 kg = 100 microg/kg q12h 10–14 kg = 1 mg q12h 15–19 kg = 2 mg q12h 20–29 kg = 2.5 mg q8h 30–59 kg = 5 mg q8h	
(SC infusion over 24 hr)	300 microg/kg	200 microg/kg (max 2 mg/24 hr)	<10 kg = 300 microg/kg 10–14 kg = 2 mg 15–19 kg = 4 mg 20–29 kg = 7.5 mg 30–59 kg = 15 mg	
metronidazole (PEG, oral)	7.5 mg/kg q12h	7.5 mg/kg q8h (max 1.2 g/24 hr)	2–12 yrs = 7.5 mg/kg q8h >12 yrs = 400 mg q8h	Doses and regimens vary with the diagnosis.
(rectal)	Not recommended	1–12 m = 125 mg q8h 1–2 yrs = 250 mg q8h	2–5 yrs = 250 mg 8-q12h 5–12 yrs = 500 mg q8–12h >12 yrs = 1 g q8–12h	Doses and regimens vary with the diagnosis.
miconazole (topical oral gel)	24 mg (1 mL) q12h	48 mg (2 mL) q12h	2–6 yrs = 120 mg (5 mL) q12h 6–12 yrs = 120 mg (5 mL) q6h >12 yrs = 240 mg (10 mL) q6h	Not licensed in children under 2 yrs.
midazolam (SC or IV infusion for sedation)	25 microg/kg/hr infusion	1–24 m = 50 microg/kg/hr infusion 6–24 m = 30 microg/kg/hr infusion	2–12 yrs = 50 microg/kg/hr infusion >12 yrs = 50 microg/kg/hr infusion	Allows more accurate titration than diazepam.
(buccal or IV for seizure)	300 microg/kg repeated once after 10 min if needed as single dose	1–6 m = 300 microg/kg 6–12 m = 2.5 mg 1–2 yrs = 5 mg Repeat after 10 min if necessary	2–5 yrs = 5 mg 5–10 yrs = 7.5 mg >10 yrs = 10 mg Repeat after 10 min if necessary	Buccal route delay is 5–10 min.
octreotide (SC)	2 microg/kg q8h	1 microg/kg q6h	1 microg/kg q6h	Higher doses needed for hyperinsulinemic hypoglycemia.

Suggested starting doses				
Drug (route)	**Neonates (under 1 month)**	**Infants (1 month to 2 years)**	**Children (2–18 years)**	**Comments**
omeprazole (PEG, oral)	700 microg/kg once daily	700 microg/kg once daily	10–20 kg = 10 mg daily >20 kg = 20 mg daily	Available as granules for suspension (US).
ondansetron (PEG, oral)	Not recommended	1–12 m = not recommended >1 yr = 4 mg q12h	4 mg q12h	Constipating.
(SC or IV)	Not recommended	1–2 yrs = 100 microg/kg q12h	100 microg/kg q12h	Not licensed in children under 2 yrs.
phenobarbital (PEG, oral, IV, SC)	2.5 mg/kg once daily	1 mg/kg q12h	2–12 yrs = 1 mg/kg q12h >12 yrs = 60 mg once daily	Plasma half-life shorter in young children. Give IV slowly.
ranitidine (PEG, oral)	2 mg/kg q8h	1–6 m = 1 mg/kg q8h 6–24 m = 2 mg/kg q12h	2–12 yrs = 2 mg/kg q12h >12 yrs = 150 mg q12h	Daily doses should not exceed 300 mg.
salbutamol (nebulized)	2.5 mg as a single dose, repeated if necessary	2.5 mg as a single dose, repeated if necessary	2–12 yrs = 2.5 mg >12 yrs = 5 mg Give as a single dose, repeated if necessary	For older children, administration through a mouthpiece is better tolerated and more effective.
senna syrup (PEG, oral)	Not recommended	0.5 mL/kg once daily (max 2.5 mL)	2–6 yrs = 2.5 mL/kg daily 6–12 yrs = 5 mL/kg daily >12 yrs = 10 mL/kg daily	Can be given once daily, but there is less chance of colic with divided doses.
spironolactone (PEG, oral)	1 mg/kg once daily	1 mg/kg once daily	2–12 yrs = 1 mg/kg q12h >12 yrs = 50 mg q12h	Monitor K^+ levels, especially in renal impairment.
sucralfate (PEG, oral)	Not recommended	250 mg q6h	2–12 yrs = 500 mg q6h >12 yrs 1 g q6h	Used as a hemostatic agent or gastric mucosal coating agent.
temazepam (PEG, oral for sedation)	Not recommended	1–12 m = not recommended 1–2 yrs = 1 mg/kg as single dose	2–12 yrs = 1 mg/kg as single dose >12 yrs = 10 mg	For sleep or procedures.
tranexamic acid (PEG, oral)	Not recommended	15 mg/kg q12h	15 mg/kg q12h	Can be used topically to stop bleeding.

NOTES

Using drugs off-label

In adult and pediatric palliative care up to a quarter of drugs are not licensed for their intended use or routes.[8] It is accepted, however, that this is a legitimate aspect of practice.[9] The following guidelines have been adapted from the UK ones:[10]

- A drug license applies to the activities of the pharmaceutical company, not the doctor's prescribing practice.
- The cost of testing new uses and routes means that they are unlikely to be tested by pharmaceutical companies to gain a license.
- Preparations that are imported or specially prepared can be prescribed for named patients.
- The responsibilities lie with the prescribing doctor.

Background to off-label prescribing

The key to safe prescribing and administration of drugs off-label is to keep risks to a minimum. Some basic rules will reduce the risks to the prescriber and person administering the preparation:[10]

- The drug or preparation should
  - be licensed for other uses and routes
  - be well known and studied
  - have previously been used by others for the intended route and purpose.
- The reasons for use should not be trivial.
- In the case of new, or little used, uses and routes:
  - the reasons should be documented in the chart
  - the patient should be asked for consent (or if the patient does not have capacity the clinical team should document why it is in the patient's best interests)
  - other professionals involved with the patient should be informed.

Basic rules for off-label prescribing

Alternative routes for drugs

ORAL ROUTE

This is preferred by most patients. When available, patients should be given a choice of preparation. This may be a tablet (plain or coated), capsule, liquid (solution or suspension), or a dispersible preparation.

High sodium containing drugs: some oral drugs and preparations contain high levels of sodium which can cause severe hypernatremia. Particular culprits are tablets that effervesce in water. Patients with conditions that can be exacerbated by sodium retention (e.g. cerebral edema, heart failure) should be switched to other preparations.

NON-ORAL ROUTES

The oral route is not always possible. The intravenous route is sometimes needed for a rapid effect in emergencies. The intramuscular route is suitable for single doses when the intravenous route is not available, but it is not suitable for repeated use because of discomfort. However, the subcutaneous, rectal, and buccal/sublingual routes provide useful alternatives. Experience and investigation have shown that many drugs can be safely and effectively given by the subcutaneous route.[10,11] Some drugs can also be given topically or through a feeding tube.[12]

CONTINUOUS SUBCUTANEOUS INFUSION (CSCI)

This route is now well known and fully described elsewhere.[10] Following some basic rules, increases the likely success of this delivery system:

- Use a plastic cannula rather than a metal butterfly.
- Choose a protected site, e.g. upper anterior chest.
- Use a pump that is familiar to you.
- Use a familiar procedure for priming the line.
- Use only drugs that are known to be safe and effective by the subcutaneous route.
- Use 0.9% saline for diluting drugs. If necessary drugs can be diluted with "water for injection," except for ketamine, ketorolac, ondansetron and octreotide, which should be diluted with 0.9%saline.
- Limit the number of drugs per syringe or bag to two.
- Check the pump sever al times in 24 hours (or instruct the patient, partner or relative to do so).
- Know the procedure needed for infusion failures (check cannula, tubing, syringe/bag, battery, and pump).

Basic rules for CSCI

GASTROSTOMY AND JEJUNOSTOMY ROUTES

Many drugs can be given this way with some precautions:

- Do not use enteric coated tablets or capsules.
- Do not use modified release tablets or capsules.
- Do not use preparations intended for buccal use.
- Avoid giving antibiotics, cytotoxics, or hormones.
- If an injection solution is used, dilute it with at least 30 mL water.

See www.palliativedrugs.com for more details.

AVAILABLE ROUTES FOR DRUGS

Abbreviations: tablet (T), capsule (C), liquid (L), powder (P), granules (G), chewable (Ch), dispersible (D), transdermal (TD), specially prepared (s) ir = immediate release, sr = sustained release, CSCI = SC infusion, bolus = bolus injection

Drug	Tablet or capsule	Liquid or dispersible preps	Buccal/ sublingual/ nasal	Gastrostomy route possible?	IV	IM	SC	Rectal	Topical
acetaminophen	Yes T (ir)	Yes L	No	Yes – use oral liquid	No	No	No	Yes	No
amitriptyline	Yes T	No	No	No	No	No	No	No	No
amoxicillin	Yes C (ir)	Yes L, P	No	Yes – oral suspension or injection solution	Yes	Yes, but not usually used	No information	No	No
amoxicillin/ clavulanic acid	Yes T (ir)	Yes L, D	No	Yes – use oral suspension but dilute to half strength and flush well	No	No	No	No	No
antacids	Yes T, C (ir)	Yes L	No	May interact with feeds	No	No	No	No	No
baclofen	Yes T (ir)	No	No	Yes – crush tablet in water (takes 5 min)	No	No	No	No	No
bulk laxatives	No	Yes P	No	No – use feed with high fiber content	No	No	No	No	No
calcitonin	No	No	Yes – nasal spray	No	No	Yes	Yes Bolus or CSCI	No	No
carbamazepine	Yes T (ir/sr)	Yes L	No	Yes – use oral liquid diluted with equal volume water (stop feed 1 hr before and after). May interact with feeds.	No	No	No	Yes, 125 mg PR = 100 mg orally[13–15]	No
ceftriaxone	No	No	No	No information	Yes	Yes	Yes. Bolus (1 mL mixed with 2 mL lidocaine)[16]		
chloral hydrate	Yes T (ir) (Canada); C (ir) (US)	Yes L	No	Yes – use oral liquid diluted with water	No	No	No	No	No
cimetidine	Yes T	Yes L	No	Yes – use oral liquid	No	No	No	No	No

Abbreviations: tablet (T), capsule (C), liquid (L), powder (P), granules (G), chewable (Ch), dispersible (D), transdermal (TD), specially prepared (s) ir = immediate release, sr = sustained release, CSCI = SC infusion, bolus = bolus injection

Drug	Tablet or capsule	Liquid or dispersible preps	Buccal/ sublingual/ nasal	Gastrostomy route possible?	IV	IM	SC	Rectal	Topical
ciprofloxacin	Yes T (ir)	Yes L	No	Use oral solution washed down with 30–50 mL *distilled* or *sterile* water. May interact with feeds.	Yes	No	No	No	No
clonazepam	Yes T (ir)	No	No	Yes – crush tablet with 30–60 mL water. May bind to tube.	No	No	No	Yes[17]	No
codeine	Yes T (ir/sr)	Yes L	No	Yes – use oral liquid diluted with equal volume of water	Yes, but not usually used	Yes, but not usually used	No information	No information	No
co-trimoxazole	Yes T(ir)	Yes L	No	Yes – dilute liquid with 3 times as much water	Yes	No	No	No	No
desmopressin	Yes T (ir)	Yes D	Yes (nasal)	No information	Yes, but not usually used	Yes, but not usually used	Yes Bolus or CSCI	No	No
dexamethasone	Yes T (ir)	Disperse or dissolve in water	Yes (topical)	Yes – disperse tablet in water	Yes over 2 min	Yes, but not usually used	Yes Bolus	Yes (local action)	Yes
diazepam	Yes T (ir)	Yes L	No	Yes – use oral liquid but dilute with equal volume water and flush well. May bind to and interact with feeds.	Yes	Yes	No	Yes	No
diclofenac	Yes T (ir/sr)	No	No	No	Yes	No	No	Yes[18]	No
docusate	Yes C (ir)	Yes L (very bitter taste)	No	Yes – dilute liquid with equal volume of water	No	No	No	Yes	No
domperidone (in US available from a compounding pharmacy)	Yes T (ir)	Yes L	No	Yes – dilute liquid with equal volume of water	No	No	No	Yes	No

Abbreviations: tablet (T), capsule (C), liquid (L), powder (P), granules (G), chewable (Ch), dispersible (D), transdermal (TD), specially prepared (s) ir = immediate release, sr = sustained release, CSCI = SC infusion, bolus = bolus injection

Drug	Tablet or capsule	Liquid or dispersible preps	Buccal/ sublingual/ nasal	Gastrostomy route possible?	IV	IM	SC	Rectal	Topical
doxepin	Yes C (ir)	No	No	Yes – disperse capsule contents in water	No	No	No	No	Yes
erythromycin	Yes T, C (ir)	Yes L	No	Dilute liquid with equal volume of water	Yes	Yes	No information	No	No
fentanyl	No	No	Yes (use injection liquid)	No	Yes, titrated	Yes, but not usually used	Yes Bolus or CSCI	Yes, but unusual	Yes (trans-dermal)
fluconazole	Yes T, C (ir)	Yes L	No	Yes – use oral liquid (do not use contents of 150 mg capsule)	Yes	No	No	No	No
fluoxetine	Yes C (ir)	Yes L	No	No information	No	No	No	No	No
furosemide	Yes T (ir)	Yes L	No	Yes – use oral liquid but flush with 30–50 mL water	Yes	Yes	Yes	No	No
gabapentin	Yes C (ir)	No	No	Yes – disperse capsule contents in water	No	No	No	No	No (Canada) Yes (from compounding pharmacy in US)
glycopyrrolate	No	No	No	Yes – use injection solution	Yes, but not usually used	Yes, but not usually used	Yes Bolus or CSCI	No	No
haloperidol	Yes T (ir)	Yes L	No	Yes – disperse tablets in water. Oral solution can cause diarrhea.	Yes, but not usually used	Yes, but not usually used	Yes Bolus or CSCI	No	No
hydromorphone	Yes T (ir) C (sr)	No	No[19]	No – blocks tube	Yes, but not usually used	Yes, but not usually used	Yes[20] Bolus or CSCI	Yes,[21] but not often used	No
hyoscine butylbromide (Canada only)	Yes but poor absorption T (ir)	No	No	Yes, but poor absorption	Yes, but not usually used	Yes, but not usually used	Yes Bolus or CSCI	No	No

Abbreviations: tablet (T), capsule (C), liquid (L), powder (P), granules (G), chewable (Ch), dispersible (D), transdermal (TD), specially prepared (s) ir = immediate release, sr = sustained release, CSCI = SC infusion, bolus = bolus injection

Drug	Tablet or capsule	Liquid or dispersible preps	Buccal/ sublingual/ nasal	Gastrostomy route possible?	IV	IM	SC	Rectal	Topical
hyoscine hydrobromide/ scopolamine	No	No	Yes (SL, buccal)[1,22]	Yes – but not usually used	Yes, but not usually used	Yes, but not usually used	Yes Bolus or CSCI	No	Yes (TD)
ibuprofen	Yes T (ir) T, C (sr)	Yes L	No	Yes – use oral liquid or granules with 20 mL water	No	No	No	No	No
ketamine	No	Yes L (use Injection liquid orally)	Yes (SL, nasal) but experience is limited	No information	Yes, but not usually used	Yes, but not usually used	Yes Bolus or CSCI	No	No
ketoconazole	Yes T (ir)	No	No	Yes – crush tablet with water (stop feed 1 hr before and after). May interact with feeds.	No	No	No	No	No
lansoprazole	Yes C (ir/sr)	No	No	Yes – use dispersible tablets in water. Oral liquid too viscous. Do not use capsule contents.	No	No	No	No	No
lactulose	No	Yes L	No	Yes – dilute with equal volume of water	No	No	No	No	No
loperamide	Yes C (ir)	Yes T (quick dissolve)	Yes – use quick-dissolve tablet	Yes – disperse capsule contents in water.	No	No	No	No	No
lorazepam	Yes T (ir)	No	Yes, SL tab but absorption may be same as oral[23,24]	Yes – dissolve SL tablet in water	No	No	No	No	No
methadone	Yes T (ir)	Yes L	Yes	No information	Yes (Special access in Canada)	Yes	Yes, but causes irritation[25–27] CSCI only	Yes	No
metho-trimeprazine (Canada only)	Yes T (ir)	No	No	Yes – crush tablet with water or use injection solution	Yes, but not usually used	Yes, but not usually used	Yes Bolus or CSCI	No	No

Abbreviations: tablet (T), capsule (C), liquid (L), powder (P), granules (G), chewable (Ch), dispersible (D), transdermal (TD), specially prepared (s) ir = immediate release, sr = sustained release, CSCI = SC infusion, bolus = bolus injection

Drug	Tablet or capsule	Liquid or dispersible preps	Buccal/ sublingual/ nasal	Gastrostomy route possible?	IV	IM	SC	Rectal	Topical
metoclopramide	Yes T (ir)	Yes L	No	Yes – use injection solution or crush tablets and disperse in water (takes 5 min). Oral liquid can cause diarrhea.	Yes, but not usually used	Yes, but not usually used	Yes[28] Bolus or CSCI	Yes,[29] but not usually used	No
metronidazole	Yes T (ir)	No	No	No	Yes	Yes, but not usually used	No	Yes	Yes
methylphenidate	Yes T (ir/sr)	No	Yes	No information	No	No	No	No	No[30]
mirtazapine	Yes T (ir)	Yes T (rapid disintegration)	No	No	No	No	No	No	No
midazolam	No	No	Yes (buccal or nasal)[31]	Yes – use diluted injection solution	Yes, but not usually used	Yes, but not usually used	Yes[32] Bolus or CSCI	Yes, but not usually used	No
morphine	Yes T (ir) T, C (sr)	Yes L, G (sr cap with granules)	SL no[33] Nasal – yes[34]	Yes – use oral liquid or mix sr granules and flush with 30 mL water	Yes, but not usually used	Yes, but not usually used	Yes Bolus or CSCI	Yes[35]	Yes[36–38]
octreotide	No	No	No	No information	Yes, but not usually used	No	Yes Bolus or CSCI	No	No
olanzapine	Yes T (ir)	Yes D	No	Mix disp. tabs with 25 mL water or use injection solution	No	Yes, but not usually used	No information	No	No
omeprazole	Yes C, T (sr)	No	No	Crush tablet and mix with 10 mL Na bicarbonate solution (1.6 g $NaHCO_3$ in 120 mL water). Administer 50 mL bicarb solution, then omeprazole solution, then 50 mL bicarb solution)	No	No	No	No	No

Abbreviations: tablet (T), capsule (C), liquid (L), powder (P), granules (G), chewable (Ch), dispersible (D), transdermal (TD), specially prepared (s) ir = immediate release, sr = sustained release, CSCI = SC infusion, bolus = bolus injection

Drug	Tablet or capsule	Liquid or dispersible preps	Buccal/ sublingual/ nasal	Gastrostomy route possible?	IV	IM	SC	Rectal	Topical
ondansetron	Yes T (ir)	Yes L	No	Yes – use oral liquid (may cause diarrhea), or injection solution mixed with 30 mL water	Yes	Yes, but not usually used	Yes Bolus or CSCI	No	No
oxycodone	Yes T (ir/sr)	No	No[19]	Yes – crush ir tablets with water. (Do not crush sr tablets.)	No	No	No	Yes[39,40]	No
oxymorphone	Yes T (ir/sr)	No	No	Yes – crush ir tablets with water. (Do not crush sr tablets.)	Available, but not commonly used	No	No	No information	No
pamidronate	No	No	No	No	Yes, with 500 mL 0.9% saline over 2–4 hours	No	Yes, diluted in 500 mL 0.9% saline over at least 4 hours[41]	No	No
pantoprazole	Yes T (sr)	No	No	No	Yes	No	No	No	No
phenobarbital	Yes T (ir)	Yes L	No	Yes – use oral liquid	Yes, but not usually used	Yes, but not usually used	Yes Bolus (keep concentration =<60 mg/mL) or CSCI	Yes[42]	No
phenytoin	Yes T (ir)	Yes L, Ch	No	Yes – dilute oral liquid by half with water, flush well. May bind to tube. May interact with feeds.	Yes (as fos-phenytoin)	Yes (as fos-phenytoin)	No	No	No
prednisolone	Yes T (ir)	Yes L	No	Yes – use liquid	No	No	No	No	No
ranitidine	Yes T (ir)	Yes L, D	No	Yes – crush tablet in water (5 min)	Yes, over 2 min	Yes, but not usually used	Yes[43,44] Bolus or CSCI	No	No
senna	Yes T (ir)	Yes L	No	Yes – use oral liquid	No	No	No	No	No
sertraline	Yes C (ir)	No	No	No information	No	No	No	No	No

Abbreviations: tablet (T), capsule (C), liquid (L), powder (P), granules (G), chewable (Ch), dispersible (D), transdermal (TD), specially prepared (s) ir = immediate release, sr = sustained release, CSCI = SC infusion, bolus = bolus injection

Drug	Tablet or capsule	Liquid or dispersible preps	Buccal/ sublingual/ nasal	Gastrostomy route possible?	IV	IM	SC	Rectal	Topical
sodium valproate	Yes C (ir)	Yes L (ir)	No	Yes – oral liquid	No	No	Yes Bolus or CSCI	Yes[45]	No
spironolactone	Yes T (ir)	No	No	Yes	No	No	No	No	No
sucralfate	Yes T (ir)	Yes L	No	Yes – dilute suspension with equal volume water. Stop feed 1 hr before and after dose	No	No	No	Yes (local action)	Yes[46,47]
temazepam	Yes C (ir)	Yes L	No	Yes – use oral liquid	No	No	No	No	No
tramadol	Yes T (ir/sr) In Canada ir form is only available with acetaminophen	No	No			No	No	No	No
tranexamic acid	Yes T (ir)	No	No			No	No	No	Yes[48,49]
warfarin	Yes T (ir)	No	No			No	No	No	No

DRUGS COMMONLY USED BY CSCI[10,50]

Drug	Local irritation*	Diluent	Compatibility — incompatible at all concs. — *may be incompatible at higher concentrations*	Alternative to CSCI
alfentanil	uncommon	saline or water	*dexamethasone*, furosemide, diclofenac	buccal alfentanil or transdermal fentanyl
fentanyl	uncommon	saline or water	furosemide, phenobarbital, diclofenac	transdermal fentanyl
glycopyrrolate	uncommon	saline or water	dexamethasone, ketorolac, furosemide, phenobarbital, diclofenac	sublingual or transdermal hyoscine hydrobromide
haloperidol	uncommon	water only	ketorolac, *dexamethasone*, furosemide, *hydromorphone*, *morphine*, phenobarbital, diclofenac	haloperidol as single SC bedtime dose
hydromorphone	uncommon	saline or water	*dexamethasone*, furosemide, *haloperidol*, *ketorolac*, phenobarbital, diclofenac	hydromorphone SC q4h
hyoscine butylbromide	uncommon	saline or water	*dexamethasone*, furosemide, phenobarbital, diclofenac	hyoscine as SC dose q4–6h
hyoscine hydrobromide	uncommon	saline or water	furosemide, phenobarbital, diclofenac	sublingual or transdermal hyoscine hydrobromide
metho-trimepromazine	occasional	saline or water	*dexamethasone*, furosemide, *ketorolac*, *octreotide*, phenobarbital, diclofenac	methotrimeprazine as single SC bedtime dose
metoclopramide	uncommon	saline or water	*dexamethasone*, furosemide, phenobarbital, diclofenac	SC dose q8h or domperidone PR
midazolam	uncommon	saline or water	dexamethasone, furosemide, *ketorolac*, *morphine*, phenobarbital, diclofenac	lorazepam SL q6–8h
morphine	uncommon	saline or water	*haloperidol*, furosemide, ketorolac, *midazolam*, phenobarbital, diclofenac	Change to hydromorphone and once daily haloperidol
octreotide	uncommon	saline or water	*dexamethasone*, furosemide, *methotrimeprazine*, phenobarbital, diclofenac	octreotide as SC dose q8h

* Information on local irritation is based only on CSCI. Bolus SC injections are more likely to cause local pain or irritation.

DRUGS WITH LIMITED EXPERIENCE IN CSCI

Drug	Local irritation*	Diluent	Compatibility — incompatible at all concs. — *may be incompatible at higher concentrations*	Alternative to CSCI
clodronate[46]	limited experience	saline (1 L/24 hr)	No experience with other drugs – use alone	IV infusion
dexamethasone	uncommon	water only	Most drugs – use alone	dexamethasone as single SC morning dose (preferred to CSCI)
ketamine	uncommon	saline only	Limited experience with other drugs	ketamine as SC dose q8h
furosemide	limited experience	saline or water	Most drugs – must be used alone	IV infusion
methadone	common	saline or water	Limited experience with other drugs – use alone	methadone as once daily SC dose
ondansetron, granisetron	uncommon	saline or water	*methotrimeprazine, metoclopramide*	give as SC injection q8h
omeprazole	may be irritant (ph >9)	saline (100 mL/3 hr)	No experience with other drugs – use alone	ranitidine CSCI
pamidronate[51]	can be irritant	saline (500 mL/24 hr	No experience with other drugs – use alone	IV infusion
phenobarbital	limited experience	saline or water	Most drugs – must be used alone	carbamazepine PR or midazolam SC
ranitidine[43]	uncommon	saline or water	Limited experience with other drugs – use alone	IM or slow IV (2 min)
valproate	uncommon	saline or water	No experience with other drugs – use alone	carbamazepine PR

*Information on local irritation is based only on CSCI. Bolus SC injections are more likely to cause local pain or irritation.

Problems with syringe pump infusions

- Syringe drivers continue to be used and manufactured. Some teams are switching to more complex, programmable pumps.
- Check pump infusions at least 6 hourly.
- If there is a problem, start from the periphery checking battery, pump type, correct placement of bag or syringe, syringe contents, line, any filters, connections, and insertion site.

Clinical decision	If YES ⇒ Action
1 Change in appearance of infusion solution?	• **Check drug compatibility:** *see* chart on pp. 321–2 and check www.palliativedrugs.com for current compatibility data. • **Reduce risk of incompatibility:** — for drugs with a long half-life give once daily (e.g. haloperidol, methotrimeprazine (Canada), dexamethasone) — dilute drugs by using a larger volume and adjusting the infusion settings accordingly — consider setting up second CSCI to reduce number of drugs in one syringe or bag — consider using water for injection as the diluting solution.
2 Excess drug effects?	• **Overinfusion:** check through the reasons for an infusion running through early, in cd-4 overleaf. • **Incorrect infusion site:** Subcutaneous: aspirate to check that the needle or cannula is not intravenous. Spinal: contact pain or palliative care specialist with experience in spinal lines. • **Administration error** in making up the drug or setting the infusion rate, *see* cd-4 overleaf.
3 Reduced drug effects?	• **Leak:** check all connections and lines for signs of leakage. If filters are being used their connectors can easily develop fine cracks. Because infusion rates are very low (0.5 mL/hr or less) leaks may not be obvious, so if a leak is suspected it is best to replace and refill all lines and filters. Many teams no longer use filters in subcutaneous infusions, but they are used in spinal infusions. • **Drug reactions (when two or more drugs used):** it is possible for a soluble, colorless and inactive product to be produced when two drugs are mixed. This risk is minimized by keeping the number of drugs in the same syringe or bag to a minimum (usually no more than two). • **Drug precipitation:** check through cd-1 and compatibility table, pp. 321–2. • **Underinfusion:** check through the reasons for an infusion running through late, in cd-5 overleaf. • **Incorrect infusion site:** Subcutaneous: check that the needle or cannula is still in place. Inject 1 mL water to exclude a blockage. Spinal: contact pain or palliative care specialist with experience in spinal lines. • **Administration error** in making up the drug or setting the infusion rate, *see* cd-5 overleaf.

cd = clinical decision

Clinical decision	If YES ⇒ Action
4 **Infusion running through early?**	• **Incorrect pump programming:** check patient for signs of overdosage and manage according to assessment. Correct the programming. • **Pump fault:** mechanical or electrical fault – replace pump.
5 **Infusion running through late?**	• **Incorrect pump programming:** check patient for signs of inadequate symptom control and manage according to assessment. Correct the programming. • **Battery low or exhausted:** replace battery and/or plug pump into power outlet. • **Blocked line:** depending on pump design, the pump will switch off or alarm. A blockage may be due to — kinked line: replace and refill the line — clamp left on the line: remove the clamp — indurated infusion site: change the infusion site (*see* cd-7) — blood in the needle/cannula: change the infusion site (*see* cd-7) — drug precipitation: *see* cd-3. NB: a blocked spinal line should only be checked by a pain or palliative care specialist with experience in spinal lines. • **Pump fault:** mechanical or electrical fault – replace pump.
6 **Site reaction?**	• **Swelling:** this is common in subcutaneous infusions and mild swellings only need observation. Infusions for hydration can cause uncomfortable swelling if the wrong sites are used such as the thigh or upper chest. The upper back is the best site for large volumes. Observe if mild, otherwise change site. • **Inflammation/pain:** Stop using highly irritant drugs, e.g. chlorpromazine, diazepam, prochlorperazine. Change to small-gauge plastic IV cannula inserted subcutaneously. Consider: — adding hydrocortisone 50 mg or dexamethasone 0.5 mg to the syringe mixture — rotating sites every 3 days — using other routes, e.g. rectal, transdermal, sublingual (*Alternative routes for drugs*, p. 314).
7 **Infusion site leaking?**	• **Leakage of drug from the infusion site:** this can happen with older sites (7 days or more) even in the absence of inflammation. Change to a new site. • **Bleeding from the infusion site:** this can occur on insertion but usually stops within minutes. If it persists this may be due to a coagulation disorder: — if bleeding stops within minutes of insertion, flush cannula with 1 mL 0.9% saline, then start infusion. — if bleeding persists or starts in an established site, exclude a coagulation disorder and consider alternative routes of drug administration (*Alternative routes for drugs*, p. 314).

cd = clinical decision

REFERENCES: DRUG INFORMATION

B = book; C = comment; Ch = chapter; CS-n = case study-no. of cases; CT-n = controlled trial-no. of cases; E = editorial; GC = group consensus; I = interviews; LS = laboratory study; MC = multi-center; OS-n = open study-no. of cases; PC = personal communication; R = review; RCT-n = randomized controlled trial-no. of cases; RS-n = retrospective survey-no. of cases; SA = systematic or meta analysis.

1 Zhang H, Zhang J, Streisand JB. (2002) Oral mucosal drug delivery: clinical pharmacokinetics and therapeutic applications. *Clinical Pharmacokinetics*. **41**(9): 661–80. (R, 101 refs)

2 Siden H, Nalewajek G. (2003) High dose opioids in paediatric palliative care. *Journal of Pain and Symptom Management*. **25**(5): 397–9. (Let, OS-80).

3 Grond S, Radbruch L, Lehmann KA. (2000) Clinical pharmacokinetics of transdermal opioids: focus on transdermal fentanyl. *Clinical Pharmacokinetics*. **38**(1): 59–89.

4 Pelham A, Regnard C. (2003) Severe respiratory depression and sedation with transdermal fentanyl: four case studies. *Palliative Medicine*. **17**(8): 714–16.

5 Chandler, S. (1999) Oral transmucosal fentanyl citrate: a new treatment for breakthrough pain. *American Journal of Hospice and Palliative Care*. **16**(2): 489–91.

6 Hanks G. (2001) Oral transmucosal fentanyl citrate for management of breakthrough pain. *European Journal of Palliative Care*. **8**(1): 6–9.

7 Cranswick N, Coghlan D. (2000) Paracetamol efficacy and safety in children: the first 40 years. *American Journal of Therapeutics*. **7**(2): 135–41.

8 Atkinson C, Kirkham S. (1999) Unlicensed uses for medication in a palliative care unit. *Palliative Medicine*. **13**: 145–52.

9 Bennett M, Simpson K. (2002) The use of drugs beyond licence in palliative care and pain management. *Palliative Medicine*. **16**: 367–8. (E)

10 *Palliative Drugs* website: www.palliativedrugs.com

11 Back IN. (2001) *Palliative Medicine Handbook, 3rd ed.* Cardiff: BPM Books. (Also available on www.pallmed.net)

12 For fuller and current information see: www.palliativedrugs.com for palliative care drugs (or *Hospice and Palliative Care Formulary USA, 2nd edition* or *Palliative Care Formulary*, Canadian Edition, both published by palliativedrugs.com). See also www.e-therapeutics.ca for licensed Canadian drug information (subscription required). In the US other useful sources include: Lexi-Drugs online (http://webstore.lexi.com/Store/Individual-Databases/Lexi-Drugs), and Epocrates (www.epocrates.com).

13 Arvidsson J, Nilsson HL, Sandstedt P, Steinwall G, *et al.* (1995) Replacing carbamazepine slow-release tablets with carbamazepine suppositories: a pharmacokinetic and clinical study in children with epilepsy. *Journal of Child Neurology*. **10**(2): 114–17. (MC, CT-31)

14 Neuvonen PJ, Tokola O. (1987) Bioavailability of rectally administered carbamazepine mixture. *British Journal of Clinical Pharmacology*. **24**(6): 839–41. (RCT)

15 Graves NM, Kriel RL, Jones-Saete C, Cloyd JC. (1985) Relative bioavailability of rectally administered carbamazepine suspension in humans. *Epilepsia*. **26**(5): 429–33. (OS)

16 Bricaire F, Castaing JL, Pocidalo JJ, Vilde JL. (1988) Pharmacokinetics and tolerance of ceftriaxone after subcutaneous administration. [French] *Pathologie et Biologie*. **36**(5 Pt. 2): 702–5. (CS-8)

17 Rylance GW, Poulton J, Cherry RC, Cullen RE. (1986) Plasma concentrations of clonazepam after single rectal administration. *Archives of Disease in Childhood*. **61**(2): 186–8. (OS-11)

18 Wennstrom B, Reinsfelt B. (2002) Rectally administered diclofenac (Voltaren) reduces vomiting compared with opioid (morphine) after strabismus surgery in children. *Acta Anaesthesiologica Scandinavica*. **46**(4): 430–4. (RCT-50)

19 Weinberg DS, Inturrisi CE, Reidenberg B, Moulin DE, *et al.* (1988) Sublingual absorption of selected opioid analgesics. *Clinical Pharmacology and Therapeutics*. **44**(3): 335–42. (OS)

20 Vanier MC, Labrecque G, Lepage-Savary D, Poulin E, *et al.* (1993) Comparison of hydromorphone continuous subcutaneous infusion and basal rate subcutaneous infusion plus PCA in cancer pain: a pilot study. *Pain*. **53**(1): 27–32. (RCT-8)

21 Parab PV, Ritschel WA, Coyle DE, Gregg RV, Denson DD. (1988) Pharmacokinetics of hydromorphone after intravenous, peroral and rectal administration to human subjects. *Biopharmaceutics and Drug Disposition*. **9**(2): 187–99. (RCT)

22 Golding JF, Gosden E, Gerrell J. (1991) Scopolamine blood levels following buccal versus ingested tablets. *Aviation Space and Environmental Medicine*. **62**(6): 521–6. (CT-18)

23 Yager JY, Seshia SS. (1988) Sublingual lorazepam in childhood serial seizures. *American Journal of Diseases of Children*. **142**(9): 931–2.

24 Gram-Hansen P, Schultz A. (1988) Plasma concentrations following oral and sublingual administration of lorazepam. *International Journal of Clinical Pharmacology, Therapy, and Toxicology*. **26**(6): 323–4.

25 Makin MK. (2000) Subcutaneous methadone in terminally-ill patients. *Journal of Pain and Symptom Management*. **19**(4): 237–8. (Let)

26 Mathew P, Storey P. (1999) Subcutaneous methadone in terminally ill patients: manageable local toxicity. *Journal of Pain and Symptom Management*. **18**(1): 49–52. (CS-6)

27 Bohrer H, Schmidt H. (1992) Comment on Bruera *et al.*, Local toxicity with subcutaneous methadone: experience of two centers. *Pain*. **50**(3): 373. (Let)

28 McCallum RW, Valenzuela G, Polepalle S, Spyker D. (1991) Subcutaneous metoclopramide in the treatment of symptomatic gastroparesis: clinical efficacy and pharmacokinetics. *Journal of*

Pharmacology and Experimental Therapeutics. **258**(1): 136–42. (CT-10)

29 Hardy F, Warrington PS, MacPherson JS, Hudson SA, *et al.* (1990) A pharmacokinetic study of high-dose metoclopramide suppositories. *Journal of Clinical Pharmacy and Therapeutics*. **15**(1): 21–4. (RCT-14)

30 Sane N, McGough JJ. (2002) MethyPatch Noven. *Current Opinion in Investigational Drugs*. **3**(8): 1222–4.

31 Lim TW, Thomas E, Choo SM. (1997) Premedication with midazolam is more effective by the sublingual than oral route. *Canadian Journal of Anaesthesia*. **44**(7): 723–6. (RCT-100)

32 Gremaud G, Zulian GB. (1998) Indications and limitations of intravenous and subcutaneous midazolam in a palliative care center. *Journal of Pain and Symptom Management*. **15**(6): 331–3. (Let, CT)

33 Coluzzi PH. (1998) Sublingual morphine: efficacy reviewed. *Journal of Pain and Symptom Management*. **16**(3): 184–92. (R, 30 refs)

34 Pavis H, Wilcock A, Edgecombe J, Carr D, *et al.* (2002) Pilot study of nasal morphine-chitosan for the relief of breakthrough pain in patients with cancer. *Journal of Pain and Symptom Management*. **24**(6): 598–602. (CS-9)

35 Moolenaar F, Meijler WJ, Frijlink HW, Visser J, Proost JH. (2000) Clinical efficacy, safety and pharmacokinetics of a newly developed controlled release morphine sulphate suppository in patients with cancer pain. *European Journal of Clinical Pharmacology*. **56**(3): 219–23, (RCT-25)

36 Krajnik M, Zylicz Z, Finlay I, Luczak J, van Sorge AA. (1999) Potential uses of topical opioids in palliative care: report of 6 cases. *Pain*. **80**(1–2): 121–5. (OS-14)

37 Twillman RK, Long TD, Cathers TA, Mueller DW. (1999) Treatment of painful skin ulcers with topical opioids. *Journal of Pain and Symptom Management*. **17**(4): 288–92. (CS-9)

38 Krajnik M, Zylicz Z. (1997) Topical morphine for cutaneous cancer pain. *Palliative Medicine*. **11**: 325–6. (CS-6)

39 Leow KP, Cramond T, Smith MT. (1995) Pharmacokinetics and pharmacodynamics of oxycodone when given intravenously and rectally to adult patients with cancer pain. *Anesthesia and Analgesia*. **80**(2): 296–302. (RCT-12)

40 Leow KP, Smith MT, Watt JA, Williams BE, Cramond T. (1992) Comparative oxycodone pharmacokinetics in humans after intravenous, oral, and rectal administration. *Therapeutic Drug Monitoring*. **14**(6): 479–84. (RCT-48)

41 Walker P, Watanabe S, Lawlor P, Bruera E. (1996) Subcutaneous clodronate (and pamidronate). *The Lancet*. **348**: 345–6. (Let, CS-2)

42 Graves NM, Holmes GB, Kriel RL, Jones-Saete C, *et al.* (1989). Relative bioavailability of rectally administered phenobarbital sodium parenteral solution. *DICP*. **23**(7–8): 565–8. (OS-7)

43 Dickman A, SC (2003) Ranitidine or omeprazole. Bulletin board on www.palliativedrugs.com (accessed 11 February). (PC)

44 Dean M. Personal communication.

45 Yoshiyama Y, Nakano S, Ogawa N. (1989) Chronopharmacokinetic study of valproic acid in man: comparison of oral and rectal administration. *Journal of Clinical Pharmacology*. **29**(11): 1048–52. (OS-8)

46 Banati A, Chowdhury SR, Mazumder S. (2001) Topical use of sucralfate cream in second and third degree burns. *Burns*. **27**(5): 465–9. (RCT-85)

47 Regnard CFB, Mannix K. (1990) Palliation of gastric carcinoma haemorrhage with sucralfate. *Palliative Medicine*. **4**: 329–30. (Let, CS-1)

48 De Bonis M, Cavaliere F, Alessandrini F, Lapenna E, *et al.* (2000) Topical use of tranexamic acid in coronary artery bypass operations: a double-blind, prospective, randomized, placebo-controlled study. *Journal of Thoracic and Cardiovascular Surgery*. **119**(3): 575–80. (RCT-40)

49 McElligot E, Quigley C, Hanks GW. (1992) Tranaxamic acid and rectal bleeding. *Lancet*. **337**: 431. (Let, CS-1)

50 Barnes L, Westmoreland J, Wilson C. (2009) Syringe drivers: standardised protocols to minims errors. *End of Life Care*. **3**(3): 43–51. (R, 34 refs)

51 Duncan AR. (2003) The use of subcutaneous pamidronate. *Journal of Pain and Symptom Management*. **26**: 592–3.

Emergencies

NOTES

CLINICAL DECISION AND ACTION CHECKLIST

1. Is comfort the only aim?
2. Is this a sudden collapse?
3. Are drugs the cause?
4. Is severe agitation present?
5. Is severe pain present?
6. Is the patient breathless?
7. Is there a metabolic cause?
8. Is there a hematological cause?
9. Is tumor causing local pressure problems?
10. Is the need for treatment uncertain?
11. Has the situation been explained?

KEY POINTS

- Several drugs and conditions can mimic the terminal phase of an illness, but causes can be reversible.
- Treating emergencies can improve comfort and reduce distress even if the prognosis is unaltered.
- When the need for treatment remains uncertain an observation period can be helpful.

INTRODUCTION

In the presence of progressive disease some drugs and medical conditions can cause unexpected but reversible deterioration. Some conditions can give the impression that a patient is dying when, in reality, the cause is reversible and the patient has the potential to recover. Examples are hypercalcemia, hypoglycemia, hyperglycemia, severe anemia, and infection. Although these conditions may reflect underlying disease, they do not necessarily reflect a terminal event. Other reversible conditions may be unrelated to the underlying disease.[1] It is usually clear from the patient or the circumstances whether treatment is appropriate. In general, if a patient was coping well before the emergency, reversal of the problem will result in a return to the previous performance status. However, other situations are more complex and decisions about treating an emergency must include consideration of the issues below:

A clear understanding of
- the patient's wishes, beliefs, and values
- the reversibility of the current problem
- any distress the treatment may cause
- the feasibility and availability of the treatment
- any ethical issues
- why estimates of previous quality of life are *not* helpful.

Issues to consider when assessing emergencies in palliative care

WHEN COMFORT IS THE ONLY AIM

In some situations the deterioration is unequivocally irreversible (e.g. massive hemoptysis), or the patient may have already been deteriorating rapidly because of their primary condition. Alternatively, the patient with capacity may refuse treatment, or in patients without capacity the clinical team and substitute decision maker/health care proxy may have decided that treatment is not in the patient's best interests (*see Making ethical choices*, p. 263, *Decisions around capacity*, p. 267, and *Issues around cardiopulmonary resuscitation*, p. 273). In these situations the treatment is aimed at relieving distress and discomfort. This does not exclude partially reversing the cause of the emergency. For example, a patient distressed with the symptoms of a chest infection may benefit from an antibiotic to improve comfort.

SUDDEN COLLAPSE

Cardiac or respiratory arrest

If no decision has been made in advance and cardiopulmonary resuscitation could succeed, treatment should start immediately. *See Issues around cardiopulmonary resuscitation*, p. 273 for further information.

Hemorrhage

Treatment of hemorrhage may be possible if the source is accessible and the rate of bleeding allows time for treatment. However, in very advanced disease, hemorrhage may be too severe or the patient too ill for treatment.[2] Hemorrhage is frightening for the patient, and those around. It may be necessary to ease the patient's distress with a benzodiazepine given by whichever accessible route will give the fastest absorption.

Major seizure

This is uncommon in advanced cancer, even in patients with cerebral metastases. However, some patients, especially neurologically impaired children, already have a history of frequent and complex seizures. In these, a change in seizure type or pattern can herald either a decline in general health or indicate a concurrent problem such as infection, or constipation. Parents and carers are sensitive to the changes in seizures and a potential cause should be sought.

A major (tonic-clonic) seizure usually resolves by itself in less than 5 minutes. If it persists the patient needs a benzodiazepine. In both adults and children midazolam is as effective in controlling seizures as rectal diazepam[3] but has a faster recovery time, is safer, and can be given IV, IM, bucally or intranasally. In children the buccal route is better tolerated and as effective.[4–9] Midazolam is rapidly absorbed through the oral or nasal mucosa in adults,[10,11] and is a useful alternative when other routes are unavailable.[12] Lorazepam IV or intranasal is an alternative.

Any seizure is a prompt to review anticonvulsant medication, but in children some seizure disorders are ultimately drug-resistant, causing significant morbidity and distress for the child and carers. In addition, adverse effects from anticonvulsant medication include behavioral changes, sleep disturbance, and drowsiness. Occasionally, status epilepticus may be a terminal event. Control may be gained using subcutaneous infusion of midazolam either on its own or in combination with phenobarbital.

Clinical decision	If YES carry out the action below
1 Is comfort the only aim?	e.g. rapid deterioration with irreversible cause (e.g. massive hemoptysis, hematemesis or pulmonary embolus), very short prognosis (hour-by-hour deterioration), or a patient refusing treatment. *See Terminal phase*, p. 211. • **Ensure the patient has company.** Keep warm if hypotensive. • **Ensure there is support** for the patient, partner, family, and staff (including you!). • **Partial reversal of the cause may still be appropriate** for comfort (e.g. furosemide in heart failure).
2 Is this a sudden collapse?	**a. Cardiac or respiratory arrest:** *Cardiopulmonary resuscitation (CPR) should start if* — there is no "Do Not Resuscitate" (DNR) order *and* successful CPR is possible *Cardiopulmonary resuscitation should not be done if* — this arrest was anticipated *and* could not succeed, or there is a valid and applicable Advance Health Care Directive indicating no resuscitation (*see Issues around cardiopulmonary resuscitation*, p. 273). **b. Drug toxicity:** *see* cd-3 on p. 333. **c. Hemorrhage:** *If treatment is possible:* obtain IV access, take blood for cross-match and start a rapid infusion of 0.9% saline, followed by a plasma substitute while awaiting blood (e.g. Dextran). Find the bleeding source visually, or using endoscopy or radiology. *If treatment is impossible (or has been refused by patient):* — give midazolam 5–15 mg IV, buccally, or IM into deltoid muscle. Diazepam IV or PR is an alternative (avoid Diazemuls because of its slow onset of action) — if the bleeding is visible (e.g. ulcer, hemoptysis, hematemesis), use dark green or blue towels to make the appearance of blood less frightening to patient, partner, and family — place warm blankets over the patient — do not leave the patient unattended. **d. Major seizure (tonic-clonic type):** Put the patient into the standard recovery position. *If the seizure does not resolve spontaneously after 5 min:* give midazolam 2.5–5 mg buccally (for doses in children, *see* p. 310). *If the seizure is persisting after a further 5 min:* repeat with 5 mg midazolam buccally, but if the seizure has not resolved, obtain IV access and titrate lorazepam 1–4 mg by slow IV into a large vein until the seizure has stopped. If IV access is not possible consider IM phenobarbital (for doses in children *see Drugs in children: starting doses*, p. 310). — exclude hypoglycemia and hypoxia — review the anticonvulsant medication. **e. Consider the following as causes:** fall (simple faint, postural hypotension, vertigo), hypoglycemia, cardiac arrhythmia, pulmonary embolus, septicemia, or a pericardial effusion (cold, pale, raised pulse rate, BP is maintained initially, poor pulse volume which reduces on inspiration – an exaggeration of normal).

cd = clinical decision

DRUGS

Many drugs have the potential to mimic deterioration due to the disease, by causing drowsiness, respiratory depression, or hypotension. If a serious adverse effect is causing the patient harm or distress, it must be treated. The drug dose should be reduced or the patient changed to a different drug. Patients have the right to be as alert and aware as possible if this is their wish. It is not acceptable to view a serious drug adverse event as inevitable.

SEVERE AGITATION

Hyperactive delirium should be managed as described in *Confusional states*, p. 245.

In most other cases of agitation, the aim is to reduce the agitation sufficiently for comfort, and to find a treatable cause if possible. Sedation is not the aim since this would make it difficult for the patient to understand what is happening and would hinder assessment. Consequently, any drug should be titrated to reduce the agitation that is distressing the patient. The intention is to enable the patient to express their distress and allow them to respond to company, empathy, and treatments such as massage and relaxation.

There are situations in which the cause of the agitation is irreversible, the agitation is causing severe distress or preventing urgent assessment or treatment. In these situations sedation will be needed.[13] The drug doses needed to control agitation may result in drowsiness.[14–20] However, the dose is titrated to the minimum dose that reduces the agitation. Used in this way there is no evidence that such drugs reduce survival.[21–23]

Requirements for treatment

- Agitation causing severe distress to the patient, risking harm to the patient or others, or agitation that prevents assessment or treatment.
- Permission from the patient (or if they lack capacity for this decision a decision made in their best interest by carer(s) and/or substitute decision makers/health care proxies).
- Documentation of treatment reasons, length, and review dates.
- Understanding of the drugs used to control severe agitation (e.g. avoiding the use of opioids).
- Willingness to ask for help if agitation persists.

Aims of treatment

- Reduce distress by more than half.
- Enable the patient to express the reasons for their distress.
- Reduce the agitation sufficiently to allow assessment.
- Keep drowsiness to a minimum if possible.

Treating severe agitation

Drugs: haloperidol is the drug of choice in hyperactive delirium.[24–26] However, haloperidol should be avoided in Lewy body dementia (because of the risk of serious adverse effects) and Parkinson's disease (because it worsens the movement disorder). In these patients a low dose of a short-acting benzodiazepine such as midazolam can be used. In delirium due to alcohol withdrawal benzodiazepines are usually first-line treatment with haloperidol as second line.[27] Opioids are contraindicated in delirium since they may make the agitation worse through the accumulation of active metabolites.

Decisions: most patients in this situation do not have capacity and it is helpful to have a clear consensus between the clinical team and the substitute decision maker/health care proxy. In all circumstances it is essential to have a clear plan (*see* table above) to avoid decisions being made on anecdotal experiences.[28]

Clinical decision	If YES carry out the action below
3 Are drugs the cause?	**a. Reduce the dose or change** to an alternative drug. **b. If ventilation has been seriously compromised** (<5 resps/min): *Opioids:* start 28% oxygen. Dilute naloxone 400 microg (0.4 mg) in 10 mL of N. saline and titrate IV in 1 mL (40 microg (0.04 mg)) boluses until respiration improves, followed by naloxone infusion using 60% per hour of the previous dose used, e.g. if 100 microg (0.1 mg) used initially, infusion should be 60 microg/hr (0.06 mg/hr). Full opioid reversal is not the aim. *Spinal local anesthetics:* ventilation may be needed for 1–2 hours. *Benzodiazepine:* start 28% oxygen. Flumazenil IV 200 microg (0.2 mg) over 15 seconds followed by 100 microg (0.1 mg)/min up to 1000 microg (1 mg). **c. If severe hypotension is present** (systolic <60 mmHg): *Spinal local anesthetics:* IV 0.9% saline 500 mL infused rapidly. If the response is brief or insufficient give ephedrine 3–9 mg IV. *Steroid withdrawal:* give hydrocortisone 100 mg IM or slow IV. Restart oral corticosteroid. *Antimuscarinic hypotension* (e.g. amitriptyline): usually postural so elevate legs and stop drug. Fit support stockings until the drug effect has reduced. **d. If anaphylaxis has occurred** (edema, stridor, hypotension): Give 1:1000 (1 mg/mL) adrenalin (epinephrine) IM every 10–15 min until the blood pressure is stable. *Dose for adults:* use Epipen or Anapen 300 microg (0.3 mg–0.3 mL) IM. *Dose for children:* for a child >30 kg use Epipen or Twinject (300 microg = 0.3 mg) IM; for a child <30 kg give 10 microg/kg (0.01 mg/kg) using 1:10 000 (100 microg/mL = 0.1 mg/mL) solution. Also give hydrocortisone 100 mg IM or IV. If bronchospasm persists give salbutamol 2.5 mg nebulized or 250 microg (0.25 mg) slow IV. **e. If drowsiness or confusion are present:** *See Fatigue, drowsiness, lethargy and weakness*, p. 149, and *Confusional states*, p. 245.
4 Is severe agitation present?	• **If this is hyperactive delirium:** *see Confusional states*, p. 245. • **If urgent control of the agitation is essential** (e.g. irreversible hemorrhage, severe breathlessness, prevention of injury to patient): — do not use opioids to treat the agitation (*see* text). — give midazolam 2–10 mg titrated IV, <u>or</u> 2.5–5 mg IM or buccal/sublingual. If necessary, repeat the dose up to three times (for IV repeat at 2 min intervals, for IM/sublingual repeat at 10 min intervals). If the agitation worsens on midazolam, *add* haloperidol 2.5 mg SC or IM q1h as required until the agitation settles (up to 10 mg/24 hr) — sedation is not the aim unless the distress is overwhelming. Using titration it is possible to settle a patient without causing respiratory depression — ensure the environment is safe (e.g. placing mattress on floor) — do not leave patient unattended since another person is comforting and makes it clear to the patient that they will not be abandoned. • **Consider the following as causes:** anger, confusional state, fear, hypoglycemia, hypoxia, pain. • **If the agitation is persistent and the patient is terminal:** consider phenobarbital SC 600–2400 mg/24 hours infusion,[29] <u>*or*</u> propofol 0.5 mg/kg by slow IV followed by a propofol IV infusion of 2 mg/kg/hr.[30–32]

SEVERE PAIN

Requirements for treatment

- Pain causing distress to the patient.
- Understanding of the drugs used to control severe pain (e.g. strong opioids do not control all pains).
- Willingness to ask for help if pain persists.

Aims of treatment

- Reduce the pain at rest by more than two-thirds.
- Reduce the pain on movement sufficiently to allow essential movements such as going to the toilet.
- Keep adverse effects to a minimum.
- Plan for medium- and long-term analgesia.

Treating severe pain

The most immediate goal is to reduce pain at rest and to allow the patient to settle sufficiently to allow adequate assessment. Check the likely cause of pain in *Diagnosing and treating pain*, p. 43. For example, colic needs to be differentiated from other causes of pain as the treatment is very different. However, for the urgent treatment of most other causes of pain a strong opioid can be used initially.

Pain on the slightest movement can be managed with positioning, padding, and splints, before excluding a fracture or vertebral collapse. Treatment for pathological fractures is best planned, rather than managed as an acute emergency. If surgery is not possible, the pain can be controlled with immobilization, ketamine, local nerve blocks, or spinal analgesia.

Peritonitis: this is a rare complication of obstruction, NSAIDs, and inflammatory bowel disease. If surgery is not an option, in our experience intraperitoneal steroid and local anesthetic can provide rapid analgesia for the last hours of a patient's life. Intraperitoneal corticosteroids have been used safely for ascites and can be used in peritonitis without compromising a possible recovery.[33]

Pleuritic pain: this may be due to a rib metastasis, or pleural inflammation due to infection, tumor, or embolus. A local intercostal block can help, as can an intrapleural infusion of local anesthetic.[34]

PERSISTENT AGITATION OR PAIN

The advice of palliative care, pain, and oncology colleagues is essential. Although the agitation or pain may settle, low mood, anxiety, and exhaustion may persist (*see Anxiety*, p. 239, *Anger*, p. 235, and *Withdrawal and depression*, p. 253). This persistence of psychological problems will delay the resolution of the agitation or pain, and to avoid disappointment this delay needs to be explained to the patient, partner, and staff. In situations when a pain-relieving procedure has to be delayed benzodiazepines can reduce anxiety and distress.

Clinical decision	If YES carry out the action below
5 Is severe pain present?	a. **Breakthrough pain:** *see* cd-2 in *Diagnosing and treating pain*, p. 45. b. **Periodic pain suggesting colic** (i.e. coming and going every few minutes): — *see* cd-4 in *Diagnosing and treating pain*, p. 49. c. **Pain worsened by the slightest passive movement:** — find a comfortable position. Use padding or splints to reduce painful movements — if two breakthrough doses of opioid have been ineffective give ketamine 5 mg buccal/sublingual 10 min before moving. *If this is back pain:* check for spinal cord compression (*see* cd-9a, p. 345) *If a pathological fracture is suspected:* — too unwell to travel: ensure the patient is on a pressure-relieving mattress, give analgesia before turning or moving (usual breakthrough opioid 30 min, or ketamine 5–10 mg buccal/sublingual 10 min before moving, or SL fentanyl or sufentanil). — well enough to travel: plan for an X-ray and orthopedic advice (best done electively, rather than as an emergency). Give analgesia as above prior to travel. d. **Peritonitis** (constant abdominal pain, pain on light percussion of abdomen, abdominal wall rigidity): *Well enough for surgery and agrees to this option:* refer urgently for a surgical opinion. Give metronidazole 400 mg as IV infusion over 20 min. *Too ill for surgery (or refuses this option):* at the site of least pain inject 20 mL 0.25% bupivacaine plus 8 mg dexamethasone intraperitoneally. If the pain is no better after 15 min, repeat at another abdominal site. *If nausea or vomiting are present:* give methotrimeprazine (Canada only) 5 mg SC. e. **Pleuritic pain:** *If two breakthrough doses of opioid have been given with no or minimal relief:* ask a pain or palliative care specialist to consider an intercostal nerve block or an intrapleural infusion of bupivacaine. — treat the underlying cause if possible, e.g. chest infection. f. **If severe pain persists** (i.e. pain remains at 50% or more of its severity at the start) — check through the clinical decisions 2–12 in *Diagnosing and treating pain*, p. 45–55 — consider anxiety, anger, or depression as factors reducing the patient's ability to cope with pain — contact a pain or palliative care specialist to consider regular ketamine, nerve block, or intraspinal analgesia — if further treatment is to be delayed for more than 2 hours, reduce anxiety and fear with lorazepam 0.5–1 mg PO or sublingually as required, or use midazolam 20–30 mg/24 hours SC infusion. Sedation is rarely needed.

cd = clinical decision

BREATHLESSNESS

Severe breathlessness is frightening and simple relief measures are important first steps. If severe hypoxia is present, the patient may be too agitated to tolerate oxygen and the agitation will need to be reduced to a level where oxygen can be tried.

Respiratory distress: occurs in keto-acidosis due to diabetes mellitus and is usually reversible. It can also occur in the presence of fear or persistent hypoxia at the end of life, requiring support for the patient and family.[35–37] Fast respiratory rates are distressing and exhausting. An opioid may help, but may also increase agitation. If there is no improvement the agitation should be treated as in cd-4, p. 333. For severe breathlessness at the end of life, sedation may be needed.[38] Terminal gasping can occur in patients who are deeply unconscious in the last minutes of life, but there is no evidence that it is distressing to the patient.

Chest pain: this may indicate acute problems such as myocardial infarction, pneumothorax, pulmonary embolism, or an acute chest infection. Cardiac ischemic pain is more likely if the pain is caused by exertion and radiates to the arms or shoulders.[39] Vertebral metastases or rib metastases can be differentiated by the presence of pain on local pressure over the ribs or gentle percussion over the spine.

Pulmonary emboli can cause distressing pain and breathlessness. D-dimers can be used as a screening test, even in cancer patients.[40,41] The standard practice is to anticoagulate,[42] but in patients with advanced malignancy full anticoagulation causes new problems with bleeding or unstable anticoagulation control.[43–46] Low molecular weight heparin which, in low doses, needs no monitoring, can be given once daily, is acceptable to most patients, and is now the preferred long-term treatment in advanced cancer.[47–50] Preventing recurrent emboli with an inferior vena cava filter can help patients who cannot receive concomitant anti-coagulation, but patients need to be carefully selected since vena cava obstruction can develop.[51,52]

Heart failure: this needs urgent treatment even when the prognosis is hours or days, since the consequent agitation and bronchial secretions will be distressing to patient, partner, relatives, and staff. A common cause is a terminally ill patient being nursed flat and such patients will be less breathless sitting upright or lying at a 45-degree angle at the hips. Initial treatment is with intravenous furosemide but, if the prognosis allows, longer-term control may be needed with ACE inhibitors, beta blockers or spironolactone, according to established guidelines.[53] The need for continuing with diuretics should be reviewed in the patient with advanced disease whose fluid intake decreases or stops.

Clinical decision	If YES carry out the action below
6 Is the patient breathless?	**a. First steps:** — sit the patient/as upright as is tolerated — ensure there is cool air over the face (fan or window) — stay with the patient. If the patient is agitated *see* cd-4, p. 333 — if available, check the oxygen saturation with a pulse oximeter. If the S_pO_2 is 90% or less, start 24% oxygen. If the S_pO_2 improves, or the patient is more comfortable, continue the oxygen. **b. Chest pain and breathlessness** Consider the following causes: *Cardiac pain:* arrange for urgent ECG — with ST elevation (STEMI): give aspirin PO 325 mg. Give 2.5 mg morphine IV if not on opioid, otherwise use equivalent of usual breakthrough dose, repeat after 5 min if necessary. Arrange for urgent cardiac intervention if the patient wishes. — with normal ST segments: give NTG for angina. *Massive pulmonary embolism* (chest pain, collapse, breathlessness which is not relieved on sitting up, chest sounds normal, gallop rhythm): — in the context of advanced disease a massive pulmonary embolism is usually a terminal event. Streptokinase is an option,[54] but is rarely indicated in palliative care. *Chest infection* causing pleurisy. *Pneumothorax* (acute breathlessness, chest pain, trachea may be deviated towards the lung collapse side, hollow chest on percussion but reduced or absent breath sounds): if the collapse is >30%, consider intercostal drainage with water seal. **c. Air hunger** (gasping type of respiration): *Diabetic ketoacidosis: see* cd-7c p. 341. *Tachypnea:* a respiratory rate of >20/min. If it is due to fear, *see Anxiety*, p. 239. Otherwise give morphine 5 mg SC and repeat after 20 min. If after three opioid doses the patient is still distressed by the tachypnea, treat as for agitation (*see* cd-4, p. 333). *Terminal gasping in last stages of life:* this is sometimes seen in the last minutes of life of a deeply unconscious patient. This can be a normal part of dying and needs no treatment, although the partner or relative will need explanation and support. Repositioning the head can reduce or stop any noise due to respiratory secretions (*see* cd-4, p. 193). **d. Acute heart failure** (acute breathlessness, pink frothy sputum, hypotension, tachycardia, third heart sound, lung crepitations, raised jugular venous pressure): — give loop diuretic such as furosemide 40 mg IV, repeat after 5 min if no better — consider giving morphine as a titrated IV injection (or IM if IV access is not possible) followed by SC infusion. Give 2.5 mg if not on opioid, otherwise use equivalent of usual breakthrough dose — consider an ACE inhibitor for long-term control (start under hospital control if creatinine >150 mmol/L, sodium <130 mmol/L, systolic BP <100 mmHg, or aged >70 years) — nurse the patient in as upright a sitting position as is tolerated.

cd = clinical decision

Acute severe asthma: generalized reversible bronchoconstriction is common. Wheeze is usually present, but will be absent in severe cases. Reversibility can be assessed by a >15% response in PEF (peak expiratory flow) after a bronchodilator. Most bronchospasm will respond to inhaled bronchodilators, but a nebulized bronchodilator and intravenous hydrocortisone may be needed in severe cases.[55] Nebulizers deliver much larger doses, which may cause adverse effects, but a nebulizer may be needed in weak patients or for severe bronchospasm. The use of mouthpieces with nebulizers is better tolerated and more effective than face masks.[56] However, if a patient's bronchospasm is extremely severe (e.g. can't manage a bronchodilator and nebulizer ineffective) this suggests urgent ventilator support is needed. Many patients with lung cancer have generalized bronchoconstriction and would benefit from bronchodilators, but have not been prescribed them.[57] However, bronchodilators will have little effect on breathlessness caused by widespread intrapulmonary cancer.

Pleural effusion: severe breathlessness due to an effusion requires rapid drainage of the effusion for comfort.

Stridor is due to obstruction of the upper trachea. In cancer, and in the absence of an inhaled foreign body, airway compression by tumor is the commonest cause. A 4:1 helium/oxygen mixture (Heliox28) has less viscosity than air and can be breathed more comfortably through an obstruction.[30–32] Dexamethasone will help reduce any edema around the tumor, reducing the obstruction. Hoarseness suggests a unilateral vocal cord paralysis, which can be treated by the ENT specialists with a Teflon injection of one cord.[61] A cough that lacks its normal force and brevity suggests a "bovine" cough caused by bilateral vocal cord paralysis with a risk of complete laryngeal obstruction by the paralyzed vocal cords. Urgent referral to the ENT specialists may be needed for surgical reconstruction.[62]

Clinical decision	If YES carry out the action below
6 Is the patient breathless? (contd.)	**e. Acute severe asthma** (unable to talk, fatigue, exhaustion, low respiratory rate, using accessory muscles of respiration, cyanosis, chest may have no wheeze) — start 28% oxygen — use oxygen-driven nebulizer to deliver salbutamol (albuterol in US) 2.5 mg. Repeat at 15–30 min intervals. If nebulizer not available use salbutamol (albuterol) inhaler 200 microg through a spacer device and repeat up to 10 times over 10 min if necessary — if no improvement give salbutamol (albuterol) 5 mg plus ipratropium 250 microg nebulized — if still no improvement give hydrocortisone 100 mg IV and admit to hospital. *Danger signs* are hypoxia S_aO_2 <92%, exhaustion, confusion, silent chest, bradycardia, or hypotension. Urgent ventilator support should be considered. **f. Pleural effusion** (acute breathlessness, trachea may be deviated away from the side of the effusion, dull percussion note and reduced or absent breath sounds) *See Respiratory problems*, p. 194 for advice on management. **g. Stridor** (rasping sound from upper airway with a sensation of suffocation) *Exclude a foreign body obstruction* (food or inhaled object). *Immediate treatment:* if available, start a 28% oxygen/72% helium mixture (Heliox28) through a high concentration mask. If a tumor is obstructing the airway give dexamethasone 16–24 mg IV as a slow injection over 2 minutes. *If a bovine cough is present* (weak, ineffectual cough): refer urgently to ear, nose, and throat specialist for assessment of vocal cord function and consideration for Teflon injection of a vocal cord. A tracheostomy is sometimes urgently required. *If radiotherapy or chemotherapy is an option:* refer to the oncologists. *If no further radiotherapy or chemotherapy possible:* refer to the respiratory physicians for consideration of a bronchial stent. Continue high-dose dexamethasone until after treatment. **h. For persistent breathlessness** *See* cd-9 in *Respiratory problems*, p. 197.

cd = clinical decision

METABOLIC PROBLEMS

Adrenocortical insufficiency: causes include adrenal damage (metastases, infection, or infarction), hypothalamic damage (brain metastases, cranial irradiation) or abrupt withdrawal of systemic corticosteroids. It may also occur during physical stress while on steroids, or soon after weaning off corticosteroids.

Hypercalcemia: this is common in some cancers (50% of myeloma, 25% of bronchial carcinomas, and 20% of breast carcinomas).[63,64] In 80% of cases the cause is the production of a parathyroid hormone-like protein by the tumor,[64–66] a process which is unrelated to the presence of bone metastases. In cancer it is associated with a poor prognosis, but the median survival is 2 months and treatment is often worthwhile.[67] Symptoms are insidious and mimic those seen in a dying patient, so that hypercalcemia is often missed or undertreated.[68] Drowsiness, nausea, vomiting, confusion, constipation, or thirst may occur, but drowsiness alone is common. Symptoms that develop unexpectedly over 2 weeks or less should arouse suspicion of a raised calcium. Patients with suspected hypercalcemia should have their serum calcium and albumin checked and the calcium corrected for a low albumin. The corrected total serum calcium may better correlate with symptoms.[69–73] Values of corrected serum calcium >2.7 mmol/L (approx. 10.6 mg/dL) are abnormal.[74] Serum chloride levels are usually unaffected, but if they are raised and combined with a low bicarbonate, this suggests primary hyperparathyroidism as a cause of the hypercalcemia.[75]

Although hydration is important, this alone will not achieve useful control of the hypercalcemia.[64,76] However, hydration is necessary if renal function has deteriorated due to dehydration. Steroids are only effective in myeloma and lymphoma.[64] For other tumors the bisphosphonates are now the most effective treatment available.[77] All bisphosphonates are potentially nephrotoxic, although the incidence is low and may be lowest with ibandronate (US only).[78-80] However, they can be used safely in patients on dialysis.

Pamidronate, zoledronic, and ibandronic acid (not Canada) can be given as a single infusion. To reduce the risk of renal impairment ensure adequate hydration and follow recommended infusion times:

Pamidronate (onset <4 days)
30 mg in 250 mL 0.9% NaCl over 1 hour
60 mg in 500 mL 0.9% NaCl over 2 hours
90 mg in 500 mL 0.9% NaCl over 4 hours

Zoledronic acid (onset <3 days)
2 mg in 100 mL 0.9% NaCl over 30 min
4 mg in 100 mL 0.9% NaCl over 45 min
6 mg in 250 mL 0.9% NaCl over 1 hour

Ibandronic acid (not Canada) (onset <4 days)
2–6 mg in 500 mL 0.9% NaCl over 1 hour

Clodronate (onset <2 days)
1500 mg in 250 mL 0.9% NaCl over 2 hours

Bisphosphonate infusions[81]

Zoledronic acid is more potent and can be used as second-line treatment,[82–84] but adverse effects are more frequent including fever, eye inflammation, and osteonecrosis of the jaw. Ibandronic acid (not Canada) may be a safer alternative to zoledronic acid.[85] Because of a 24–48 hour delay in effect the bisphosphonate should be given at the outset of treatment. Calcitonin can be useful in resistant cases.[86] Following IV bisphosphonate, re-treatment may be needed in 2–4 weeks,[87] but the patient is now alert to the symptoms and treatment can begin before the calcium level is high. Oral

Clinical decision	If YES carry out the action below
7 Is there a metabolic cause?	a. **Adrenocortical insufficiency** (lethargy, nausea, vomiting, abdominal pain, diarrhea, hypotension, low sodium, raised potassium): — if the symptoms are severe and adrenal failure is suspected take blood for cortisol level and give a trial dose of hydrocortisone 100 mg IV. An immediate improvement supports the diagnosis. — maintain on hydrocortisone PO 20 mg on waking and 10 mg early evening. It is often necessary to add fludrocortisone 50–200 microg PO once daily. b. **Hypercalcemia** (drowsiness, nausea, confusion, corrected serum calcium >2.7 mmol/L (10.4 mg/dL)). Obtain serum calcium and albumin then calculate the corrected serum calcium in mmol/L from the formula: [(40-serum albumin) × 0.02] + serum calcium.[88] (or [(4.4-serum albumin in g/dL) × 0.8] + serum calcium in mg/dL). *Immediate treatment:* Hydrate until a bisphosphonate can be started: either 60–90 mg pamidronate as 2- or 4-hour IV infusion in 500 mL 0.9% saline; or zoledronic acid 2–4 mg IV infusion over 30–45 minutes; or ibandronic acid 2 mg IV in 500 mL 0.9% saline over 2 hours (not Canada). Add regular acetaminophen to prevent bisphosphonate pyrexia. *Use bisphosphonates cautiously if renal function is at risk*, but they can be used in patients on dialysis. *Encourage calcium loss:* encourage oral fluids, but if unable to drink continue to hydrate parenterally IV or SC (especially if renal function is abnormal). *If no response (or worse) after 72 hours:* repeat pamidronate dose. If this is still ineffective after a further 72 hours start calcitonin 100–400 units SC q6h. *Prevent recurrence:* recheck corrected serum calcium at first sign of symptoms returning, or monthly. Review antitumor treatment. c. **Hyperglycemia** (thirst, polyuria, lethargy, glucose >15 mmol/L (270 mg/dL)): *Immediate treatment:* — start 24% oxygen (20% have a low O_2 saturation) — check electrolytes, blood glucose, and urinary ketones — start an IV infusion of 0.9% saline at 500 mL/hour. Give 500 mL 0.9% saline hourly until BP and signs of dehydration have resolved — insulin: give short-acting insulin 6 units IV <u>or</u> 20 units IM (the SC route cannot be used until peripheral circulation improves) — if hyperventilating or low potassium: the patient needs admission to hospital for close monitoring of potassium, blood gases, and correction of acidosis. *Keep glucose under control:* check blood glucose hourly, repeat electrolytes 1 and 5 hours after starting. Establish 24-hour requirement of insulin. *Prevent recurrence:* maintain glucose to whatever range controls symptoms (usually 8–15 mmol/L (144–270 mg/dL)). Convert to once daily (long-acting) insulin. Exclude drug causes of hyperglycemia (corticosteroids, octreotide, diuretics). d. **Hypoglycemia** (pale, sweaty, drowsiness, coma, glucose <2.5 mmol/L (45 mg/dL) *Immediate treatment:* give sugar in water orally, but if too sleepy give 20–50 mL 50% glucose IV (flush needle afterwards with 0.9% saline to clear all glucose from the vein and prevent local thrombosis). If IV access is not available give glucagon 1 mg IM. *Maintain glucose levels:* ensure glucose is being maintained above 5 mmol/L (90 mg/dL). Repeat IV 20 mL 50% glucose if necessary. Glucagon 1 mg is an alternative but will be less effective in cachectic patients or with repeated doses. Monitor glucose q4h until 3 normal levels obtained. *Prevent recurrence:* reduce the dose of insulin or hypoglycemics. Exclude other causes of hypoglycemia (e.g. adrenocortical insufficiency).

cd = clinical decisions

bisphosphonates are an alternative, but they delay rather than prevent the need for an infusion. Most patients return to their pre-hypercalcemic state with a good quality of life. However, hypercalcemia is an indicator of disease progression, and cancer patients may require a change in their anticancer treatment.

Severe hyperglycemia:[89] drowsiness, confusion, or coma require urgent treatment. The main goals are to rehydrate, restore a normal blood pressure, treat hypoxia, and reduce blood glucose while maintaining potassium levels, but this often needs inpatient admission. Avoiding hypoglycemia is more important than the tight control of blood glucose.[90] Patients who have a history of hyperglycemia may tolerate blood glucose levels of 20 mmol/L (360 mg/dL).

Severe hypoglycemia: it is common for existing diabetics with advanced disease to require less insulin or oral hypoglycemics as their oral intake and activity reduce. Consequently, these patients are at a risk of hypoglycemia. Symptoms will normally occur at glucose levels of less than 2 mmol/L (36 mg/dL), although some patients with diabetes-induced autonomic failure may show few symptoms before they collapse.[91] In a diabetic with advanced disease it is safer to plan for a blood glucose range of 8–15 mmol/L (144–270 mg/dL).

Syndrome of inappropriate ADH (SIADH): this can be caused by malignancy (especially small cell lung cancer and head and neck cancers), brain damage (e.g. meningitis, tumor, injury), respiratory conditions (e.g. pneumonia, tuberculosis, empyema), and drugs (e.g. antidepressants, carbamazepine, cytotoxics, methotrimeprazine, NSAIDs, thiazide diuretics).[92–95] It causes severe fluid retention which results in a very low plasma sodium (usually <120 mmol/L (120 mEq/L)), but a normal potassium and high urinary sodium.[96] Demeclocycline (US only) blocks the action of ADH on the kidney and is a simple and effective treatment.

Children with inborn errors of metabolism: these may become acutely unwell with concurrent infection, especially if they have been unable to tolerate their normal feeds. The child will look unwell with cool peripheries and an increased respiratory rate due to acidosis. To avoid irreversible neurological damage urgent treatment is needed with high energy feeds or infusion. An emergency feeding regime usually involves rehydration with a high energy feed such as "Resource 2," or dextrose 10% should be administered either via the gastrostomy tube, nasogastric tube, or intravenously. Specialist advice is often needed.

HEMATOLOGICAL PROBLEMS

Disseminated intravascular coagulation (DIC): this condition is a paradoxical combination of bleeding and clotting that damages vital organs.[97] It occurs in up to 10% of cancer patients and in its acute form in patients with advanced cancer it is often fatal.[98] It is caused by the depletion of clotting factors due to microscopic clotting. It is secondary to many conditions including metastatic carcinoma, sepsis, myeloproliferative disorders, liver failure, transfusion reactions, and rheumatological disease. It is diagnosed by the simultaneous presence of prolonged bleeding times and evidence of clotting shown by the presence of D-dimer, a breakdown product of blood clots.[99] Measuring D-dimers is a useful diagnostic test of clotting in both cancer and non-cancer patients.[100]

Treatment will depend on the cause, since DIC in the presence of advanced cancer is likely to be a terminal event, whereas DIC due to a treatable infection may be reversible.[101] For those patients

Clinical decision	If YES carry out the action below
7 Is there a metabolic cause? (contd.)	**e. Syndrome of Inappropriate ADH (SIADH)** (lethargy, drowsiness, confusion, headache, sodium <120 mmol/L (120 mEq/L), urine osmolality >300 mosmol/kg). Treat causes of SIADH such as drugs (reduce drug dose or change to alternative) or chest infection. Demeclocycline (not Canada) 150–600 mg PO q12h is simple, effective, and convenient for many patients. **f. Crisis in children with inborn errors of metabolism:** if this is felt to be a metabolic crisis (*see* text opposite) start urgent rehydration and high energy feed, e.g. Resource 2. Ask for specialist help.
8 Is there a hematological cause?	**a. Disseminated intravascular coagulation (DIC)** (bruising, mucosal bleeding, prolonged prothrombin time, low platelets, low fibrinogen <1 g/L, raised D-dimer). — *if the symptoms are mild* (bruising, occasional bleeds): start low-dose, low molecular weight heparin 100–150 units/kg SC once daily and tranexamic acid PO 1 g q8 — *if the symptoms are severe* (hemorrhage, thrombosis): consider urgent admission to an inpatient unit with facilities for close hematological control, but if this is inappropriate *see* cd-2c in *Emergencies*, p. 331. **b. Neutropenia** (4–15 days post chemotherapy, fever, low neutrophils <1 × 10^9/L) *If no fever and no risk factors* (*see* text below): observe, checking neutrophils daily. *If a fever is present, but no risk factor* (*see* text below): start a broad-spectrum antibiotic according to local antimicrobial policy. *If the fever persists >24 hours despite antibiotics or one risk factor is present:* discuss with the oncologists and/or consider admission to an air-filtered isolation room and supportive treatment in hospital.

where transfer to an acute unit is inappropriate, low molecular weight heparin can help.[102] The difficulty in diagnosis and treatment means that the advice of a hematologist is essential.

Neutropenia: The risk of infection depends on several factors:

Neutrophil count <1 × 10^9/L
High-dose corticosteroids
Indwelling venous catheter
Invasive procedure (e.g. urinary catheterization)
Chronic infection (TB, herpes simplex, fungal infection)
Immunodeficiency (e.g. HIV)
Age <1 year
Fever persisting more than 24 hours after starting antibiotic
Poor home conditions

High risk factors for infection[103,104]

Neutrophil count <0.5 × 10^9/L
Presence of one or more risk factors:

- symptoms persisting more than 24 hours after starting antibiotic (fever, sore throat, mouth ulcers, diarrhea, cough, breathlessness, dysuria, skin rash, cold sore)
- bruising or bleeding
- hypotension
- sudden onset of confusion or drowsiness.

Indicators for hospital admission for neutropenia

Neutropenia is usually seen 4–15 days after chemotherapy (especially with intensive regimes for Hodgkin's disease), but it can also occur after radiotherapy to large areas of bone marrow or in some leukemias. Ninety percent of patients with neutropenia are at low risk of infection,[105] and these are best managed in their existing place of care.[106] Ten percent of patients need to be admitted to hospital because of persisting neutropenia and at least one risk factor. Such patients may need parenteral, broad-spectrum antibiotics. Complications are due to infection with fungi, viruses or multi-drug resistant bacteria. If the neutropenia is persisting or worsening, such patients will need admission to an air-filtered isolation room, and administration of granulocyte stimulating factor.[107]

PROBLEMS CAUSED BY TUMOR PRESSURE

Spinal cord compression: patients deserve to be spared the distress of paraplegia if possible and cord compression requires urgent treatment.[108] Six-month survival rates in cancer patients with cord compression vary from 4% in those with widespread and rapidly progressive disease, to 99% in those with localized, slow growing and treatable disease,[109] with a median survival of 4 months.[110] Up to 5% of cancer patients may develop compression, but the proportion is higher in myeloma and prostatic carcinoma.[111] Back pain has been present for many months in up to 95% of patients, and in a patient with cancer this should alert the carer to the risk of compression.[108,112,113] Radiating pain can mask the source of the pain,[114] and this may be unilateral in cervical or lumbar compression, bilateral and encircling in thoracic compression. It is often accompanied by sensory changes in limbs. Pain on small movements such as coughing or straining suggests the presence of a spinal instability. Sensory and motor loss occurs initially but sphincter disturbance is a late sign. The final stage is rapid cord ischemia. Slow progression of weakness over 14 days or more has a much higher chance of recovery after treatment while deterioration 48 hours before treatment has the lowest chance of recovery.[115,116] Magnetic resonance imaging (MRI) is a key investigation to determine the presence and extent of compression.[117] Bone scans and X-rays localize the area of damage in only 21% of patients.[109]

The patient should be nursed with the spine in a neutral position (including "log-rolling" the patient when turning) until imaging confirms bony and neurological stability.[108] High-dose dexamethasone given immediately will reduce cord edema and may delay the onset of cord ischemia. Radiotherapy is the definitive treatment.[118] Surgery is worthwhile in suitable patients if radiotherapy is not possible, skeletal instability is present, or if the patient deteriorates while receiving dexamethasone and radiotherapy.[119,120] In sensitive tumors, chemotherapy can be effective.[121] Dexamethasone alone is suitable for patients for whom radiotherapy, chemotherapy, or surgery is not possible.[122] Any patients with partial or complete motor loss will require assessment by the physiotherapist and occupational therapist.

Some patients develop an autonomic dysreflexia with raised blood pressure, pounding headache, flushing, sweating, or blotching skin above the injury level, pallor, feeling cold, and goose bumps. These often need their BP to be reduced urgently and advice from a spinal injury unit can be invaluable.

Raised intracranial pressure: in palliative care this is usually due to intracranial tumor or metastases. If a patient responds to dexamethasone, radiotherapy is the treatment of choice.[123] Steroids should be continued for at least 3 weeks before deciding they are ineffective. Chemotherapy has a role in sensitive tumors.[124,125] Occasionally, a tumor causes hydrocephalus which may need excision or an intracranial shunt.

Clinical decision	If YES carry out the action below
9 Is tumor causing local pressure problems?	**a. Spinal cord compression** (early signs and symptoms: mild weakness or sensory change with vertebral pain, especially on coughing or lying; late: clear sensory or motor changes; very late: sphincter disturbance. Sensory changes are usually one or two dermatomes below site of compression, except in cauda equina lesions where changes are often asymmetrical). — nurse patient flat with neutral spine alignment until spinal stability is confirmed with imaging — treat pain (*see* cd-2, *Diagnosing and treating pain*, p. 45). Avoid spinal analgesia. *If neurological signs or symptoms are present:* give dexamethasone 16 mg IV as slow injection over 2 minutes, then 16 mg PO once daily. Higher doses can be used but adverse effects are more likely and more likely to be severe *If the prognosis allows*, arrange an urgent MRI and refer for radiotherapy. *Consider referral for surgical decompression* if the patient has late signs, the symptoms are worsening despite radiotherapy, further radiotherapy not possible, or investigations have shown an unstable spine. *If permanent cord damage has occurred: see Constipation*, p. 107, *Urinary problems and sexual difficulties*, p. 223, and *Skin problems*, p. 203. Arrange for physiotherapy and occupational therapy. Contact rehabilitation medicine team for help and advice. Reduce and stop dexamethasone unless this is required for pain control. Consider prophylactic heparin. *If autonomic dysreflexia is present* (*see* text opposite for symptoms): check BP (usually 20–40 mmHg higher than normal). Check for full bladder or rectum. Consider 10 mg sublingual nifedipine. If severe ask for advice from spinal injury unit. **b. Raised intracranial pressure** (headache, vomiting, drowsiness, papilledema). — arrange for a CT or MRI scan to assess the cause. *If cerebral metastases are the cause:* start dexamethasone 6 mg PO on waking, if necessary titrating up to 24 mg. Treatment should continue for at least 3 weeks. If a response is seen, refer for radiotherapy. *If hydrocephalus is the cause:* refer for neurosurgery. **c. Stridor:** *see* cd-6g, p. 339. **d. Vena cava obstruction:** SVCO (edema of face or arms, stridor, distended neck, chest and arm veins, headache, dusky color to skin in chest, arms, and face); IVCO (edema of genitals and legs, distended abdominal and leg veins, dusky color to legs). *If a venous thrombosis is suspected:* arrange urgent ultrasound and start low molecular weight heparin if a thrombus is confirmed. *If tumor is the cause:* give dexamethasone 16 mg IV as a slow injection over 2 minutes and start dexamethasone 16 mg PO once daily, reducing to the lowest dose that controls symptoms. If the prognosis allows, refer to the oncologists for urgent investigation and radiotherapy or chemotherapy. Consider referral for vena cava stent.

cd = clinical decision

Vena cava obstruction: the superior vena cava (SVC) drains the upper half of the body, while the inferior vena cava (IVC) drains the lower half and the symptoms of vena cava obstruction reflect which half of the body is affected (*see* cd-9d, p. 345). Obstruction of the SVC is often caused by tumor in the mediastinum (usually due to lung cancer). IVC obstruction can be caused by abdominal tumor, but also may be caused by thrombosis. Vena cava obstruction usually occurs slowly over weeks or months, allowing alternative (collateral) drainage to develop. Occasionally, the obstruction occurs rapidly over days and needs urgent treatment.

In SVCO, dexamethasone is still useful first-line treatment if the symptoms are severe. Radiotherapy relieves symptoms in 50–95% within the first two weeks of treatment, but chemotherapy is useful in SVCO due to small cell lung cancer.[126,127] In IVCO, a thrombus needs to be excluded with ultrasound or CT scan. If tumor obstruction is the cause, dexamethasone may be helpful. If radiotherapy is ineffective or cannot be used, a stent can be inserted into the SVC or IVC as an interventional radiology technique.[128–130] In acute SVCO the symptoms can include distressing headache and anxiety which will need treatment.

IS THE NEED FOR TREATMENT UNCERTAIN?

Even after taking all the details into consideration, including discussions with the patient and partner or relatives, it can still be difficult to know how appropriate it is to treat the cause of the deterioration. Waiting a short time will often resolve the situation since the new circumstances will make the situation clearer. Continuing deterioration suggests treatment should be for comfort only. Partners and relatives find that such changes make them much less likely to request treatment interventions other than for comfort.[131] If the situation remains unchanged this suggests the patient has sufficient reserves to undergo treatment of the primary cause of the deterioration.

AN OPPORTUNITY FOR DISCUSSION

After an emergency is over there is an important opportunity for discussing the current progression of the illness with the patient and with the partner and relatives (if the patient agrees). If the emergency reflects disease progression, some will not want to discuss the situation and this needs to be respected, while others will find this an opportunity for open sharing of information and feelings (*see Breaking difficult news*, p. 23). Because these discussions can involve difficult news, the individual may become distressed, although many have already suspected progression of the disease and are not surprised by the news (*see Helping a person with the effects of difficult news*, p. 27).

Clinical decision	If YES carry out the action below
10. Is the need for treatment uncertain?	• **If the patient has capacity for this decision:** ask the patient. • **If the patient does not have capacity for this decision:** Consult with the partner or relatives as they may offer useful information (e.g. previously stated refusal of a specific treatment in specific circumstances). — any stated refusals of treatment only apply to the circumstances anticipated by the patient (or agreed with the clinical team in the case of a non-competent patient) — partners or relatives of adults do not have the right to demand, for a patient without capacity, non-beneficial or ineffective treatment. They can give helpful information on the patient's previously stated preferences, and a substitute decision maker or health care proxy can make decisions based on those preferences. • **Consult with the clinical team** taking into account the history, rate of deterioration, and the availability of treatment. *See also Making ethical choices*, p. 263, and *Decisions around capacity*, p. 267. • **If the need is still unclear agree an observation period using the rule of 3:** Hour-by-hour deterioration: review in 3 hours. Day-by-day deterioration: review in 3 days. *If further deterioration has occurred:* treat for comfort. *If no further deterioration:* consider treating or set another review time or date.
11 Has the situation been explained?	• Explain the circumstances to the patient, if they want to discuss the emergency. • If the patient agrees, explain the situation to the partner or family.

cd = clinical decision

REFERENCES: EMERGENCIES

B = book; C = comment; Ch = chapter; CS-n = case study-no. of cases; CT-n = controlled trial-no. of cases; E = editorial; G = Guideline; GC = group consensus; I = interviews; LS = laboratory study; MC = multi-center; OS-n = open study-no. of cases; R = review; RCT-n = randomized controlled trial-no. of cases; RS-n = retrospective survey-no. of cases; SA = systematic or meta analysis.

1 Taube AW, Jenkins C, Bruera E. (1997) Is a "palliative" patient always a palliative patient? Two case studies. *Journal of Pain and Symptom Management.* **13**(6): 347–51. (R)

2 Prommer E. (2005) Management of bleeding in the terminally ill patient. *Hematology.* **10**(3): 167–75. (R)

3 Scott RC, Besag FM, Neville BG. (1999) Buccal midazolam and rectal diazepam for treatment of prolonged seizures in childhood and adolescence: a randomised trial. *Lancet.* **353**(9153): 623–6. (RCT-42)

4 Appleton R, Macleod S, Martland T. (2008) Drug management for acute tonic-clonic convulsions including convulsive status epilepticus in children. *Cochrane Database of Systematic Reviews.* **3**: CD001905. (SA, R-11 refs)

5 McIntyre J, Robertson S, Norris E, Appleton R, *et al.* (2005) Safety and efficacy of buccal midazolam versus rectal diazepam for emergency treatment of seizures in children: a randomised controlled trial. *Lancet.* **366**(9481): 205–10. (RCT-177)

6 Holsti M, Sill B, Firth S, Filloux F, *et al.* (2007) Prehospital intranasal midazolam for the treatment of pediatric seizures. *Pediatric Emergency Care.* **23**(3): 148–53. (RCT-857)

7 McGlone R, Smith M. (2001) Intranasal midazolam: an alternative in childhood seizures. *Emergency Medicine Journal.* **18**(3): 234. (Let)

8 Fisgin T, Gurer Y, Senbil N, Tezic T, *et al.* (2000) Nasal midazolam effects on childhood acute seizures. *Journal of Child Neurology.* **15**(12): 833–5. (OS-16)

9 Geldner G, Hubmann M, Knoll R, Jacobi K. (1997) Comparison between three transmucosal routes of administration of midazolam in children. *Paediatric Anaesthesia.* **7**(2): 103–9. (RCT-47)

10 Scott RC, Besag FM, Boyd SG, Berry D, Neville BG. (1998) Buccal absorption of midazolam: pharmacokinetics and EEG pharmacodynamics. *Epilepsia.* **39**(3): 290–4. (CT-10)

11 Scheepers M, Scheepers B. (1998) Midazolam via the intranasal route: an effective rescue medication for severe epilepsy in adults with a learning disability. *Seizure.* **7**: 509–12. (CS-2)

12 Arif H, Hirsch LJ. (2008) Treatment of status epilepticus. *Seminars in Neurology.* **28**(3): 342–54. (R, 62 refs)

13 Cherry N. (2009) Recommended organisational guidelines for the use of sedation in palliative care. *In press.*
14 Morita T, Tsuneto S, Shima Y. (2002) Definition of sedation for symptom relief: a systematic literature review and a proposal of operational criteria. *Journal of Pain and Symptom Management.* **24**(4): 447–53. (SA, 32 refs)
15 Beel A, McClement SE, Harlos M. (2002) Palliative sedation therapy: a review of definitions and usage. *International Journal of Palliative Nursing.* **8**(4): 190–9. (R, 43 refs)
16 Cowan JD, Palmer TW. (2002) Practical guide to palliative sedation. *Current Oncology Reports.* **4**(3): 242–9. (R, 65 refs)
17 Cowan JD, Walsh D. (2001) Terminal sedation in palliative medicine: definition and review of the literature. *Supportive Care in Cancer.* **9**(6): 403–7. (SA, 41 refs)
18 Quill TE, Byock IR. (2000) ACP–ASIM End-of-Life Care Consensus Panel. American College of Physicians-American Society of Internal Medicine. Responding to intractable terminal suffering: the role of terminal sedation and voluntary refusal of food and fluids. *Annals of Internal Medicine.* **132**(5): 408–14. (GC, 65 refs)
19 Chater S, Viola R, Paterson J, Jarvis V. (1998) Sedation for intractable distress in the dying: a survey of experts. *Palliative Medicine.* **12**(4): 255–69. (Q-61)
20 Fainsinger RL, Waller A, Bercovici M, Bengston K, *et al.* (2000) A multicentre international study of sedation for uncontrolled symptoms in terminally ill patients. *Palliative Medicine.* **14**: 257–65. (OS-287)
21 Morita T, Tsunoda J, Inoue S, Chihara S. (2001) Effects of high dose opioids and sedatives on survival in terminally ill cancer patients. *Journal of Pain and Symptom Management.* **21**(4): 282–9. (OS-209)
22 Sykes N, Thorns A. (2003) Sedative use in the last week of life and the implications for end-of-life decision making. *Archives of Internal Medicine.* **163**: 341–4.
23 Sykes N, Thorns A. (2003) The use of opioids and sedatives at the end of life. *Lancet Oncology.* **4**: 312–8.
24 Gagnon PR. (2008) Treatment of delirium in supportive and palliative care. *Current Opinion in Supportive and Palliative Care.* **2**(1): 60–6. (R, 61 refs)
25 Michaud L, Bula C, Berney A, Camus V, *et al.* (2007) Delirium Guidelines Development Group. Delirium: guidelines for general hospitals. *Journal of Psychosomatic Research.* **62**(3): 371–83. (R, 148 refs)
26 Meagher D, Leonard M. (2008) The active management of delirium: improving detection and treatment. *Advances in Psychiatric Treatment.* **14**: 292–301.
27 Bayard M, McIntyre J, Hill KR, Woodside J Jr. (2004) Alcohol withdrawal syndrome. *American Family Physician.* **69**(6): 1443–50. (R, 29 refs)
28 Morita T, Akechi T, Sugawara Y, Chihara S, Uchitomi Y. (2002) Practices and attitudes of Japanese oncologists and palliative care physicians concerning terminal sedation: a nationwide survey. *Journal of Clinical Oncology.* **20**(3): 758–64. (I-697)
29 Stirling LC, Kurowska A, Tookman A. (1999) The use of phenobarbitone in the management of agitation and seizures at the end of life. *Journal of Pain and Symptom Management.* **17**(5): 363–8. (OS-60)
30 Mercadante S, De Conno F, Ripamonti C. (1995) Propofol in terminal care. *Journal of Pain and Symptom Management.* **10**(8): 639–42. (CS-1)
31 Moyle J. (1995) The use of propofol in palliative medicine. *Journal of Pain and Symptom Management.* **10**(8): 643–6. (CS-1)
32 Cheng C, Roemer-Becuwe C, Pereira J. (2002) When midazolam fails. *Journal of Pain and Symptom Management.* **23**(3): 256–65. (CS-2)
33 Mackey JR, Wood L, Nabholtz J, Jensen J, Venner P. (2000) A phase II trial of triamcinolone hexacetanide for symptomatic recurrent malignant ascites. *Journal of Pain and Symptom Management.* **19**(3): 193–9. (OS-15)
34 Paniagua P, Catala E, Villar Landeira JM. (2000) Successful management of pleuritic pain with thoracic paravertebral block. *Regional Anesthesia and Pain Medicine.* **25**(6): 651–3. (CS-1)
35 Tarzian AJ. (2000) Caring for dying patients who have air hunger. *Journal of Nursing Scholarship.* **32**(2): 137–43. (I-12)
36 Tripodoro VA, De Vito EL. (2008) Management of dyspnea in advanced motor neuron diseases. *Current Opinion in Supportive and Palliative Care.* **2**(3): 173–9. (R, 29 refs)
37 Shumway NM, Wilson RL, Howard RS, Parker JM, Eliasson AH. (2008) Presence and treatment of air hunger in severely ill patients. *Respiratory Medicine.* **102**(1): 27–31. (OS-98)
38 Rietjens JA, van Zuylen L, van Veluw H, van der Wijk L, *et al.* (2008) Palliative sedation in a specialized unit for acute palliative care in a cancer hospital: comparing patients dying with and without palliative sedation. *Journal of Pain and Symptom Management.* **36**(3): 228–34. (RS-157)
39 Goodacre S, Locker T, Morris F, Campbell S. (2002) How useful are clinical features in the diagnosis of acute, undifferentiated chest pain? *Academic Emergency Medicine.* **9**(3): 203–8. (OS-893)
40 King V, Vaze AA, Moskowitz CS, Smith LJ, Ginsberg MS. (2008) D-dimer assay to exclude pulmonary embolism in high-risk oncologic population: correlation with CT pulmonary angiography in an urgent care setting. *Radiology.* **247**(3): 854–61. (OS-531)
41 Righini M, Le Gal G, De Lucia S, Roy PM, *et al.* (2006) Clinical usefulness of D-dimer testing in cancer patients with suspected pulmonary embolism. *Thrombosis and Haemostasis.* **95**(4): 715–9. (MC, OS-1721)
42 Tai NR, Atwal AS, Hamilton G. (1999) Modern management of pulmonary embolism. *British Journal of Surgery.* **86**(7): 853–68. (R, 145 refs)
43 Johnson MJ. (1997) Problems of anticoagulation

within a palliative care setting: an audit of hospice inpatients taking warfarin. *Palliative Medicine*. **11**: 306–12.

44 Weber C, Merminod T, Herrmann FR, Zulian GB. (2008) Prophylactic anti-coagulation in cancer palliative care: a prospective randomised study. *Supportive Care in Cancer.* **16**(7): 847–52. (CT-20)

45 Noble S. (2007) Management of venous thromboembolism in the palliative care setting. *International Journal of Palliative Nursing*. **13**(12): 574–9. (R, 39 refs)

46 Noble S. (2007) The challenges of managing cancer related venous thromboembolism in the palliative care setting. *Postgraduate Medical Journal*. **83**(985): 671–4. (R, 32 refs)

47 Nazario R, Delorenzo LJ, Maguire AG. (2002) Treatment of venous thromboembolism. *Cardiology in Review*. **10**(4): 249–59. (R, 66 refs)

48 Noble SI, Nelson A, Turner C, Finlay IG. (2006) Acceptability of low molecular weight heparin thromboprophylaxis for inpatients receiving palliative care: qualitative study. *British Medical Journal*. **332**: 577–80. (OS-28)

49 Noble SI, Hood K, Finlay IG. (2007) The use of long-term low-molecular weight heparin for the treatment of venous thromboembolism in palliative care patients with advanced cancer: a case series of sixty-two patients. *Palliative Medicine*. **21**(6): 473–6. (OS-62)

50 Noble SI, Shelley MD, Coles B, Williams SM, Wilcock A, Johnson MJ. (2008) Association for Palliative Medicine for Great Britain and Ireland. Management of venous thromboembolism in patients with advanced cancer: a systematic review and meta-analysis. *Lancet Oncology*. **9**(6): 577–84. (R, 55 refs)

51 Ray CE, Prochazka A. (2008) The need for anticoagulation following inferior vena cava filter implacement: systematic review *Cardiovascular and Interventional Radiology*. **31**(2): 316–24.

52 Kalva SP, Chlapoutaki C, Wicky S, Greenfield AJ, *et al.* (2008) Suprarenal inferior vena cava filters: a 20-year single-center experience. *Journal of Vascular and Interventional Radiology*. **19**(7): 1041–7. (OS-70)

53 NHS Clinical Knowledge Summaries (CKS). (2009) Heart failure – chronic. Available at: www.cks.nhs.uk/heart_failure_chronic. (G)

54 Jerjes-Sanchez C, Ramirez-Rivera A, Arriaga-Nava R, Iglesias-Gonzalez S, *et al.* (2001) High dose and short-term streptokinase infusion in patients with pulmonary embolism: prospective with seven-year follow-up trial. *Journal of Thrombosis and Thrombolysis*. **12**(3): 237–47. (CT-40)

55 Canadian Asthma Consensus Report. (1999) *Canadian Medical Association Journal*. **161**(Suppl. 1): S1–62.

56 Ahmedzai S. (1997) Palliation of respiratory symptoms. In: Doyle D, Hanks GWC, MacDonald N, eds. *The Oxford Textbook of Palliative Medicine, 2nd ed.* Oxford: Oxford Medical Publications. pp. 583–616. (Ch)

57 Congleton J, Muers MF. (1995) The incidence of airflow obstruction in bronchial carcinoma, its relation to breathlessness, and response to bronchodilator therapy. *Respiratory Medicine*. **89**(4): 291–6. (RCT-57)

58 Hansen JJ, Jepsen SB, Lund J. (2000) Symptomatic helium treatment of upper and lower airway obstruction. *Ugeskrift for Laeger.* **162**(49): 6669–72. (R, 22 refs)

59 Laude EA, Ahmedzai SH. (2007) Oxygen and helium gas mixtures for dyspnoea. *Current Opinion in Supportive and Palliative Care*. **1**(2): 91–5. (R, 31 refs)

60 Gainnier M, Forel JM. (2006) Clinical review: use of helium-oxygen in critically ill patients. *Critical Care* **10**(6): 241. (R, 62 refs)

61 Hillel AD, Benninger M, Blitzer A, Crumley R, *et al.* (1999) Evaluation and management of bilateral vocal cord immobility. *Otolaryngology – Head and Neck Surgery*. **121**(6): 760–5. (R, 34 refs)

62 Sapundzhiev N, Lichtenberger G, Eckel HE, Friedrich G, *et al.* (2008) Surgery of adult bilateral vocal fold paralysis in adduction: history and trends. *European Archives of Oto-Rhino-Laryngology*. **265**(12): 1501–14. (R)

63 Heath DA. (1989) Hypercalcaemia of malignancy. *Palliative Medicine*. **3**: 1–11. (R)

64 Bower M, Cox S. (2009) Endocrine and metabolic complications of advanced cancer. In: Hanks G, Cherney NI, Christakis NA, Fallon M, Kaasa S, Portenoy RK, eds. *Oxford Textbook of Palliative Medicine, 4th ed*. Oxford: Oxford University Press. (Ch)

65 Kovacs CS, MacDonald SM, Chik CL, Bruera E. (1995) Hypercalcaemia of malignancy in the palliative care patient: a treatment strategy. *Journal of Pain and Symptom Management*. **10**: 224–32. (R, 51 refs)

66 Rabbani SA. (2000) Molecular mechanism of action of parathyroid hormone related peptide in hypercalcemia of malignancy: therapeutic strategies (review). *International Journal of Oncology*. **16**(1): 197–206. (R, 54 refs)

67 Penel N, Dewas S, Doutrelant P, Clisant S, *et al.* (2008) Cancer-associated hypercalcemia treated with intravenous diphosphonates: a survival and prognostic factor analysis. *Supportive Care in Cancer*. **16**(4): 387–92. (RS-260)

68 Lamy O, Jenzer-Closuit A, Burckhardt P. (2001) Hypercalcaemia of malignancy: an undiagnosed and undertreated disease. *Journal of Internal Medicine*. **250**(1): 73–9. (OS-71)

69 Riancho JA, Arjona R, Sanz J, Olmos JM, *et al.* (1991) Is the routine measurement of ionized calcium worthwhile in patients with cancer? *Postgraduate Medical Journal*. **67**(786): 350–3. (OS-188)

70 Nussbaum SR, Younger J, Vandepol CJ, Gagel RF, *et al.* (1993) Single-dose intravenous therapy with pamidronate for the treatment of hypercalcemia of malignancy: comparison of 30-, 60-, and 90-mg dosages. *American Journal of Medicine*. **95**(3): 297–304. (RCT-50)

71 Nussbaum SR, Warrell RP Jr., Rude R, Glusman J, *et al.* (1993) Dose-response study of alendronate sodium for the treatment of cancer-associated

hypercalcemia. *Journal of Clinical Oncology*. **11**(8): 1618–23. (RCT-59)

72 Thode J, Juul-Jorgensen B, Bhatia HM, Kjaerulf-Nielsen M, *et al*. (1989) Comparison of serum total calcium, albumin-corrected total calcium, and ionized calcium in 1213 patients with suspected calcium disorders. *Scandinavian Journal of Clinical and Laboratory Investigation*. **49**(3): 217–23. (OS-1213)

73 Payne RB, Carver ME, Morgan DB. (1979) Interpretation of serum total calcium: effects of adjustment for albumin concentration on frequency of abnormal values and on detection of change in the individual. *Journal of Clinical Pathology*. **32**(1): 56–60. (OS-1693)

74 Lum G. (1996) Evaluation of a laboratory critical limit (alert value) policy for hypercalcemia. *Archives of Pathology and Laboratory Medicine*. **120**(7): 633–6. (OS-191)

75 Lind L, Ljunghall S. (1991) Serum chloride in the differential diagnosis of hypercalcemia. *Experimental and Clinical Endocrinology*. **98**(3): 179–84. (OS-221)

76 Gucalp R, Theirault R. (1994) Treatment of cancer-associated hypercalcaemia. *Archives of Internal Medicine*. **154**: 1935–44. (RCT-46)

77 Body JJ. (2000) Current and future directions in medical therapy: hypercalcemia. *Cancer*. **88**(Suppl. 12): S3054–8. (SA, 23 refs)

78 Perazella MA, Markowitz GS. (2008) Bisphosphonate nephrotoxicity. *Kidney International*. **74**(11): 1385–93. (R, 65 refs)

79 McDermott RS, Kloth DD, Wang H, Hudes GR, Langer CJ. (2006) Impact of zoledronic acid on renal function in patients with cancer: clinical significance and development of a predictive model. *The Journal of Supportive Oncology*. **4**(10): 524–9. (RS-446)

80 Bergner R, Diel IJ, Henrich D, Hoffmann M, Uppenkamp M. (2006) Differences in nephrotoxicity of intravenous bisphosphonates for the treatment of malignancy-related bone disease. *Onkologie*. **29**(11): 534–40. (R, 51 refs)

81 Bisphosphonates. In www.palliativedrugs.com

82 Major P, Lortholary A, Hon J, Abdi E, *et al*. (2001) Zoledronic acid is superior to pamidronate in the treatment of hypercalcemia of malignancy: a pooled analysis of two randomized, controlled clinical trials. *Journal of Clinical Oncology*. **19**(2): 558–67. (RCT-287)

83 Major PP, Coleman RE. (2001) Zoledronic acid in the treatment of hypercalcemia of malignancy: results of the international clinical development program. *Seminars in Oncology*. **28**(2 Suppl. 6): S17–24. (R, 30 refs)

84 Neville-Webbe HL, Coleman RE. (2003) The use of zoledronic acid in the management of metastatic bone disease and hypercalcaemia. *Palliative Medicine*. **17**: 539–53. (R, 61 refs).

85 Bobba RS, Beattie K, Parkinson B, Kumbhare D, Adachi JD. (2006) Tolerability of different dosing regimens of bisphosphonates for the treatment of osteoporosis and malignant bone disease. *Drug Safety*. **29**(12): 1133–52. (R, 82 refs)

86 Diskin CJ, Stokes TJ, Dansby LM, Radcliff L, Carter TB. (2007) Malignancy-related hypercalcemia developing on a bisphosphonate but responding to calcitonin. *Clinical Lung Cancer*. **8**(7): 434–5. (CS-1)

87 Wimalawansa SJ. (1994) Optimal frequency of administration of pamidronate in patients with hypercalcaemia of malignancy. *Clinical Endocrinology*. **41**: 591–5. (RCT-34)

88 Iqbal SJ, Giles M, Ledger S, Nanji N, Howl T. (1988) Need for albumin adjustments of urgent total serum calcium. *Lancet*. **332**(8626): 1477. (OS)

89 Poulson J. (1997) The management of diabetes in patients with advanced cancer. *Journal of Pain and Symptom Management*. **13**: 339–46. (R, 26 refs)

90 Ford-Dunn S, Smith A, Quin J. (2006) Management of diabetes during the last days of life: attitudes of consultant diabetologists and consultant palliative care physicians in the UK. *Palliative Medicine*. **20**(3): 197–203. (Q)

91 Cryer PE. (2001) Hypoglycemia risk reduction in type 1 diabetes. *Experimental and Clinical Endocrinology and Diabetes*. **109** (Suppl. 2): S412–23. (R, 67)

92 Flombaum CD. (2000) Metabolic emergencies in the cancer patient. *Seminars in Oncology*. **27**(3): 322–34. (R, 110 refs)

93 Ferlito A, Rinaldo A, Devaney KO. (1997) Syndrome of inappropriate antidiuretic hormone secretion associated with head neck cancers: review of the literature. *Annals of Otology, Rhinology and Laryngology*. **106**(10 Pt. 1): 878–83. (R, 30 refs)

94 Woo MH, Smythe MA. (1997) Association of SIADH with selective serotonin reuptake inhibitors. *Annals of Pharmacotherapy*. **31**(1): 108–10. (R, 32 refs)

95 Chan TY. (1997) Drug-induced syndrome of inappropriate antidiuretic hormone secretion: causes, diagnosis and management. *Drugs and Aging*. **11**(1): 27–44. (R, 211 refs)

96 Decaux G, Musch W. (2008) Clinical laboratory evaluation of the syndrome of inappropriate secretion of antidiuretic hormone. *Clinical Journal of the American Society of Nephrology*. **3**(4): 1175–84. (R, 66 refs)

97 Stewart C. (2001) Disseminated intravascular coagulation (DIC). *Australian Critical Care*. **14**(2): 71–5. (R, 14 refs)

98 Maxson JH. (2000) Management of disseminated intravascular coagulation. *Critical Care Nursing Clinics of North America*. **12**(3): 341–52. (R, 14 refs)

99 Horan JT, Francis CW. (2001) Fibrin degradation products, fibrin monomer and soluble fibrin in disseminated intravascular coagulation. *Seminars in Thrombosis and Hemostasis*. **27**(6): 657–66. (R, 58 refs)

100 ten Wolde M, Kraaijenhagen RA, Prins MH, Buller HR. (2002) The clinical usefulness of D-dimer testing in cancer patients with suspected deep venous thrombosis. *Archives of Internal Medicine*. **162**(16): 1880–4. (OS-1739)

101 Bick RL, Arun B, Frenkel EP. (1999) Disseminated intravascular coagulation: clinical and

pathophysiological mechanisms and manifestations. *Haemostasis.* **29**(2–3): 111–34. (R, 179 refs)

102 Hofmann M, Rest A, Hafner G, Tanner B, Brockerhoff P, Weilemann LS. (1997) D-dimer, thrombin-antithrombin III-complex (TAT) and prothrombin fragment 1+2 (PTF): parameters for monitoring therapy with low molecular-weight heparin in coagulation disorders. *Anaesthesist.* **46**(8): 689–96. (RCT-30)

103 Price CGA, Price P. (1995) Acute emergencies in oncology. In: *Oxford Textbook of Oncology on CD-ROM.* Oxford: Oxford University Press and Optimedia Ltd. (Ch)

104 Castagnola E, Paola D, Giacchino R, Viscoli C. (2000) Clinical and laboratory features predicting a favorable outcome and allowing early discharge in cancer patients with low-risk febrile neutropenia: a literature review. *Journal of Hematotherapy and Stem Cell Research.* **9**(5): 645–9. (R, 35 refs)

105 Innes H, Lim SL, Hall A, Chan SY, Bhalla N, Marshall E. (2008) Management of febrile neutropenia in solid tumours and lymphomas using the Multinational Association for Supportive Care in Cancer (MASCC) risk index: feasibility and safety in routine clinical practice. *Supportive Care in Cancer.* **16**(5): 485–91. (OS-100)

106 Orudjev E, Lange BJ. (2002) Evolving concepts of management of febrile neutropenia in children with cancer. *Medical and Pediatric Oncology.* **39**(2): 77–85. (SA, 51 refs)

107 Tigue CC, McKoy JM, Evens AM, Trifilio SM, *et al.* (2007) Granulocyte-colony stimulating factor administration to healthy individuals and persons with chronic neutropenia or cancer: an overview of safety considerations from the Research on Adverse Drug Events and Reports project. *Bone Marrow Transplantation.* **40**(3): 185–92. (R, 64 refs)

108 NICE (National Institute for Health and Clinical Excellence). (2008) *Metastatic Spinal Cord Compression: diagnosis and management of adults at risk of, or with, metastatic cord compression (Clinical Guideline 75).* London: NICE (www.nice.org.uk/G75) (G, GC)

109 Rades D, Dunst J, Schild SE. (2008) The first score predicting overall survival in patients with metastatic spinal cord compression. *Cancer.* **112**(1): 157–61. (OS-1852)

110 Rades D, Fehlauer F, Veninga T, Stalpers LJ, *et al.* (2007) Functional outcome and survival after radiotherapy of metastatic spinal cord compression in patients with cancer of unknown primary. *International Journal of Radiation Oncology, Biology, Physics.* **67**(2): 532–7. (RS-143)

111 Kramer JA. (1992) Spinal cord compression in malignancy. *Palliative Medicine.* **6**: 202–11.

112 Levack P, Graham J, Collie D, Grant R, *et al.* (2002) The Scottish Cord Compression Study Group. Don't wait for a sensory level – listen to the symptoms: a prospective audit of the delays in diagnosis of malignant cord compression. *Clinical Oncology.* **14**: 472–80. (OS-319)

113 Loblaw DA, Perry J, Chambers A, Laperriere NJ. (2005) Systematic review of the diagnosis and management of malignant extradural spinal cord compression: the Cancer Care Ontario Practice Guidelines Initiative's Neuro-Oncology Disease Site Group. *Journal of Clinical Oncology.* **23**: 2028–37. (SA)

114 Abrahm JL, Banffy MB, Harris MB. (2008) Spinal cord compression in patients with advanced metastatic cancer: "all I care about is walking and living my life". *Journal of the American Medical Association.* **299**(8): 937–46. (R, 101 refs)

115 Rades D, Heidenreich F, Karstens JH. (2002) Final results of a prospective study of the prognostic value of the time to develop motor deficits before irradiation in metastatic spinal cord compression. *International Journal of Radiation Oncology, Biology, Physics.* **53**(4): 975–9. (CT-98)

116 Chaichana KL, Woodworth GF, Sciubba DM, McGirt MJ, *et al.* (2008) Predictors of ambulatory function after decompressive surgery for metastatic epidural spinal cord compression. *Neurosurgery.* **62**(3): 683–92. (RS-77)

117 Rankine JJ, Gill KP, Hutchinson CE, Ross ER, Williamson JB. (1998) The therapeutic impact of lumbar spine MRI on patients with low back and leg pain. *Clinical Radiology.* **53**(9): 688–93. (CT-72)

118 Rades D, Hoskin PJ, Karstens JH, Rudat V. (2007) Radiotherapy of metastatic spinal cord compression in very elderly patients. *International Journal of Radiation Oncology, Biology, Physics.* **67**(1): 256–63. (RS-308)

119 Penas-Prado M, Loghin ME. (2008) Spinal cord compression in cancer patients: review of diagnosis and treatment. *Current Oncology Reports.* **10**(1): 78–85. (R, 54 refs)

120 Chen YJ, Chang GC, Chen HT, Yang TY, *et al.* (2007) Surgical results of metastatic spinal cord compression secondary to non-small cell lung cancer. *Spine.* **32**(15): E413–8. (OS-31)

121 Schmidt MH, Klimo P Jr., Vrionis FD. (2005) Metastatic spinal cord compression. *Journal of the National Comprehensive Cancer Network.* **3**(5): 711–9. (R, 103)

122 Falk S, Fallon M. (1997) ABC of palliative care: emergencies. *British Medical Journal.* **315**(7121): 1525–8. (R)

123 Newton HB. (2007) Symptom management and supportive care of the patient with brain metastases. *Cancer Treatment and Research.* **136**: 53–73. (R, 89 refs)

124 Davey P. (2002) Brain metastases: treatment options to improve outcomes. *CNS Drugs.* **16**(5): 325–38. (R, 102 refs)

125 Grossi F, Scolaro T, Tixi L, Loprevite M, Ardizzoni A. (2001) The role of systemic chemotherapy in the treatment of brain metastases from small-cell lung cancer. *Critical Reviews in Oncology-Hematology.* **37**(1): 61–7. (R, 44 refs)

126 Donato V, Bonfili P, Bulzonetti N, Santarelli M, *et al.* (2001) Radiation therapy for oncological emergencies. *Anticancer Research.* **21**(3C): 2219–24. (OS-43)

127 Rowell NP, Gleeson FV. (2001) Steroids, radiotherapy, chemotherapy and stents for superior vena caval obstruction in carcinoma of the

bronchus. *Cochrane Database of Systematic Reviews.* **4**: CD001316. (SA, 99 refs)

128 Fletcher WS, Lakin PC, Pommier RF, Wilmarth T. (1998) Results of treatment of inferior vena cava syndrome with expandable metallic stents. *Archives of Surgery.* **133**(9): 935–8. (RS-28)

129 Barshes NR, Annambhotla S, El Sayed HF, Huynh TT, *et al.* (2007) Percutaneous stenting of superior vena cava syndrome: treatment outcome in patients with benign and malignant etiology. *Vascular.* **15**(5): 314–21. (OS-56)

130 Nagata T, Makutani S, Uchida H, Kichikawa K, *et al.* (2007) Follow-up results of 71 patients undergoing metallic stent placement for the treatment of a malignant obstruction of the superior vena cava. *Cardiovascular and Interventional Radiology*. **30**(5): 959–67. (OS-71)

131 Mezey M, Kluger M, Maislin G, Mittelman M. (1996) Life-sustaining treatment decisions by spouses of patients with Alzheimer's disease. *Journal of the American Geriatrics Society.* **44**(2): 144–50. (I-50)

Index

cd = clinical decision **Bold = emergencies**